Photographic Atlas of Pediatric Disorders and Diagnosis

Photographic Atlas of Pediatric Disorders and Diagnosis

Ralph R. Salimpour, MD, DCH, FAAP
Clinical Professor of Pediatrics
UCLA School of Medicine
Los Angeles, CA

Pedram Salimpour, MD, MPH
Associate Clinical Professor of Pediatrics
UCR School of Medicine
Riverside, CA

Pejman Salimpour, MD, FAAP
Clinical Professor of Pediatrics
UCLA School of Medicine
Los Angeles, CA

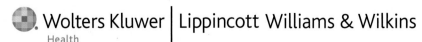
Wolters Kluwer | Lippincott Williams & Wilkins
Health

Philadelphia • Baltimore • New York • London
Buenos Aires • Hong Kong • Sydney • Tokyo

Executive Editor: Rebecca S. Gaertner
Product Manager: Ashley Fischer
Production Project Manager: Marian Bellus
Manufacturing Manager: Beth Welsh
Senior Marketing Manager: Kimberly Schonberger
Design Coordinator: Holly McLaughlin
Production Services: Aptara, Inc.

Printed in China

Library of Congress Cataloging-in-Publication Data

CIP data available on request.

Care has been taken to confirm the accuracy of the information presented and to describe generally accepted practices. However, the authors, editors, and publisher are not responsible for errors or omissions or for any consequences from application of the information in this book and make no warranty, expressed or implied, with respect to the currency, completeness, or accuracy of the contents of the publication. Application of the information in a particular situation remains the professional responsibility of the practitioner.

The authors, editors, and publisher have exerted every effort to ensure that drug selection and dosage set forth in this text are in accordance with current recommendations and practice at the time of publication. However, in view of ongoing research, changes in government regulations, and the constant flow of information relating to drug therapy and drug reactions, the reader is urged to check the package insert for each drug for any change in indications and dosage and for added warnings and precautions. This is particularly important when the recommended agent is a new or infrequently employed drug.

Some drugs and medical devices presented in the publication have Food and Drug Administration (FDA) clearance for limited use in restricted research settings. It is the responsibility of the health care provider to ascertain the FDA status of each drug or device planned for use in their clinical practice.

To purchase additional copies of this book, call our customer service department at (800) 638-3030 or fax orders to (301) 223-2320. International customers should call (301) 223-2300.

Visit Lippincott Williams & Wilkins on the Internet: at LWW.com. Lippincott Williams & Wilkins customer service representatives are available from 8:30 am to 6 pm, EST.

10 9 8 7 6 5 4 3 2 1

LWW.COM

About the Author and Photographer

My journey here—to this day, and this moment—is nothing short of miraculous. I was born to a 15-year-old mother whose labor was attended by an illiterate midwife in a small port city in the southern Iran of the early 1930s.

Growing up, I survived a virtual catalog of childhood diseases: Measles, mumps, rubella, varicella, typhoid fever, whooping cough, dysentery (three times), ascariasis, tuberculosis, and malaria,—a disease that to this day takes 1 million lives per year, most of them, children. I survived;, but two of my siblings were less fortunate and succumbed to measles and tetanus.

Since then, over the past six decades as a pediatrician and having practiced during that time on three continents, I have seen countless other youngsters suffering from those same diseases. As a young physician, I saw once-lively toddlers suddenly unable to walk due to polio. I saw children so malnourished; they no longer looked like children at all, but like the skeletal remains of prisoners of war. I saw almost 1,000 infants with tetanus, most of whom died. I had to tell countless anguished parents that their babies had departed due to conditions that I know now and knew then, might have been easily managed or prevented even, through timely access to a doctor, education, and immunizations. And I was as powerless in the face of their tears.

In 1979, when turmoil in our homeland led us to flee to America, truly, that "a mighty woman with a torch, whose flame is the imprisoned lightning, and her name, Mother of Exiles," embraced us in every conceivable way. Back then it was our dream—and a sweet one—to send our children to those famed American Universities. That dream came true and all four of our children graduated from among the best institutions of this wonderful land. Today, as grown women and men, they serve their country and communities, two of them as pediatricians and co-authors here.

In my career, I feel blessed to have realized my goals. Over 60 years after starting medical school, I believe what I believed then, that there is no higher calling than that of a doctor. In medical school and residency, I grew to consider that to be truest in service to those most vulnerable amongst us, our children. And I began to document the most interesting disease states and patient cases through another passion of mine, photography. Perhaps it could be said that the photographic atlas of pediatrics you hold in your hands, is the photo album of my career.

Today, three continents, six decades, and thousands of patients later, I am a thankful man who wishes each one of you scholars the same satisfaction and joy throughout your clinical careers, and lives.

Ralph R. Salimpour, MD, DCH, FAAP

Preface

"The only way to do great work is to love what you do."

Steve Jobs

Passion for the practice of pediatrics and of teaching has enabled us to assemble an Atlas of images that is vast in its breadth and depth. They are presented herein for maximum utility using an interactive multimedia approach, through the presentation of close to 1,000 vivid images, accompanied by a brief history of the actual patient seen in the accompanying images.

Of course, there is no substitute for direct patient—physician interaction. But this book is the next best alternative. Here, the diseased state is shown in all of its manifestations, not just its most common form. The purpose of this book is the *visual* teaching of pathology in pediatrics. Visual inspection is the first component of the physical examination and fundamental to diagnosis. It is important for students and clinicians to access the breadth of presentations of complicated illnesses, particularly since some of these disorders are only rarely encountered in the developed world. This posture on instruction enables the reader to acquire an important and implicit awareness that there are as many expressions of disease as there are patients who suffer from them. But that understanding those features most fundamental to each, will guide the astute physician to the correct diagnosis and treatment.

A few diseases are discussed in detail, in view of the specialized experience of the authors either with individual and unique patients or with specific diseases. One example is that of senior author, Dr. Ralph Salimpour. Dr. Salimpour has treated over a thousand cases of tetanus and is considered a world authority. The text that accompanies images of this terrible affliction is thus as personal as it is clinical. Special attention is also paid to rickets where Dr. Salimpour has the largest ever published series on the ailment. And malnutrition, where Dr. Salimpour identified for the first time the significance of purpura in this avertable condition, is deliberated in some detail. With these and several other of the conditions herein portrayed and discussed where the authors' personal perspectives on the disease and its manifestations are intimate and exceptional, there is elaboration that is more familiar than commonly encountered in an academic textbook. We believe this feature supplements the distinctive nature of the Atlas.

And while diseases and their manifestations remain generally constant over time, the treatment modalities deployed to prevent and fight them change continuously. Our understanding of not just a particular disease, but of disease itself, of the basic sciences and their clinical applications, and of etiology and pathophysiology, constantly improve. With this advancement in knowledge, so changes the physician's armamentarium. But, symptoms and signs do not change. It follows that these images, which are the expressions of symptoms and signs, make the utility of this book to the clinician, enduring. It is the hope of the authors that the Atlas' clinical usefulness persists.

Several pictorial views of each condition, supplemented by online access to many more ever increasing images, will enable the physician to gain an appreciation for the many ways that each disease state can present. The scholar who has read about herald patch in pityriasis rosea thus can see what many of these look like, what to look for in impetigo neonatorum, and why prune belly has earned its name. All of this is accomplished through illustrations that are vivid and in their aggregate, truthful.

For centuries, students and physicians have seen patients in hospitals and clinics. They have then referred back to their books to learn what condition the rash they had observed represented, why that thick calf boasted no power, why that child's ribs were swollen, or questioned the awkward positioning of the febrile baby's extremities. This functional Atlas is a practical and effective approach to answering their questions, enhancing the diagnostic armamentarium of physicians.

It is the authors' hope that this Atlas will as well inspire a new generation of physician—scientists to further ask and to gather even better diagnostic information. And ultimately, of finding novel ways of presenting that information to the reader. For as long as the eyes see before the mind reads, we believe this Atlas will serve as a useful tool for the physician, making him or her, a more astute diagnostician.

Pedram Salimpour, MD, MPH
Pejman Salimpour, MD, FAAP
Ralph R. Salimpour, MD, DCH, FAAP

Acknowledgments

This Atlas could not have been created without the help of many dedicated colleagues and friends. They worked tirelessly, late into evenings and on holidays on the details of this book, when I know they would rather have been with their families. Their work and commitment to this seemingly insurmountable task ensured that we would present to you, the reader, the best possible format and clinical basis for the diagnosis and treatment of childhood diseases.

Our consultants were Dr. Daniel Gross in dermatology; Dr. Roger Friedman and Dr. Tali Kolin in ophthalmology; Dr. Parvaneh Vossough in hematology, and oncology; Dr. Gary Rachelefsky in allergy, and immunology; Dr. Lori Taylor in radiology; Dr. Haleh Shaheedy in dentistry; Dr. Arash Moghimi as editor of several of the chapters; and Ms. Mary Ann Milbert, NPN in data collection.

Mr. Allen Nikka, Ms. Ariella Salimpour, Mr. Anthony Lee, Mr. Luis Carlos Prada, and Mr. Hiran Jayasinghe gave us the help we needed in technology and research. The publishing of this Atlas would likely have taken years longer if not for the skillfulness with which they brought computers and imaging technology in photography to the undertaking. It was their work that helped close the gap between academic precision and visual understanding through the use of these nearly 1,000 images. The authors would like to acknowledge Mr. Branden Nikka for his contribution and commitment to the programs in childhood development and Ms. Gabriella Salimpour whose assistance with the final editing of the manuscript helped us reach aggressive timeline milestones.

We also wish to thank Ms. Sonya Seigafuse and Ms. Ashley Fischer of Lippincott Williams & Wilkins for their patience, kindness, and close co-operation. Their gentle guidance through the many sequential processes of development necessary to publishing made our work on the clinical and visual content, possible.

We are thankful to the authors of the numerous textbooks, dictionaries, journals, and articles that we have drawn on to prepare this book. To mention each reference here would further increase the literary volume of this book, something which we have done our best to keep to the absolute minimum.

We also wish to thank Dr. Abolghassem Najafian and the late Ms. Nayereh Shiva, whose encouragement for this work is beyond words and my expression of thanks, beyond measure. My gratitude will never equal their generosity of warmth and friendship.

We wish to thank Dr. Lee Miller and Dr. Edward McCabe for their incomparable leadership in medical education over the course of the past several decades and of their recognizing the value of such an Atlas in the armamentarium of the medical educator and of the physician. We are grateful for their facilitating that vision for us.

Our families made the greatest possible sacrifice in allowing us to spend the little time we had for them, on this book. I would like to thank, especially, my wife of nearly 55 years, the partner who has come along with me every step of the way, in places—too hot and too cold, in towns—large and small, and with life's turbulence and eventual stability, on this clinical journey, and on the life that we led side by side, alongside it, Farah.

To my beautiful wife, Farah,
who has made everything possible for me,
and for our family.

Introduction

It is a wonderment of the human mind the astonishing particularity with which we may recall an especially ghastly wound, a deformed chest, or a misshaped head we may have observed in medical school or residency. It is less wonderful to reflect on the forgotten features of an equally engaging lecture from the same period of one's training or career. During the course of our medical education, we have listened to hundreds of lectures and read countless pages of text. But in the end, when faced with a challenging clinical scenario, it is the images that stare back at us.

Technology in its most recent forms has brought us vast volumes of information, but even that enormous power has failed to expand by a second an hour in a single day. We have kept these two principles, growing volumes of information and the near correspondent shrinking of time, firmly in mind in preparing this book. To that end, the text is brief, easy to read and to the point. Efficiency of teaching and of learning being thus paramount, corresponding images are representations of what the doctor ought to see in a patient once and evermore remember. It is the purpose of the authors that you will be able to draw on these in the diagnosis and treatment of patients in a manner that is meticulous and exacting, as was we are certain the expectation of all of your mentors, and the hope of all of us who are forever in the *practice* of medicine.

It is thus our desire here to take readers on a *visual* journey into the children's wards of hospitals and our pediatrics offices from Tehran, Iran to Manchester, England to Los Angeles, California. To share with you the 100 years of combined medical practice of the authors, a father and both sons, all of whom are pediatricians. To show at a glance, what would otherwise require hours to appreciate through recitation of text. And to recall in your own patients the images of clinical features seen and learned in this book, together with the clinical scenarios of the actual patients pictured.

It is the sincere hope of the three of us that with inventive ideas that are elemental and strong, uncompromising hard work, and leadership that is at once demanding and sympathetic, the reader will capitalize on this information to build future volumes of images along with novel ways of delivering that knowledge, to yet to come generations of doctors.

Contents

Contents

by ANATOMICAL SPECIFIC FEATURES

Skin

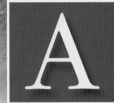

ABSCESS (L. abscessus; From: Ab, away; cedero, to go)

Definition
- Localized collection of pus in a cavity formed by the disintegration of tissue.

Etiology
- Almost any organism or foreign body can cause an abscess, but it is frequently related to coagulase positive staphylococci.

Symptoms and Signs
- Depends on the anatomic location.
- A brain abscess has symptoms and signs related to increased intracranial pressure.
- Pain is more severe when there is no room for expansion of the abscess (i.e., dental abscess).
- Figures A–E.

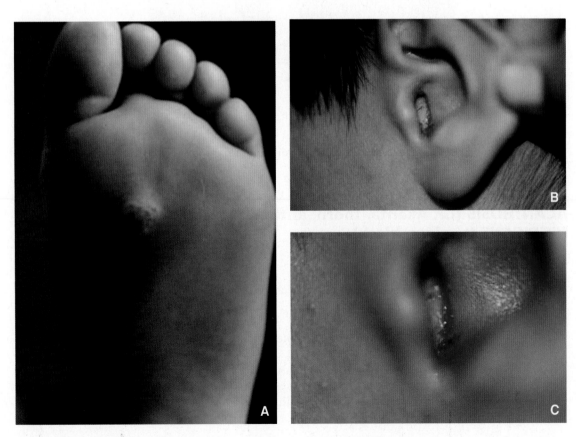

Figure A: Abscess of the foot. Four-year-old boy with 4 days of increasing pain and swelling in the foot. Erythema of the plantar surface of the left foot, black and fluctuant in the center, diffusely tender. Relief followed incision and drainage.

Figures B–C: Abscess of the ear canal. Eleven-year-old boy with 3 days of increasing ear ache. No fever. The patient felt "something popped up" in his ear. The abscess naturally drained and relief followed.

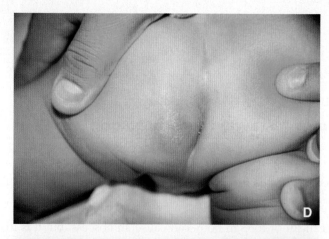

Figure D: Abscess, perianal. Nine-month-old female brought in for "a ball in her butt, increasing in size." The abscess was incised and drained.

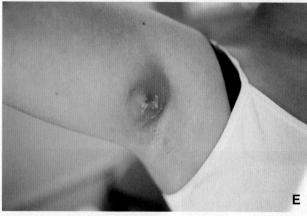

Figure E: Abscess, axilla. Teenage girl who regularly shaves her axillae. She had a large umbilicated abscess in the axilla, with some exudate.

Treatment
- Drainage is essential for healing, although antibiotics alone may be sufficient in smaller abscesses.

ACANTHOSIS (Gr. Akanta, thorn; anthos, flower)
NIGRICANS (L. niger, black)

Definition
- Acanthosis nigricans is a diffuse, dark, velvety hyperplasia of the spinous layer of the skin.

Etiology
- Acanthosis is frequently related to obesity, but it can be a sign of insulin resistance or diabetes.
- Less commonly, this condition may be inherited (benign form).
- Rarely it could be related to a pituitary tumor or other malignancies.
- It can also be associated with a syndrome, such as Bloom's syndrome, Crouzon's syndrome, Seip syndrome, or Addison's disease.

Symptoms and Signs
- Common findings are hyperpigmentation and hyperkeratosis in the axillae, intertriginous regions, and over prominences with rough surfaces, flexors of the limbs, and back of the hands and neck.

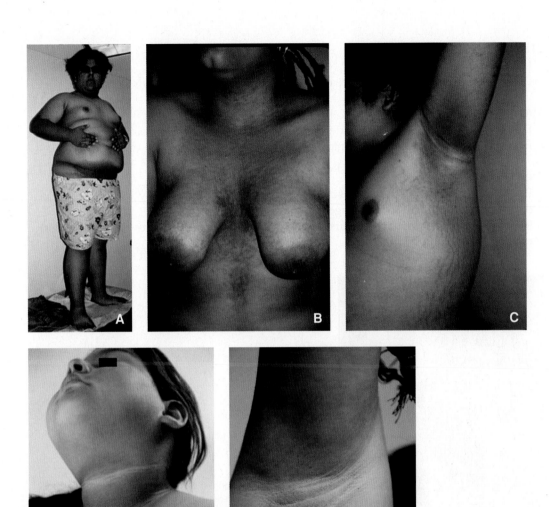

Figures A–D: The hyperpigmented, velvety, leathery changes of acanthosis nigricans in four obese children.

Figure E: Acanthosis nigricans in a 14-year-old girl with normal weight, blood sugar, and lipid profile. She has juvenile idiopathic arthritis and the same skin changes in her neck.

- Accentuation of skin lines may occur.
- Involved skin may be velvety, leathery, or warty.
- Figures A–E.

Treatment
- This condition may improve or resolve completely with weight loss, if the cause is obesity.

ACHALASIA (Gr. Chalasis, relaxation)

Definition
- Achalasia, a primary esophageal motor disorder, representing incomplete relaxation of the smooth muscle fibers of the gastrointestinal tract, and the lower esophagus in particular, during swallowing.

Etiology
- Unknown.
- Ganglion cells are frequently decreased.

Symptoms and Signs
- Dysphagia, which may lead to undernutrition or malnutrition.
- Retained food, may cause esophagitis and aspiration.

Treatment
- Pneumatic dilation, where the muscle fibers are stretched and torn by inflating a ballon that is placed in the lower esophageal sphincter.
- Heller myotomy, a cut along the first layer of the esophageal wall provides permanent relief in the majority of patients.

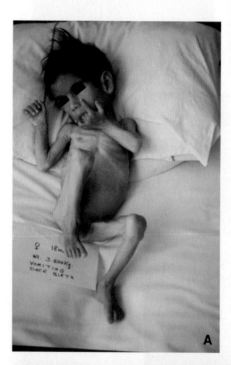

Figure A: This 18-month-old girl presented with difficulty feeding, vomiting and severe malnutrition. Her chest film and barium swallow prior to surgery are displayed in **Figures B** and **C**.

Figure B: Single frontal view of the chest demonstrates a dilated esophagus in the upper mediastinum (*curved black line*). **Figure C:** Single fluoroscopic view of the chest during an esophagram demonstrates smooth dilation of the esophagus with characteristic "bird-beak" configuration at the gastro-esophageal junction (*arrow*).

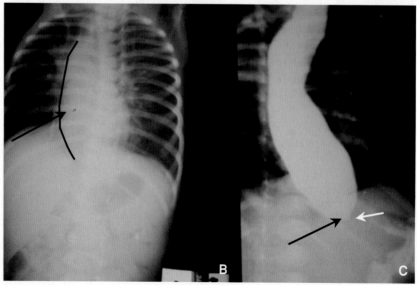

ACNE VULGARIS (Acne Gr., point; Vulgaris L., common)

Definition
- Acne vulgaris is a disorder of the pilosebaceous apparatus and the 3 most common skin disorder of the second and third decades of life.

Etiology
- The role of diet in acne is under debate. Recent studies indicate a possible relationship to ingestion of milk. However, more work in the area is needed.
- It appears mostly during the second decade of life, more commonly in boys than girls and less frequently in Asians and African Americans.
- It is more common in some families, which points to the possibility of an inheritance pattern, likely, as an autosomal dominant trait.

Symptoms and Signs
- Micro comedones may represent the earliest type of acne lesions. Subsequently, closed comedones, papules, pustules, nodules, and cysts may occur.
- Figures A–F.

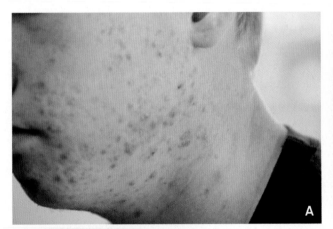

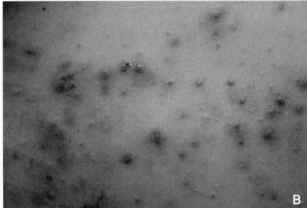

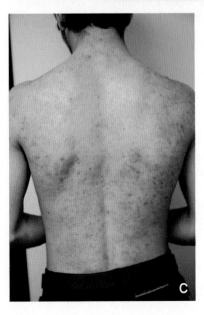

Figures A and **B** show acne on the face and neck of a 14-year-old boy. Note comedonal acne with closed comedones or white heads and pustules. In **Figure C**, the distribution pattern of acne on a 16-year-old boy's back, comedonal acne with open comedones (black heads), and closed comedones (white heads).

figures continues

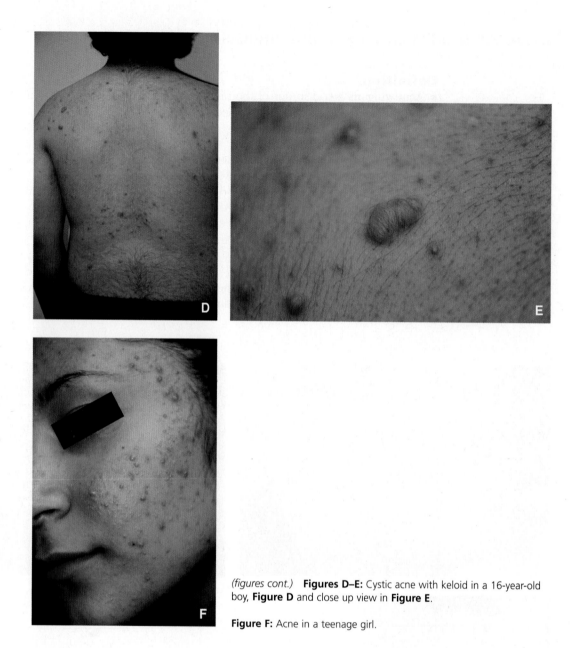

(figures cont.)   **Figures D–E:** Cystic acne with keloid in a 16-year-old boy, **Figure D** and close up view in **Figure E**.

Figure F: Acne in a teenage girl.

Treatment

- Should be individualized.
- Today's understanding of the effective treatment regiments for acne should be deployed in order to avoid the emotional burden commonly associated with this treatable problem as well as to prevent scarring of the skin.
- Benzoyl peroxide, salicylic acid, tretinoin (Retin-A), systemic antibiotics, estrogens, and oral retinoids are drugs available in the pediatricians' armamentarium for the treatment of acne.

ACRAL LICK DERMATITIS

(See Atopic Dermatitis)

ACROMEGALOGIGANTISM

Definition
- Overproduction of growth hormone in individuals with open epiphyses causes gigantism. The same problem in patients with closed epiphyses results in acromegaly. Acromegalogigantism is a rare phenomenon characterized by hypersecretion of growth hormone before puberty with continuation into adulthood.

Etiology
- A primary pituitary tumor.
- Also, deletion of the 11q13 region of chromosome 11 can cause somatotrophs adenomas.

Symptoms and Signs
- The main clinical finding in gigantism is longitudinal growth, accelerated secondary to excessive production and release of growth hormone.
- Enlarging hands and feet, as well as coarse features, are common.
- In children head growth may be conspicuous.
- The nose grows and broadens, the tongue is enlarged, the mandible grows excessively, and the teeth become separated.
- There may be some dorsal kyphosis, thickening of the fingers and toes, and vision problems due to optic nerve compression.
- The test to show the failure to suppress serum growth hormone levels is the gold standard for diagnosis.
- Figures A and B.

Treatment
- Surgery and radiation.

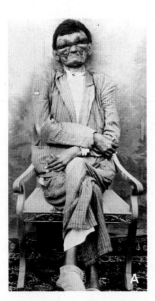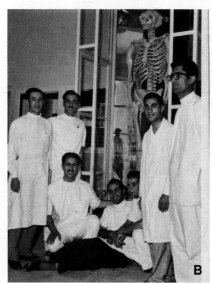

Figures A–B: The patient at the age of 10 years **(Figure A)**, and his skeleton at the entrance of Shiraz Medical School, University of Shiraz, Iran **(Figure B)**. One of the medical students is the author (RS) and the first seated from left **(Figure B)**. This patient was born to an underprivileged family and had an unremarkable medical history until the age of 6 years. His growth accelerated from that point, and he had many adult features by the age of 9 years. It was at this age that he was brought to the attention of an internist in 1940 in a rural city in Iran with the limited available medical resources. The patient was noted to have had some degree of mental retardation, was emotionally labile and bursting into tears easily, had an excessive appetite, poor vision, and was hypersexual. His weight was 245 kg (539 lbs) and his height was 259 cm (8'6"). His head was heavy for his body and he could not hold it up straight. He had some scoliosis to the left. He died of pneumonia at the age of 18 years. On autopsy, his sella turcica was wider than normal, but had no signs of erosion.

ADENOID HYPERTROPHY (Aden Gr., gland)

Definition
- Adenoids are lymphoid tissue, consisting of mostly B lymphocytes, some T lymphocytes, and plasma cells that surround the opening of the oral and nasal cavities into the pharynx.

Etiology
- Adenoids induce secretory immunity, control the production of secretory immunoglobulins, and provide primary defense against foreign materials.
- In the majority of children, adenoids and tonsils grow until the age of 8 to 9 years, and then gradually shrink in size.
- In a small number of children, adenoids remain hypertrophied and become symptomatic.

Symptoms and Signs
- Difficulty breathing through the nose, causing mouth breathing, snoring, and recurrent upper respiratory infections.
- A cephalometric lateral neck x-ray is a good diagnostic tool (Figure).

Treatment
- Adenoidectomy can help, only when medical management has failed.

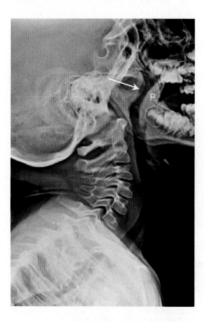

Soft tissue neck x-ray. (*Arrow*) Convex soft tissue density of the posterior nasopharynx corresponding to enlarged adenoid tonsils. Palatine tonsils (P) are not markedly enlarged.

ALBINISM (L. albus, white)

Definition
- Albinism is a congenital hypopigmentation of the skin, hair, and eyes.

Etiology
- Ocular albinism is a rare, x-linked or autosomal recessive trait with photophobia and mild depigmentation of the skin.
- The oculocutaneous form is more generalized to the skin and is inherited as autosomal recessive.

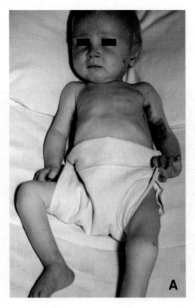 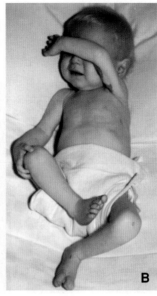

Figures A–B: This 8-month-old boy was admitted for impetigo and diarrhea. His parents had dark skin and black hair and there was no known albinism in the family. Note depigmentation of the skin, hair, and eyes and the photophobia.

Symptoms and Signs
- Photophobia, central scotoma, habitual squinting, and nystagmus.
- These children and adults learn to avoid sunlight and wear sunglasses and contact lenses.
- The skin in Caucasians with oculocutaneous albinism can be milky white, the irides are gray or blue, the pupils are pink, and the hair is white to yellow.
- The skin in people of African descent is much lighter in color, the hair is red to blonde, and the eyes are blue to hazel.
- Figures A and B.

Treatment
- Tinted glasses and contact lenses to ameliorate photophobia, protective clothing and sunscreen to protect from the sun and reduce the risk of skin cancer.

ALOPECIA

ALOPECIA AREATA
(Gr. alopekia a disease in which the hair falls out.) (Occurring in patches.)

Definition
- A common problem in pediatrics. Sudden oval or round area of hair loss.

Etiology
- Unknown. But dysregulation of the immune system with the target organ being the hair roots may be a factor. The concept of stress-induced alopecia areata is controversial.

Symptoms and Signs
- Patchy hair loss can occur anywhere on the scalp, the bearded area, and eyebrows or eyelashes. This sudden change in appearance, without any other signs or symptoms, is often of great concern to children and to their parents.
- There may be several bald patches.
- Discrete islands of noninflammatory hair loss.

Treatment

■ The hair may regrow in 2 to 3 months in the majority of cases. Topical corticosteroids and intralesional dilute steroid injections may be helpful.

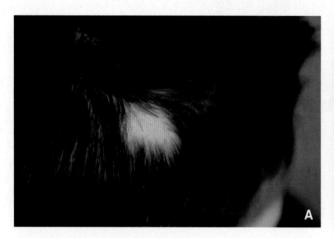 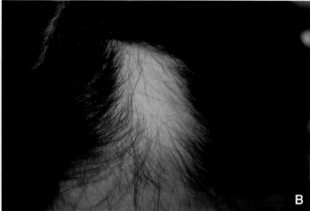

Figures A–B: Alopecia in the parietal area of an 8-year-old boy, present for 2 months **(Figure A)**. A 2-month history of hair loss in an 11-year-old girl **(Figure B)**.

ALOPECIA TOTALIS AND ALOPECIA UNIVERSALIS

■ Alopecia totalis is when the hair loss expands to the entire scalp. Total body hair loss is called alopecia universalis. The etiology in both phenomena is unknown, although autoimmunity is a probable factor in this disease. The value of local steroid treatment is questionable.

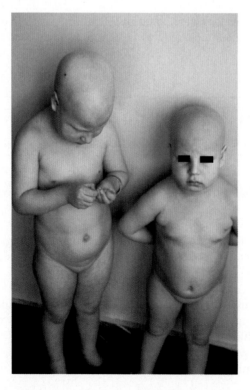

Two sisters with total body hair loss. Each lost her hair around the age of 18 months, without any preceding disease.

ALOPECIA DUE TO FRICTION

Definition
- A common finding in infants, where the head (occipital area) rubs on the bed or pillow.

Etiology
- Mechanical, constant friction.

Symptoms and Signs
- An area of hair loss on the scalp, where the friction is most intense.

Treatment
- The hair regrows when the baby lies less on her/his back and spends time crawling, sitting, and running.
- Reassurance to the parents is all that is often needed.

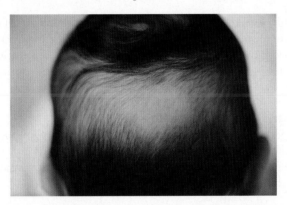

Hair loss due to friction in a 5-month-old.

AMNIOTIC BAND

Definition
- Amniotic bands are constrictive tissue bands.

Etiology
- Primary amniotic rupture, possibly due to abdominal trauma, amniocentesis, and hereditary defects of collagen such as osteogenesis imperfecta and Ehlers–Danlos syndrome.

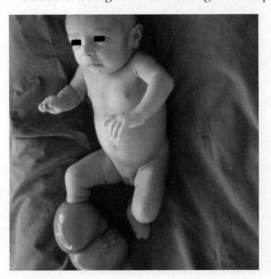

This baby was born with this isolated deformity. Her mother denied having taken any prescription or herbal medication during her pregnancy. Amniotic band was the presumed etiology.

Symptoms and Signs
- It depends on the entangled part of the fetus by the band; mostly extremities.

Treatment
- Timely removal of the band if known.

ANEMIA (Iron deficiency)

Definition
- A reduction below normal in the concentration of erythrocytes or hemoglobin in the blood. Iron-deficiency anemia is the most common hematologic disease of infancy and childhood.

Etiology
- Low-birth weight and perinatal hemorrhage can cause anemia in infancy. Bleeding from a Meckel diverticulum, peptic ulcer, polyp, or inflammatory bowel disease are the common etiologies in toddlers and older children. Consumption of large amounts of cow's milk is the common dietary cause of anemia during the second year of life.

Symptoms and Signs
- Pallor, irritability, pagophagia (the desire to ingest extraordinary amounts of ice or other substances such as clay and lead-containing paint).
- Tachycardia, systolic murmur (hemic murmur), and poor attention span. Low serum ferritin, serum iron, and hemoglobin.

Treatment
- Dietary iron supplementation.

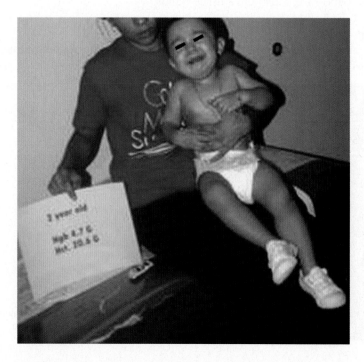

A 2-year-old boy, raised on cow's milk alone. He was seen for ear infection, had a temperature of 100°F (37.8°C), his right tympanic membrane was inflamed and pale. His hemoglobin was 4.7 g/dL and hematocrit was 19.6%.

A

ANGIOEDEMA (Angio Gr., Vessel—blood vessel)

Definition
- A subcutaneous or submucosal tissue edema causing a sudden swelling manifested in different parts of the body, but often around the eyes and lips. This type of edema is deeper than urticaria.

Etiology
- Hereditary angioedema has an autosomal dominant pattern of inheritance.
- An IgE-mediated allergic reaction to food, medication, pollen, animals, sunlight, or even water can cause angioedema. The etiology often remains unknown.

Symptoms and Signs
- The swelling may be felt as a "heavy" eyelid or lip with some associated pain and itching.
- Figures A–E.

Treatment
- Epinephrine, antihistaminics, and corticosteroids can be used in the management of angioedema.

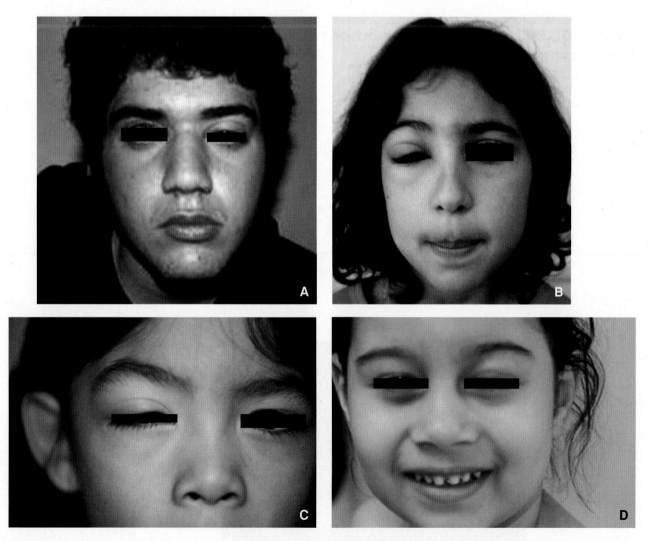

Figures A–D: The four children had a sudden onset of swelling, mostly when they woke up in the morning.

figures continues

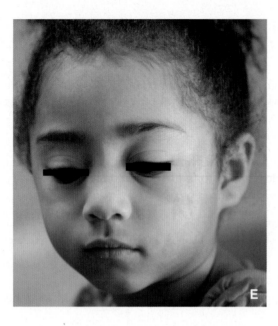

(figures cont.) **Figure E:** A 4-year-old girl woke up one morning with a rash and slight itching on her face. She had had a few such episodes for which her mother had previously taken her to the emergency department. There was mild edema around the eyes and mouth, more prominent on the left and extending to the left upper cheek. No rash elsewhere on the body.

ANKYLOGLOSSIA (Gr. Ankylos, bent or crooked; Glossa, tongue), TONGUE TIE

Definition
- Ankyloglossia is an abnormally short lingual frenum.

Etiology
- Unknown.

Symptoms and Signs
- It may rarely interfere with feeding or tongue movements (in speech).

Treatment
- The frenum grows as the tongue grows and the problem self resolves. In severe cases when it causes serious problems with speech or feeding, surgical treatment may be considered.

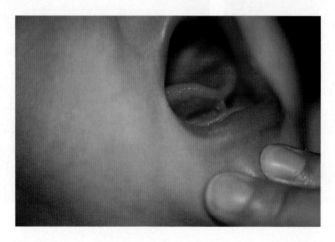

Ankyloglossia in an infant.

ANTHRAX (Gr. Coal)

A

CUTANEOUS ANTHRAX

Definition
- Anthrax is a serious disease with manifestations in the skin, respiratory tract, or gastrointestinal tract.
- The skin ulcer is black, hence the name anthrax or charbone (French, meaning coal).

Etiology
- Anthrax is caused by an anaerobic, gram-positive, encapsulated spore-forming, nonmotile rod with two exotoxins called lethal edema toxin and an antiphagocytic capsule.
- The spores can remain viable for many years.
- The source of infection is infected animals and their products; that is, carcasses, hide, wool, hair, meat, and bone.

Symptoms and Signs
- Anthrax can present in three major forms: Cutaneous, which is easily treatable; systemic or inhalation, which is lethal; and gastrointestinal.
- Cutaneous anthrax begins with a papule that ulcerates with a central black eschar.
- Figures A–D.

Treatment
- Cutaneous anthrax can be treated with penicillin, tetracycline, or ciprofloxacin.
- For bioterrorism-associated cutaneous disease in adults and children, ciprofloxacin, levofloxacin, or doxycycline is recommended.

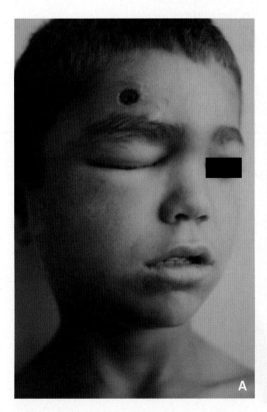
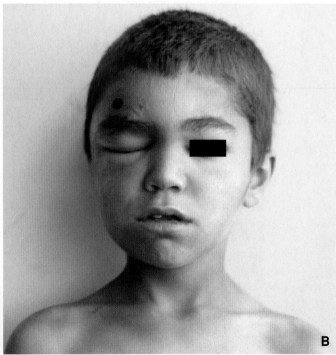

Figures A–B: This 9-year-old boy, the son of an animal skinner, used to spend his summer vacations in his father's workshop. His mother noted a black sore on his forehead and brought him to the hospital. Note the black sore and the edema of the right eye lid.

figures continues

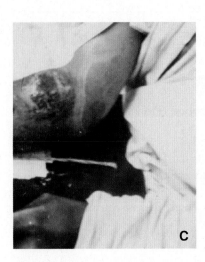

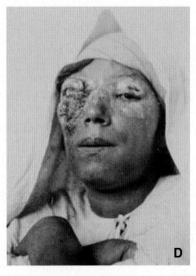

(figures cont.)   **Figures C–D:** Advanced cutaneous anthrax on the left forearm of a young man and the face, mainly the right eye, of a young woman. Both were treated successfully and discharged home. The woman sustained total destruction of her eyeball **(Figure D)**.

APHTHOUS STOMATITIS (Gr. Aphtha, ulcer)

Definition
- This is a recurrent problem and it has been aptly termed "recurrent aphthous stomatitis," with painful ulcerations, mainly of the oral mucosa.

Etiology
- Unknown.
- Trauma and stress may be the most common contributing factors.
- Some families are more prone to aphthous ulcers than others.
- The prevalence is as high as 25% in the general population at some point. It can present at any age and is rare during infancy and more common among teenagers and young adults.

Symptoms and Signs
- Each aphtha is a painful ulcer anywhere on the oropharyngeal mucosa, particularly on the tongue, and varies in size from 1 to >10 mm with a pseudomembrane and an erythematous halo with central white crater-like lesions.
- There can be one (aphtha) or many (aphthae). Eating, drinking, or even talking may be quite painful.
- Aphthous stomatitis in several children of varying ages and genders in different anatomical locations (Figures A–I).

Treatment
- Treatment is symptomatic.
- Complete recovery without any scar within 2 weeks is common.

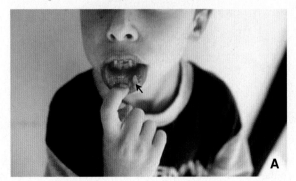

Figure A

figures continues

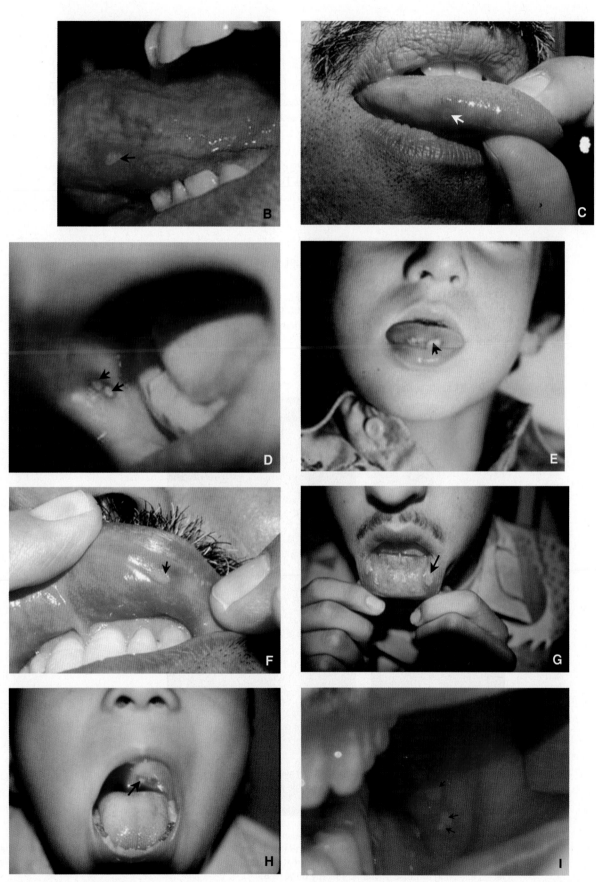

APLASTIC ANEMIA

Definition
- Aplastic anemia can be the result of bone marrow failure with reduction of hematopoietic cells and their replacement by fat, resulting in pancytopenia, often accompanied by granulocytopenia and thrombocytopenia.

Etiology
- It can be hereditary or acquired. Drugs such as chloramphenicol, benzene, and antiepileptic drugs, viruses (Epstein-Barr, hepatitis A, B, C, and nonhepatitis A, B, C, human immunodeficiency), and radiation can cause aplastic anemia, as can pregnancy and leukemia.

Symptoms and Signs
- Aplastic anemia can present with fatigue, bleeding, infection, or cardiac failure.

Treatment
- Comprehensive supportive care, treatment of underlying bone marrow failure, and selective bone marrow transplantation are some of the treatment options for acquired aplastic anemia.

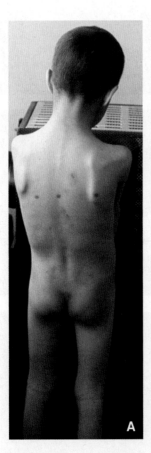 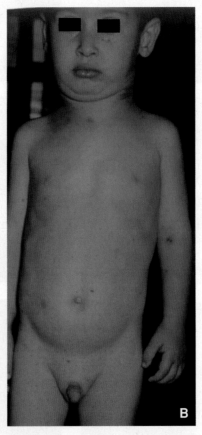

Figures A–B: A 7-year-old boy with aplastic anemia. Etiology unknown. Note the purpura and ecchymosis on the back **(Figure A)**. A 5-year-old boy who presented with a "rash" diagnosed as secondary to aplastic anemia. He had a history of chloramphenicol use for treatment of a skin infection. Note the purpura and the cushingoid facies following a course of steroid therapy **(Figure B)**.

ARACHNOID CYST (Leptomeningeal cyst)

Definition
- An arachnoid cyst is a collection of cerebrospinal fluid lined by arachnoid that does not directly communicate with the ventricular system or subarachnoid space.

Etiology
- A developmental abnormality present at birth or due to a head injury, meningitis, brain tumor, or surgery later in life.

Symptoms and Signs
- These cysts are most commonly found in the middle cranial fossa are largely asymptomatic and are generally found incidentally. Symptoms are mostly due to increased intracranial pressure and include headache, nausea, vomiting, hearing and visual disturbances, and vertigo.
- Figures A–C.

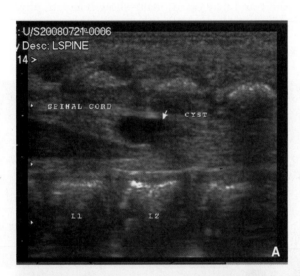

Figures A: A teenage girl ran into a metallic gate and sustained a head injury. Sagittal sonographic image demonstrates normal location of the conus medullaris above the L2/L3 disc level. There is a small ovoid cyst not centered within the filum terminalis. Appearance is favorable for a small arachnoid cyst **(Figure A)**.

Figures B–C: Axial CT images of the brain demonstrate a large fluid density cyst expanding the sylvian fissure and extending to the middle cranial fossa (*arrows*).

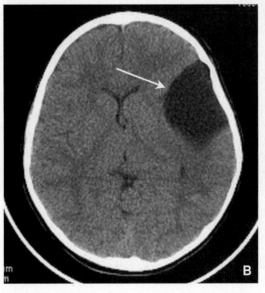

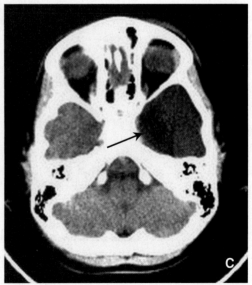

Treatment

- Will depend on the location, size, and symptoms. When asymptomatic, often no treatment is needed. Surgery is an option.

ARTHROGRYPOSIS MULTIPLEX

Definition

- Arthrogryposis multiplex is a progressive, congenital disorder.

Etiology

- Etiology is unknown.

Symptoms and Signs

- It can present with joint contractures, secondary deformities, and limited motion, and can involve from one to all four extremities.
- Lower extremities are more commonly involved. Club foot, dislocated hip, contractures of the wrist, knee, elbow, and hands, mostly in flexion and with limited motions, are common findings. The skin appears thickened and muscle fibers are atrophied (Figures A–C).
- X-rays are mostly negative and may occasionally show bone atrophy.

Treatment

- Orthopedic referral is necessary to correct deformities.

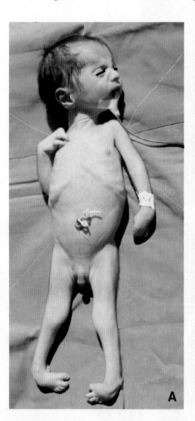
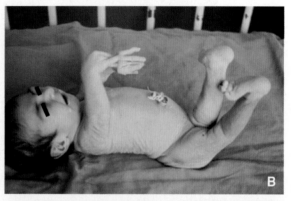
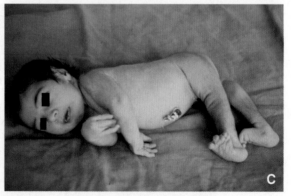

Figure A: A 10-day-old baby with multiple joint deformities; contracture and flexion of the wrist and ankles with club feet. He also had bilateral hip dislocation. His knees were swollen with limited mobility. All four extremities are involved in this child: Quadrimelic.

Figures B–C: A 2-week-old girl with congenital joint contracture and limited movement. Note the oral thrush and the gentian violet on her lips to treat the thrush. Her eyebrows are colored by a dye for cosmetic reasons (by her parents).

ASTHMA

Definition
- Asthma is a chronic pulmonary airway disease caused by inflammation and hypersensitivity.
- Allergic rhinitis or hay fever, atopic dermatitis, and asthma, in that order of frequency, are collectively known as atopic diseases.
- Atopic diseases may coexist.
- Some infants with atopic dermatitis develop allergic rhinitis and asthma, the so called "atopic march."

Etiology
- Interaction of genetics and environmental factors such as common cold viruses and allergies are believed to cause asthma.

Symptoms and Signs
- Asthma is marked by recurrent attacks of paroxysmal airflow obstruction, dyspnea, and expiratory wheezing.
- Exertion or irritants such as tobacco, dust, or cold air lead to wheezing, coughing, and dyspnea.

Treatment
- Should mostly be aimed at maintaining sleep and normal activity, preventing chronic asthma symptoms, normal lung function and minimizing treatment side effects, as well as

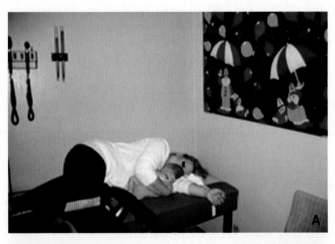

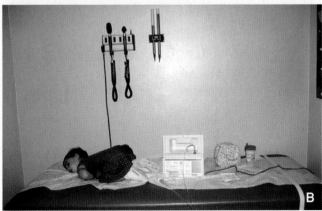

Figures A–B: Both infants presented with coughing and wheezing all night. Both mother and baby fell asleep after two treatments with nebulized albuterol (both had been up all night). Normal PO2.

regular assessment and monitoring to control the factors contributing to asthma severity, pharmacotherapy, and patient education. Clearing the environment from possible trigger factors is essential.

ATOPIC DERMATITIS (Gr. Atopy—different, out of place)

Definition
- Atopic dermatitis is a recurrent, chronic, and pruritic skin disorder and is one of the most common skin pathologies found in children.
- Approximately 30% to 50% of children with atopic dermatitis will develop another form of atopy such as allergic rhinitis, asthma, or food allergy.

Etiology
- Genetics is presumed to play a role.
- Environmental factors such as food allergies contact with certain allergens such as nickel and some fabrics.

Symptoms and Signs
- A tendency toward dry skin, lower threshold for itching stimuli, increased palmar markings, and keratosis pilaris.
- The skin may be worse during the winter, when there is a lower relative humidity.
- Excessive bathing removes lipoprotein complexes that hold water in the stratum corneum. But bathing is essential to remove bacteria and the overgrowth of staphylococci, which are common in atopic dermatitis.
- The face in infants, flexor surfaces of the arms and legs in older infants, antecubital and popliteal fossae, face and neck in older children are the sights of predilection, and pruritus which is worse at night are common signs and symptoms.
- Constant rubbing and scratching of the highly sensitive skin predisposes skin for infections.
- These children are more active, restless, irritable, have generalized pallor, and susceptibility to unusual cutaneous infections, especially viral ones such as disseminated vaccinia and herpes simplex. They also have a tendency for spreading molluscum contagiosum (Figures A–T).

Treatment
- Reduction of dryness and itching through lubrication, wet compresses, tacrolimus ointment, and topical steroids.
- Antihistamines to reduce the itching and to interrupt the itch-scratch–itch cycle.
- Antibiotics, to control the overgrowth of staphylococci on the skin and nares.
- To minimize infection, dilute Clorox soaks are recommended.
- Steroids should be used short term, the strength of the steroids depends on the severity of the dermatitis.

A

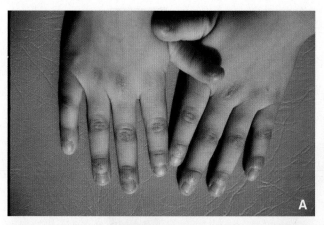

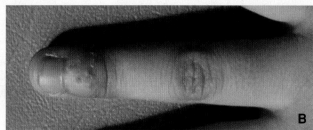

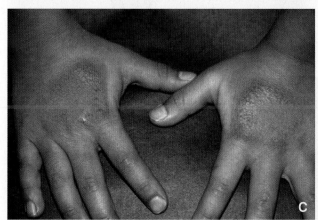

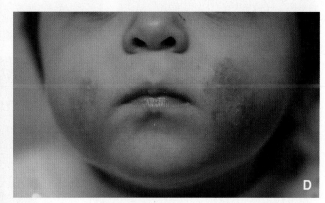

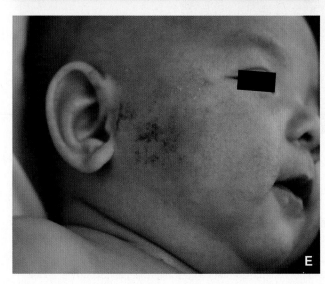

Figures A–B: *Acral lick dermatitis:* This 7-year-old boy was brought in for a rash on his fingers for a "couple of years." No itching. He has a habit of licking on his fingers. Constant wetting and drying created the dermatitis.

Figure C: *Sucking dermatitis,* on the skin of a 7-year-old boy who had a habit of sucking his hand. Constant wetting and drying caused the dermatitis.

Figures D–E: *Infantile atopic dermatitis* in two children. Note the erythema, oozing, and some scaling and crusting. All these signs resolved with moisturizers and 1% hydrocortisone cream.

figures continues

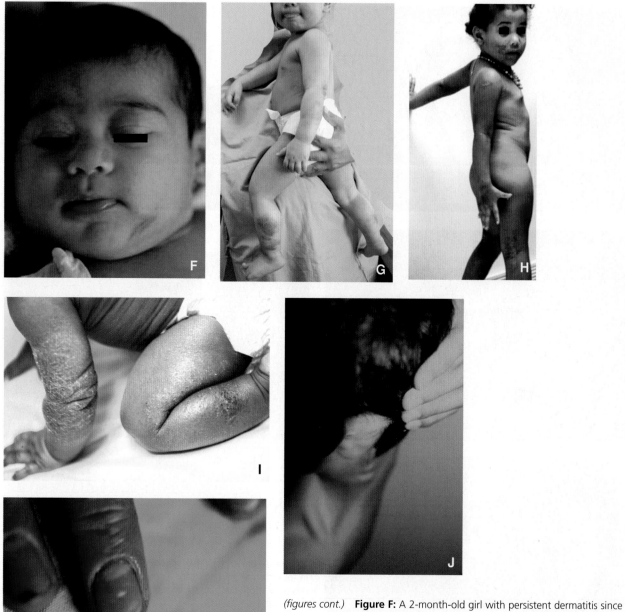

(figures cont.) **Figure F:** A 2-month-old girl with persistent dermatitis since she was a newborn. Note the scratching mark below the left cheek. She had fully recovered by 6 months of age with moisturizers and 1% hydrocortisone cream.

Figure G: Severe generalized eczema in a 1-year-old boy. Erythema, papules, and plaques can be seen on the legs and arms. There is oozing on the face.

Figure H: This child had infantile eczema when a few weeks old; improved after her first birthday. The eczema soon evolved into a more severe form, with intense itching and difficulty sleeping at night for her and her parents. Constant aggressive itching and scratching added several skin infections. Dry, erythematous papules, excoriated oozing skin on the cheeks, hands, upper arms, and flexural folds of the extremities. Treatment of her skin infection was the first step in her management. A bath with half a cup of bleach in 40 gallons (150 liters) of water, oral cephalexin, emollients, steroid cream, and antihistamines helped to treat this longstanding problem.

Figure I: Dry, excoriated, erythematous, and lichenified skin (thickened skin with accentuated surface markings) in a 10-month-old boy.

Figure J: Atopic dermatitis with regional adenopathy in a teenage boy.

Figure K: Thickened nail with ridges and pitting, in chronic atopic dermatitis.

figures continues

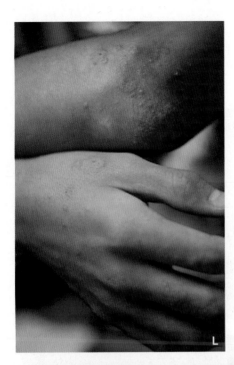

(figures cont.)   **Figure L:** Erythema and papules with some lichenification on the extensor aspect of the elbow and dermatitis of the hand of a teenager boy.

Figures M–N: Nickel induced dermatitis in a teenage girl. The button on the jeans was made of nickel. But cobalt is used in the dye of the fabric itself, another irritant allergenic material.

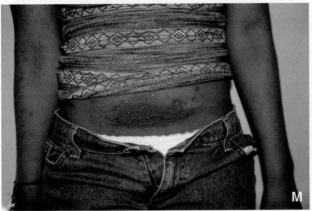

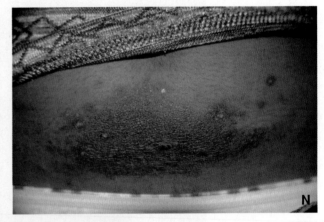

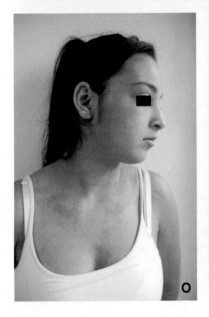

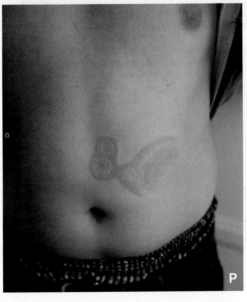

Figure O: This teenage girl developed a rash with itching following a face wash with a cleanser for acne. The liquid ran onto her neck and chest at times, irritating the skin, causing her symptoms and signs.

Figure P: Red overlapping rings seen in atopic dermatitis.

figures continues

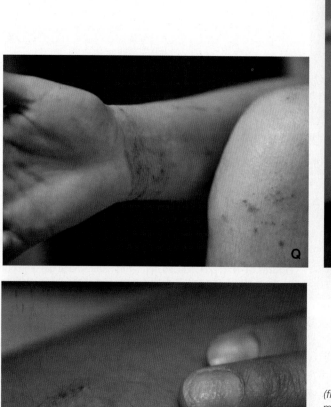

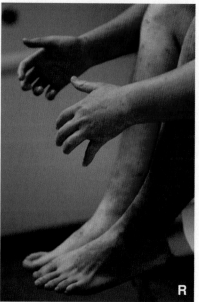

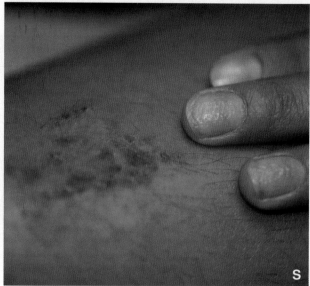

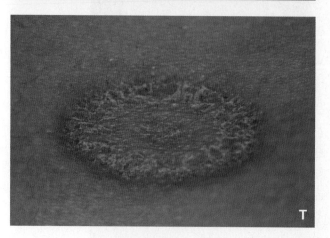

(figures cont.)   **Figures Q–R:** Contact dermatitis. This 14-year-old boy had severe itching and rash for 2 weeks. No history suggestive of any specific allergies. Note the erythema, pink macules, and plaques.

Figure S: A 9-year-old boy with 1-year history of itching and a rash on the shins and elbows. This was a healthy boy who had no other medical problems. His skin was macerated with eczematous shins and involvement of the extensor aspect of the elbows. Also note the pitting of the fingernails.

Figure T: Close-up view of a single plaque of atopic dermatitis on the abdominal wall of a young girl.

BALANOPOSTHITIS (AND INCIDENTAL FINDING OF VARICOCELE)

Definition
- Balanoposthitis is the inflammation of prepuce and glans of the penis.

Etiology
- Candida albicans, staphylococcus aureus, group B streptococcus, and Malassezia are among the possible infective organisms. Poor hygiene in uncircumcised men is usually the cause.

Symptoms and Signs
- Pain and swelling of the penis.

Treatment
- Hygiene, topical antibiotics (metronidazole), and topical steroids.

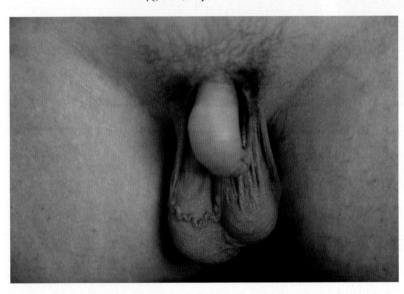

A 16-year-old sexually inactive boy with a 1-day history of pain and swelling of the penis. No fever or urinary symptoms. Swollen, erythematous, tender penis. He also has varicocele, an incidental finding. Varicocele is the varicosity of the veins of the scrotum, looking like a bag of worms, a bluish tint throughout the skin.

BEALS SYNDROME

Definition
- A rare syndrome with abnormalities in the extremities and kyphosis.

Etiology
- Unknown. Autosomal dominant inheritance.

Symptoms and Signs
- The hallmarks of this disease are abnormalities in the extremities and kyphosis.
- Other possible abnormalities are micrognathia, mitral valve prolapse, and other congenital abnormalities.
- Scoliosis may worsen with time but the joints may improve.

Treatment
- Possible corrective surgeries of the congenital deformities.

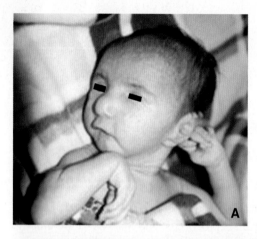
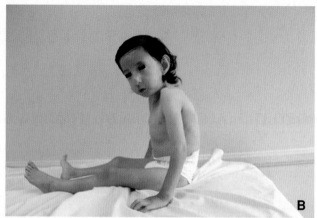
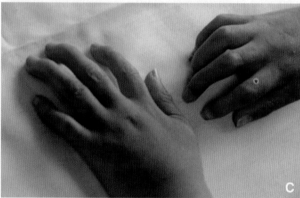
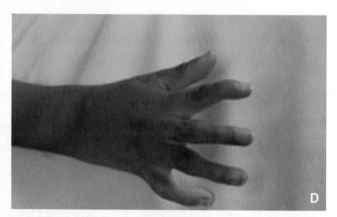

Figures A–D: This is a 1-month-old infant born at Term, SGA (IUGR) and infant of a mother with gestational diabetes. Head circumference and weight are at the 10th percentile, height is at the 50th percentile. Prominent ear crus, short palpebral fissures, epicanthic folds, prominent bulbous nose, high nasal bridge, and micrognathia are prominent features. His karyotype was normal **(Figure A).** The following features are more prominent in the patient who is 3-years old in **Figures B, C, and D:** Arachnodactyly (abnormally long, slender fingers), clinodactyly (permanent lateral or medial deviation or deflection of one or more fingers), camptodactyly (fixed flexion deformity of the interphalangeal joints of the little finger), and pectus carinatum (pigeon chest). Decreased range of motion at the hips, knees, and ankles; abducted thumbs and decreased muscle mass are marked in the extremities.

BELL'S PALSY

Definition
- Bell's palsy is a sudden unilateral paralysis due to a lesion of the facial nerve and without any other cranial neuropathy.

Etiology
- The viruses most often involved are Epstein-Barr, herpes simplex, Lyme disease, and the mumps virus.
- It may be seen at any age and is often preceded by an acute viral infection, which is believed to cause an allergic reaction or immune demyelinating process of the facial nerve.

Symptoms and Signs
- There is a characteristic distortion of the face. The upper and lower parts of the face are paralyzed, the corner of the mouth is drooped, and the lips are pooled to the opposite side.
- Patients may not be able to close the eye on the affected side and develop an exposure keratitis.

Treatment
- Research does not support steroids in the treatment of Bell's palsy.

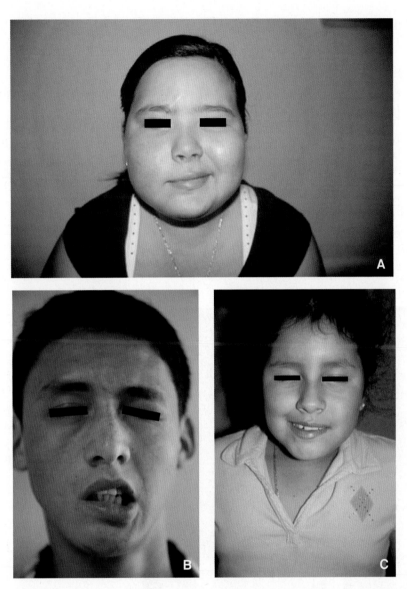

Figures A–C: Bell's palsy. Note the inability to close the right eye, drooped right cheek, and lips; and nose pulled to the left. She also complained of a diminished sense of taste, and food remaining in the right side of her mouth **(Figure A)**. Note the right facial palsy, inability to close the right eye, and lips pulled to the left in **Figure B**; and left facial palsy, inability to close the left eye, lips and lower part of the nose pulled to the right in **Figure C**.

- Protection of the cornea with a lubricant is important.
- Prognosis is good with over 85% of patients experiencing complete recovery.

BENIGN NONOSSIFYING FIBROMA

(See Fibroma).

BILIARY ATRESIA

Definition
- A progressive obliterative cholangiopathy. The most common type of biliary atresia is obliteration of the entire extrahepatic biliary tree at or above porta hepatis.

Etiology
- Unknown.

Symptoms and Signs
- Progressive, prolonged jaundice in the newborn, conjugated hyperbilirubinemia, and pale stools are suggestive but not diagnostic.
- It is important to rule out neonatal hepatitis as it may present much the same way.
- Any baby with more than 2 weeks of jaundice should be thoroughly investigated for biliary atresia.
- Abdominal ultrasound, hepatobiliary scintigraphy, and above all percutaneous liver biopsy are helpful in the diagnosis.
- Figures A–C.

Treatment
- Direct drainage of the bile will help temporarily.
- Surgery is required in the surgically correctable cases.

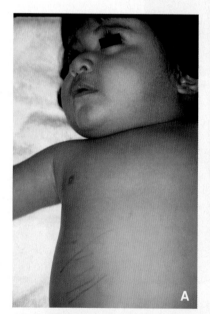
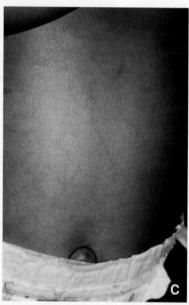
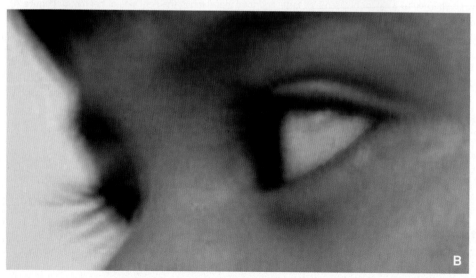

Figures A–C: Increasing jaundice and hepatosplenomegaly, in a female infant, with rising liver enzymes and bilirubin (mostly direct). Yellow sclera and skin, liver enlargement and dilated abdominal wall veins are seen here at the age of 5 months. *Liver biopsy report:* Micro nodular cirrhosis and diffuse cholestasis. Extrahepatic biliary atresia, inflammation and repair of biliary tree in distal hepatic segments, no evidence of bile duct paucity. Severe portal bridging fibrosis. Hepatocellular collapse.

BITES, ARTHROPOD

Definition
■ Arthropod bites are common in children; especially in children returning from camping trips and vacation.

Etiology
■ Spiders, mites, ticks, mosquitoes, flies, fleas, wasps, bees, ants, lice, bed bugs, and beetles are some of the arthropods that cause human skin disease.

Symptoms and Signs
■ Individual reaction to bites and stings can vary, and depend on the species (venom), age of the patient, and her/his reactivity.
■ Fleas, flies, and mosquitoes rarely have a systemic allergic reaction and a local response to the venom with pain, burning, and itching; a localized wheel and papule is more common.
■ Systemic reactions are often IgE mediated.
■ Delayed reactions are larger and may be confused with cellulitis.
■ Urticaria, angioedema, laryngeal edema, bronchospasm, and a complete anaphylactic reaction are rare.
■ Figures A–M.

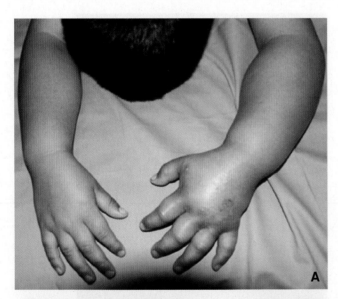

Figure A: A 3-year-old boy was stung by a bee, he developed pain and swelling in his hand and forearm, with blisters on the dorsum of the hand the following day.

Figure B: Pain and swelling of the left hand, a few hours after a bee sting.

Figure C: Pain, fever, and swelling of the left eye a few hours following a bee sting in a 6-year-old.

figures continues

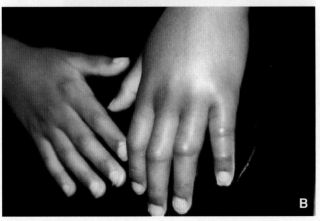

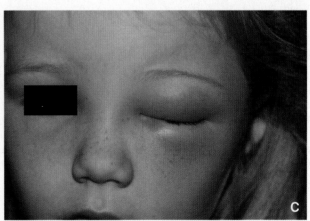

Treatment

- Cold compress, antihistamines, and oral analgesics are all that is needed in the majority of cases.
- Corticosteroids may be rarely necessary.
- Anaphylactic reactions should be treated accordingly, and self injectable epinephrine should be prescribed for possible future use.

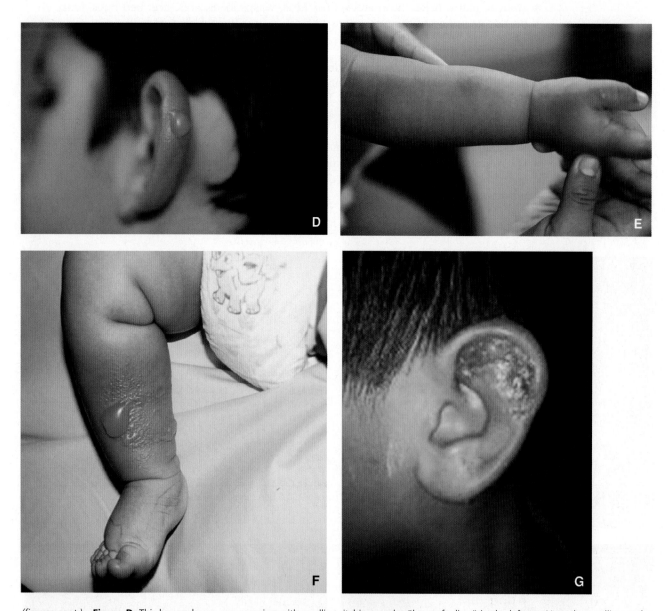

(figures cont.) **Figure D:** This boy woke up one morning with swelling, itching, and a "heavy feeling" in the left ear. Note the swelling and erythema of the left auricle, with a blister.

Figure E: This 11-month-old boy was found in his bed with numerous insect bites, all over his arms and legs.

Figures F–G: Insect bite (possible spider) in an otherwise healthy 6-month-old. Note the edema of the leg and foot, erythema, and blistering **(Figure F)**. An insect bite on the ear of a boy who fell on the grass while playing in the park the day before. Note, swelling of the auricle and the vesicles **(Figure G)**.

figures continues

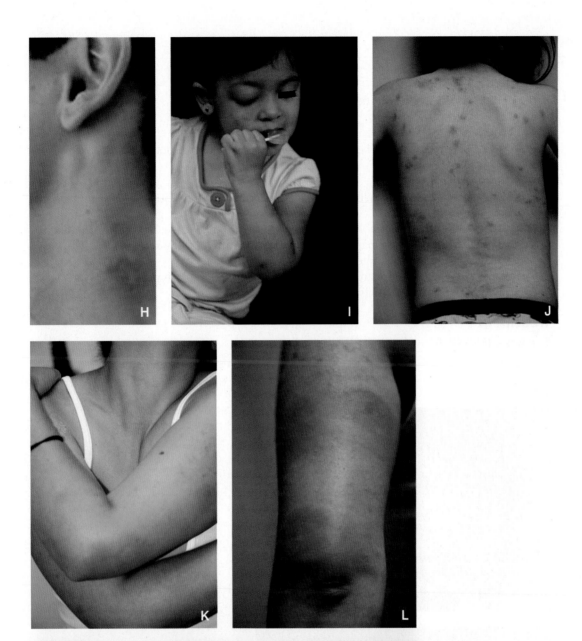

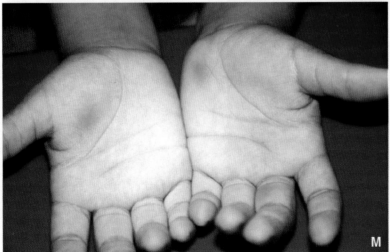

(figures cont.) **Figures H–J:** Insect bite on the neck of a teenager with regional lymphadenopathy **(Figure H)**. Severe skin reaction to insect bites **(Figure I)**. This young girl spent a night in her father's home, who has a few cats and dogs, and returned to her mother's home the next day with numerous insect bites (clearly a cause of some family anxiety) **(Figure J)**.

Figures K–L: Insect bites in a teenager, back from the Yosemite National Park in California.

Figure M: Roly polies (Armadillidiidae) are used by some children as pets and are considered harmless. But, this 5-year-old boy developed a rash and slight itching on the palms of his hands after playing with them.

BLEPHAROPHIMOSIS AND PTOSIS

Definition
- Blepharophimosis is a rare genetic disease.

Etiology
- Unknown. Blepharophimosis is often inherited as an autosomal dominant trait.

Symptoms and Signs
- It is characterized by abnormally narrow eye lids horizontally, ptosis and epicanthus inversus.
- Other associated signs are amblyopia, refractory errors, strabismus, and abnormalities of lacrimal or tear ducts, broad nasal bridge, short philtrum, and low-set ears.
- These children have normal intelligence.
- There are two types of blepharophimosis and ptosis: type 1 and type 2. Type 1 is associated with female infertility.

Treatment
- Surgical correction.

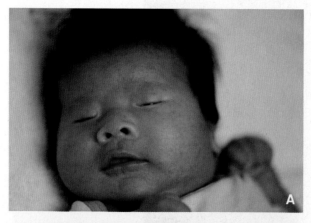

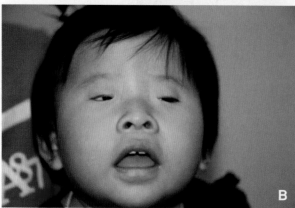

Figures A and B: A 1-month-old baby girl, born to healthy parents, who is unable to open her eyes, has narrow eye lids, ptosis, and a broad nasal bridge. The anatomy of her eyes is normal **(Figure A)**. The same baby at 6-months of age, feeding well and growing normally, but with continuing difficulty attempting to open her eyes **(Figure B)**. She has learned to look up to be able to see. She will have corrective blepharoplasty at the age of 7 years.

BLOODY NIPPLE DISCHARGE IN INFANCY

(See Mammary Duct Ectasia).

BOHN NODULE

Definition
- Bohn nodules are small pearl-shaped, mucous gland cysts.

Etiology
- Unknown.

Symptoms and Signs
- Small pear- shaped nodules found on the buccal and lingual aspect of mandibular and maxillary ridges.
- Also called gingival cyst.

Treatment
- Self limited. They fade within a few weeks.

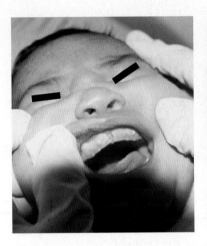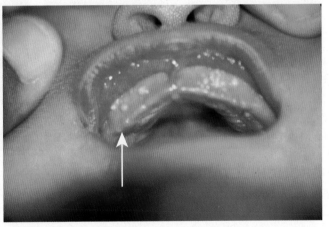

A 3-week-old, healthy asymptomatic newborn with many whitish gray nodules on the maxillary ridges.

BRANCHIAL CLEFT ANOMALY

Definition
- A congenital anomaly of branchial clefts.

Etiology
- The result of improper closure during embryonic life.

Symptoms and Signs
- Branchial cleft cysts are mostly unilateral, at times inherited as an autosomal dominant trait, and asymptomatic unless they become infected (Figures A–C).

Treatment
- Treatment is surgical.

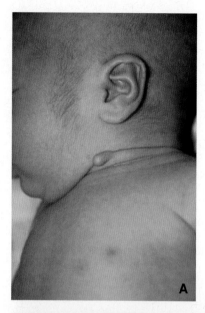

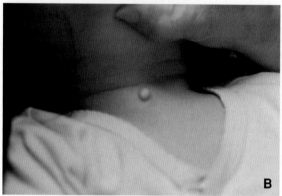

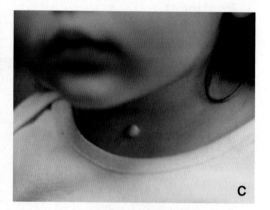

Figures A–C: Asymptomatic branchial cleft in three children. Ten-day-old boy, 2-year-old girl, and a 3-year-old girl **(Figures A, B, and C)**.

BRONCHIECTASIS

Definition
- Bronchiectasis is a chronic dilatation of the bronchi.

Etiology
- Bronchiectasis can be congenital, but it is often an acquired condition.
- Cystic fibrosis in the Western World and measles and pertussis in the developing countries are the main etiologies of this pathology.
- Pneumonia, aspiration of a foreign body, neoplasm, sarcoidosis, and lung abscess are among other causes of bronchiectasis.

Symptoms and Signs
- Cough, mostly with copious fetid sputum, offensive breath, recurrent lower respiratory infections, hemoptysis, loss of appetite, and failure to gain weight are some symptoms and signs of bronchiectasis.
- Children mostly swallow their sputum.
- Figures A–C.

Treatment
- Postural drainage and antibiotics are the mainstay of treatment in children.

B

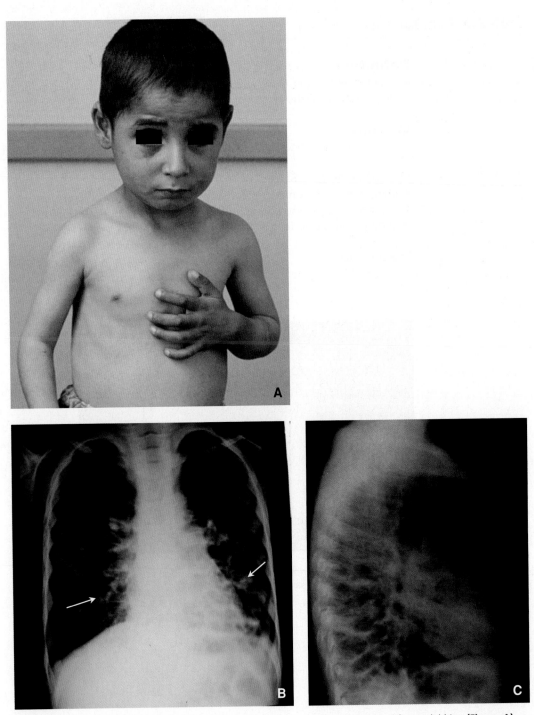

Figure A: An 8-year-old boy with bronchiectasis following pertussis. Note the marked finger clubbing **(Figure A)**. X-rays in Figures B and C are the same patient.

Figures B–C: Chest x-rays: Coarsened lung markings are seen within the bilateral lower lobes with dilated airways and peribronchial thickening, with relative sparing of the apices.

BUNION (Gr. Turnip)

Definition
- A deformity of the inner aspect of the first metatarsal head, resulting in lateral displacement of the great toe.

Etiology
- It is more common in girls, familial at times, and found more with flat feet.

Symptoms and Signs
- Many are asymptomatic; the visible deformity is a problem.
- Flat feet, narrow-toe shoes, and high heels contribute to bunions.
- Radiograph of the feet is necessary in evaluation of the problem.

Treatment
- Surgery is rarely needed. More comfortable shoes suffice in the majority of cases.

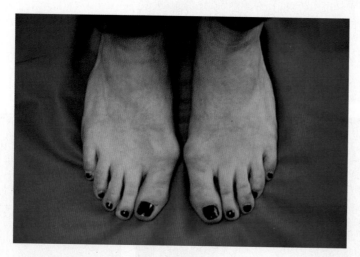

An asymptomatic 20-year-old female who has had bunion since 7-years of age. Her mother has the same condition.

CANDIDIASIS (CUTANEOUS)

Definition
- Cutaneous candidiasis can be acute or chronic. Candidal diaper dermatitis is common in children who are in diaper.

Etiology
- The wet, warm diaper mixed with feces and urine creates the environment for irritants to injure the baby's sensitive skin.
- Infrequent diaper change aggravates the problem.
- *Candida albicans* is the most common cause of this skin disorder. *C. albicans,* a part of the microflora of the oral cavity, gastrointestinal tract, and vagina, becomes aggressive whenever there is a change in the defense mechanism and can then cause the skin infection.
- Cutaneous candidiasis may follow oral thrush or the use of systemic antibiotics.

Symptoms and Signs
- Cutaneous candidiasis is characterized by a confluent, erythematous, weeping rash, and scaling edge.
- The intertriginous areas of the perineum, lower abdomen, inner aspect of the thighs, and the interdigital spaces can be affected.
- Figures A and B.

Treatment
- It is best to prevent this infection by frequent airing of the skin, particularly in the diaper areas, and by more frequent diaper changes. Use of moisturizers to protect the vulnerable areas of the skin can be helpful in prevention.
- Treatment is with antimonilial creams such as nystatin and clotrimazole.

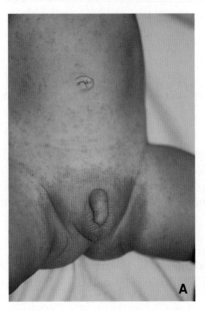

Figure A: Candida diaper dermatitis in a 10-month-old bottle-fed infant. A vivid beefy-red-rash on the diaper area and numerous satellite lesions scattered around the central lesion.

Figure B: Candida diaper dermatitis in a 6-month-old infant. Note the erythema, denuded skin, and the satellite lesions.

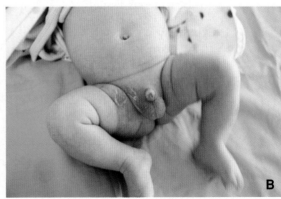

A

B

CANDIDIASIS, ORAL

(See Thrush).

CATARACT, CONGENITAL

Definition
- Any opacity present in the lens at birth is referred to as a congenital cataract.

Etiology
- Idiopathic. A metabolic work-up should be done to rule out disorders such as galactosemia, hypoparathyroidism, and homocystinuria.

Symptoms and Signs
- Opacity of the lens at birth. Absent red pupillary reflex, nystagmus, strabismus, and white fundus reflex.

Treatment
- Treatment of the underlying disease. Larger opacities that obstruct the visual axis may require cataract surgery.

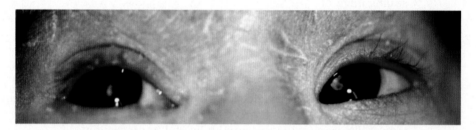

Congenital cataract in a 6-day-old female with Down syndrome and ventricular septal defect (VSD).

CELLULITIS

Definition
- Cellulitis is the infection and inflammation of loose connective tissue and the deeper subcutaneous tissue.

Etiology
- Any injury or trauma to the skin, cracks or peeling of the skin, or insect bite can cause cellulitis. In younger children, the etiology is often hematogenous.
- *Streptococcus pyogenes* and *Staphylococcus aureus* are the main pathogens. Other less common pathogens: *Streptococcus pneumoniae, Escherichia coli,* and *Haemophilus influenzae* type b.

Symptoms and Signs
- They mostly present as red, tender nodules, which enlarge to a diameter of 1 to 5 cm. And then become fluctuant, and may spontaneously drain, if left untreated.
- Figures A–C.

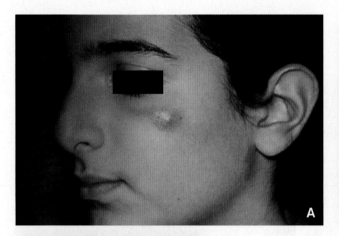

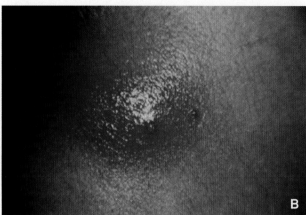

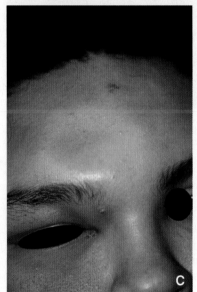

Figure A: A 10-year-old female with swelling and pain on the left cheek following an insect bite a day earlier. Note the lymphatic streak, extending proximally.

Figure B: A close-up view of the above skin lesion.

Figure C: A pimple followed by pain, swelling, and erythema in a 16-year-old girl. Note the original furuncle and the pitting edema above the right eyebrow.

Treatment
- Treatment is with the appropriate antibiotic.

CEPHALHEMATOMA

Definition
- Cephalhematoma is a localized collection of blood under the periosteum.

Etiology
- Birth trauma and occasionally linear skull fractures.

Symptoms and Signs
- It is mostly unilateral and has distinct edges, which do not cross the suture lines.
- They may calcify after 2 weeks, leading to a palpable hard rim and a central depression.

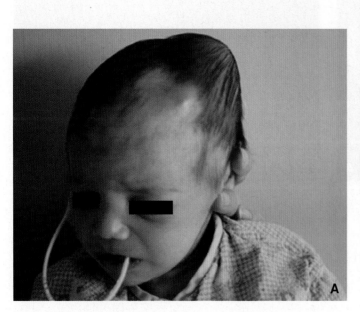
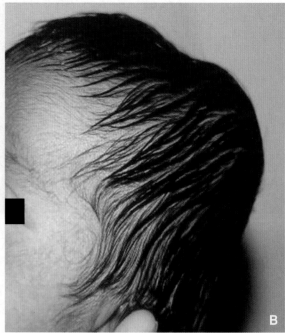

Figure A: A 21-day-old boy, still on gastric tube feeding, who has survived neonatal tetanus. His cephalhematoma has not resolved. Part of his head was shaved for IV access. Note a small swelling at the site of the old IV, which has now hardened.

Figure B: A large cephalhematoma in a 4-day-old boy, the first child of a young mother, born by normal, spontaneous vaginal delivery. His jaundice was exacerbated by the cephalhematoma. His bilirubin did not rise above 12 mg/dL.

Treatment
- They often resolve spontaneously within a few weeks and imaging studies rarely become necessary.
- Resorption of a large cephalhematoma can exacerbate or be the cause of neonatal jaundice.

CEPHALIC PUSTULOSIS, BENIGN (Acne of the newborn)

Definition
- Acne of the newborn face is a common condition in the newborn period.

Etiology
- Unknown, but possibly due to maternal androgens, baby's hyperactive adrenal glands, and neonatal hypersensitive end organ.
- Also, maternal use of hydantoin or lithium.

Symptoms and Signs
- Approximately 20% of newborns develop some acne on the face, neck, and chest during the first 2 weeks of life. The acne often resolves by 2 months of age (can last up to 6 months).
- Neonatal acne consists mostly of papules and papulopustules instead of comedones in older children.

Treatment
- Cephalic pustulosis is self-limited and treatment is rarely needed.
- Figures A–C.

C

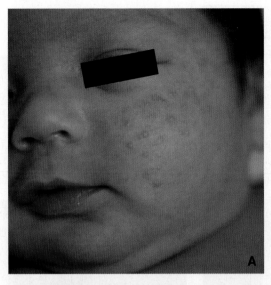

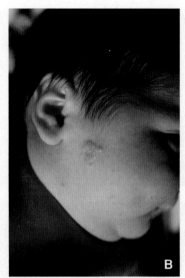

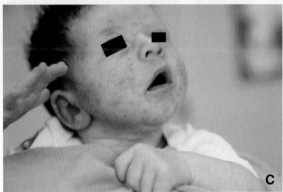

Figures A–C: Newborn Acne.

CHALAZION (Gr. Chalasions, small lump)

Definition
- Chalazion is a localized lipogranuloma.

Etiology
- Chalazion is caused by the obstruction of a meibomian gland by desquamated epithelial cells and/or lipid inspissation in the eyelid.

Symptoms and Signs
- The initial presentation is a cystic lesion usually in the middle of the eyelid. The chalazion may become inflamed and increase in size.
- Figures A–D.

Treatment
- Treatment is warm compress, eyelid hygiene, gentle lid massage in the direction of eyelashes, and possibly steroid–antibiotic eye drops.
- Surgery may be necessary when chalazion does not respond to conservative management.

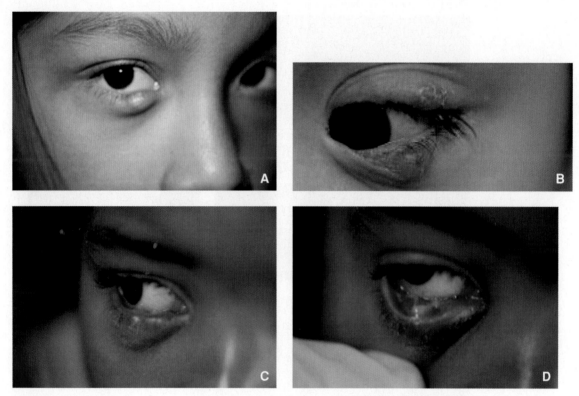

Figures A–B: Chalazion.

Figures C–D: Inflamed internal chalazion **(Figure C)** with purulent discharge from the Meibomian glands on the lower eyelid in **Figure D**.

CHILD ABUSE (Nonaccidental trauma)

Definition
- Nonaccidental infliction of physical injury resulting from punching, beating, kicking, biting, shaking, throwing, stabbing, choking, hitting, or otherwise harming a child; intention not relevant.
- Abuse can be physical, emotional, or sexual.

Etiology
- The etiology is often multifaceted. Perpetrator can be an adult or child of any age and socioeconomic and ethnic background.

Symptoms and Signs
- Physical injuries may or may not be visible, and whole body x-rays may be needed in younger children to evaluate the extent of the injuries. Psychological and physical scars may affect the child for many years after the initial abuse.

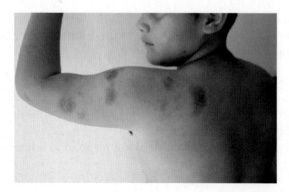

This 16-year-old boy was beaten-up at his school and by his classmates as a "birthday gift."

Treatment

- Child abuse should be reported to the local Child Protective Services (CPS).
- Appropriate, medical, and surgical treatments and psychological counseling are necessary.

SHAKEN BABY SYNDROME

Definition

- A traumatic brain injury due to violently shaking an infant.

Etiology

- Rotation, acceleration–deceleration that follows a violent head shaking is damaging and causes injuries that are different from other head traumas.

Symptoms and Signs

- A triad of subdural hematoma, retinal hemorrhage, and cerebral edema.
- Skull and long bone fractures, nerve injury causing anoxia, and leading to cerebral edema.
- Failure to thrive, anorexia, vomiting, seizure, lethargy, dilated pupil or pupils, and bulging fontanelle.
- Shaken baby syndrome's injuries are different from other types of injury in children in that they are due to rotational acceleration of the head.

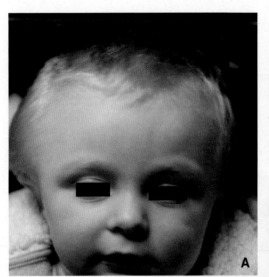
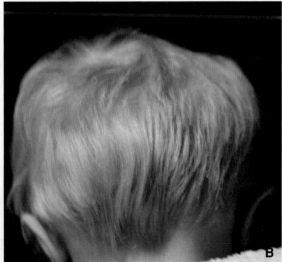
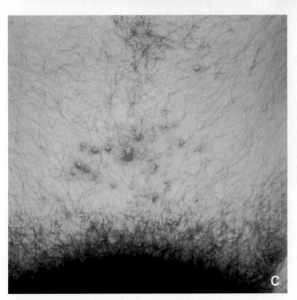

Figure A–B: This previously healthy 15-month-old girl, developed vomiting, lethargy, and seizure and was taken to an ED. She was found to have a right-sided, fixed and dilated pupil, and retinal hemorrhages. A CT scan of the head showed right-sided subdural hematoma, with severe and diffuse cerebral edema, and a significant midline shift. Patient had craniotomy and the subdural hematoma was evacuated. She now has high level cognitive impairment, communication deficit, dysphagia, and left hemiparesis, more severe in the left upper extremity. Note the right pseudomeningocele that has been tapped several times and the scar of the craniotomy.

Figure C: This 18-year-old boy was repeatedly sexually abused by the closest friend of the family. He now has herpes genitalia which he has passed on to his girl friend as well as molluscum contagiosum. His lower abdominal molluscum is visible in this picture.

- Retinal eye examination and CT scan of the head are the most valuable tests available to confirm the diagnosis.
- Bloody, xanthochromic CSF.
- Intentional head traumas carry the highest rate of mortality in cases of child abuse.

Treatment
- Treatment depends on the type and extent of the injury.

CHONDRODYSPLASIA PUNCTATA

(See Rhizomelic Chondrodysplasia Punctata).

CHOTZEN SYNDROME

Definition
- A genetic disorder characterized by asymmetric craniosynostosis.

Etiology
- Unknown. It is inherited as autosomal dominant.

Symptoms and Signs
- Craniosynostosis, plagiocephaly, facial asymmetry, ptosis of the eyelids, short fingers, and syndactyly of the second and third fingers.

Treatment
- Reconstructive surgery, if necessary.

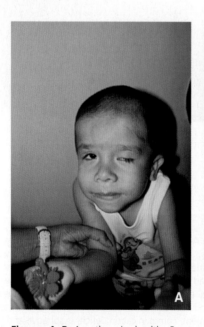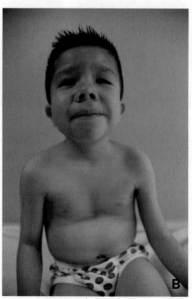

Figures A–B: An otherwise healthy 3-year-old was brought in for "droopy left eyelid" **(Figure A)**. He had slight developmental delay, plagiocephaly, large patent anterior fontanelle, ptosis of the left upper lid, long straight eyelashes, hypertelorism, low-set ears, prominent creases, simple ear lobes, low nasal bridge, and a broad nose. He had a large capillary hemangioma on his forehead, distal flaring of the rib cage, bilateral single palmar creases with slight cutaneous webbing, bilateral clinodactyly, and short broad distal phalanges of the fifth toe. He is 6 years old now in **Figure B** and postsurgery on his left upper lid. He has mild ptosis and pectus excavatum.

figures continues

C

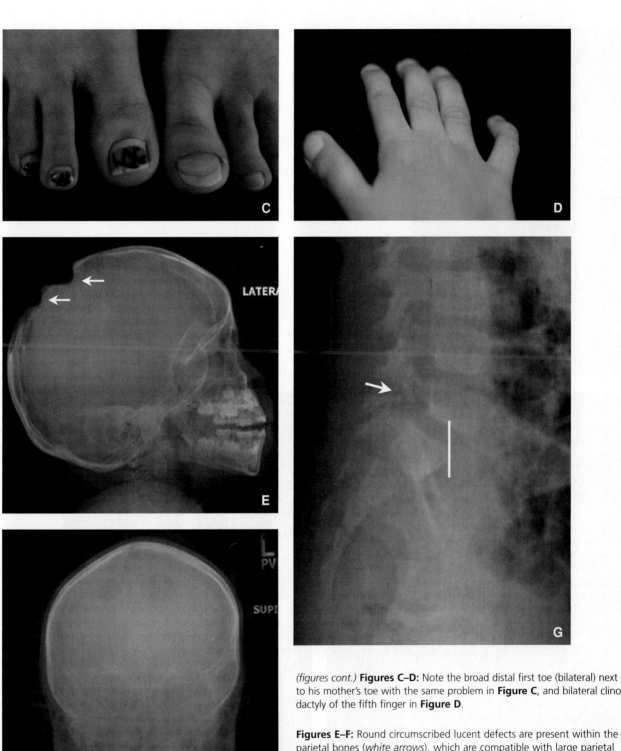

(figures cont.) **Figures C–D:** Note the broad distal first toe (bilateral) next to his mother's toe with the same problem in **Figure C**, and bilateral clinodactyly of the fifth finger in **Figure D**.

Figures E–F: Round circumscribed lucent defects are present within the parietal bones (*white arrows*), which are compatible with large parietal foramina. In addition, the coronal, lambdoid, squamosal, and sagittal sutures are not visualized (fused) compatible with craniosynostosis.

Figure G: Single lateral x-ray of the lumbar spine demonstrates a linear defect through the pars interarticularis of the L5 vertebra compatible with spondylolysis (*white arrow*). In addition, there is associated anterior displacement of the L5 vertebral body relative to the anterior margin of the sacrum (*vertical white line*) compatible with spondylolisthesis.

figures continues

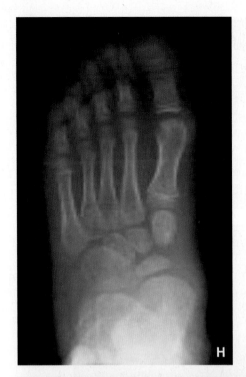

(figures cont.) **Figure H:** Single frontal x-ray of the left foot demonstrates short broad-based distal phalanges with widening of the great toe.

Figures I–J: Bilateral frontal x-rays of the hands demonstrate a mild bending or curvature of the fifth finger compatible with clinodactyly.

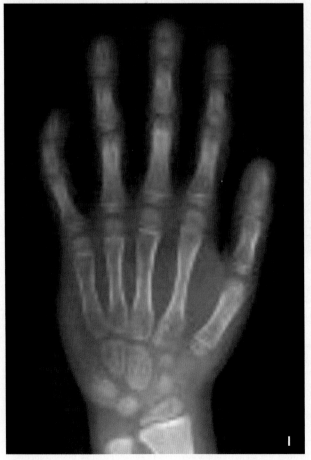

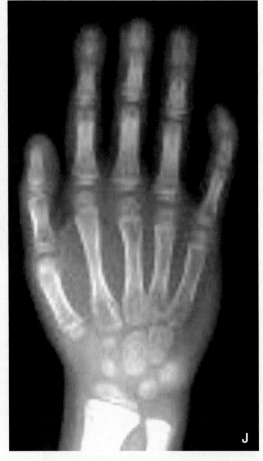

C

CIRRHOSIS OF THE LIVER (Cirrhosis, Gr. Kirhos, orange)

Definition
■ Liver disease associated with distinct pathologic and clinical manifestations, irreversible liver injury, and clinical symptoms and signs related to that pathology.

Etiology
■ Cirrhosis can be as a result of an infection such as hepatitis A, B, C (or other) or postnecrotic, following a toxic injury, or due to chronic biliary obstruction (biliary cirrhosis).

Symptoms and Signs
■ The majority of manifestations of this disease originate from its pathology; mainly the increasing, progressive scarring, which results in diminished blood flow; and damage to the liver cells, which ultimately increases the intrahepatic resistance and portal hypertension.
■ Liver enlargement, jaundice, intense itching associated with conjugated hyperbilirubinemia, palmar erythema, mostly on the thenar and hypothenar areas, pale stools (acholic), and spider angiomas or telangiectasias; central pulsating arterioles with several venules radiating from it.
■ Loss of appetite, failure to thrive, abdominal pain, and bleeding.

Treatment
■ Supportive and management of complications such as bleeding and ascites and surgery.

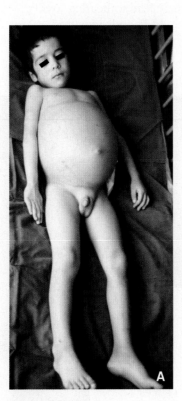 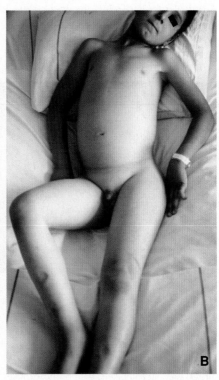

Figures A–B: Distended abdomen filled with ascites, bulging umbilicus, and dilated veins running on the abdominal wall due to portal hypertension in a boy with liver cirrhosis **(Figure A)**. Viral hepatitis is endemic in the developing countries, which can lead to liver cirrhosis. Distended abdomen due to ascites, pitting edema, purpura, and large areas of ecchymosis in a boy with liver cirrhosis **(Figure B)**.

CLEFT LIP AND CLEFT PALATE

Definition
- Cleft lip and cleft palate are congenital abnormalities that are closely related genetically, embryologically, and functionally.
- A cleft lip is an abnormality of the upper lip from skin to bone, unilateral or bilateral.
- Folic acid and Vitamin B6 supplementation have lowered the incidence of cleft lip, cleft palate, and neural tube defects.

Etiology
- Maternal drug exposure (methotrexate, isotretinoin, alcohol, smoking during pregnancy, and some of the anticonvulsants mainly phenytoin) and genetic factors.
- Cleft lip, palate, or both are inherited in some families as autosomal dominant.

Symptoms and Signs
- Cleft lip is obvious at birth but cleft palate can be missed if the newborn is not thoroughly examined.
- Cleft lip is about 30 times more common than cleft palate.
- Cleft lip is more common in boys, and is found more in Asians, and least in Blacks (Figures A and B).

Treatment
- Requires a multidisciplinary approach by a team of plastic surgeon, pediatric dentist, prosthodontist, orthodontist, geneticist, otolaryngologist, speech therapist, social worker, and pediatrician.
- The immediate problem is feeding and plastic obturators are a great help.
- Recurrent otitis media is common and may lead to hearing loss.
- Surgical repair of cleft lip and palate should be individualized.
- Cleft lips are mostly corrected by 3 months of age. Cleft palates are often corrected surgically by 1 year of age.

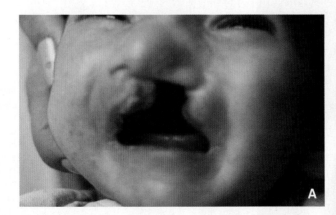

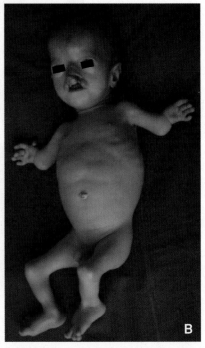

Figure A: Cleft lip and palate, with his nose, pulled to the right.

Figure B: A male infant with multiple congenital abnormalities including bilateral cleft lip and cleft palate.

CLOACAL EXSTROPHY

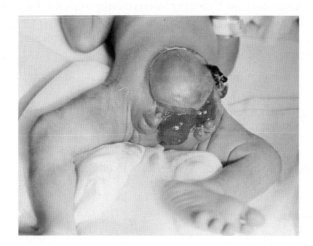

This is a classic appearance of a cloacal exstrophy in a male. The primary features are an omphalocele, pubic diastasis with the exposed split bladder place the opened up hindgut segment, the intussuscepted terminal ileum and epispadias and separated phallus, and complete separation of the scrotum into two segments.

CLUB FOOT

(See Talipes).

COLD INJURY IN THE NEWBORN

NEONATAL HYPOTHERMIA

Definition
■ Damage inflicted on the body as the direct or indirect result of exposure to low temperature, with or without structural damage.

Etiology
■ It occurs in cold weather in inadequately protected infants.

Symptoms and Signs
■ Apathy, refusal to feed, oliguria, redness, edema, hypothermia, bradycardia, and apnea may be seen. High risk of mortality and brain injury.

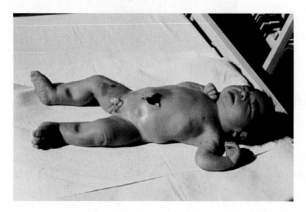

A 6-day-old male infant was brought into the Hospital in Tehran during snow storm for "not feeding." He was lethargic, was diffusely erythematous, and edematous. His temperature was 34 degrees centigrade, had a heart rate of 89, and blood sugar of 48.

Treatment
- Prevention.
- Children loose approximately 30% of their internal heat from the head, therefore covering the head in cold weather is important.
- Gradual warming by different means, a warm drink if the patient is conscious and a warm bath are helpful.

COLOBOMATA OF THE IRIS (Gr. Koloboma, defect)

Definition
- A developmental defect located inferiorly looking like a key hole.

Etiology
- Mostly an autosomal dominant trait.

Symptoms and Signs
- Asymptomatic.
- An incidental finding in most cases.

Treatment
- Needs a full ophthalmologic examination.

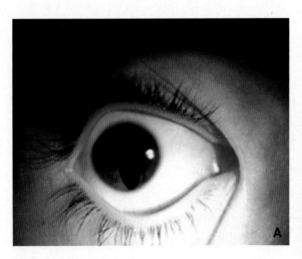
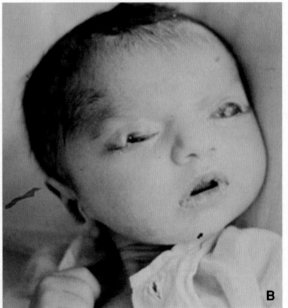

Figure A: A 12-year-old girl with dropped iris or colobomata. She had no other abnormality.

Figure B: A 9-month-old girl with colobomata of the eyelids and cornea with complete loss of vision.

CONGENITAL ADRENAL HYPERPLASIA (CAH)

Definition
- The congenital adrenal hyperplasias are a group of diseases transmitted by autosomal recessive inheritance and manifested by decreased glucocorticoid biosynthesis.

Etiology

- The synthesis of cortisol and aldosterone is disrupted in CAH due to 21-hydroxylase deficiency, which is the cause in 90% of the cases.
- The incidence of the classic 21-hydroxylase deficiency is 1 in 15,000 to 20,000 births, except in some ethnic groups where the incidence is higher.

Symptoms and Signs

- Anorexia, dehydration, hyponatremia, hypoglycemia, weight loss, progressive weakness, and shock. If not treated, can progress to cardiac arrhythmias and death.
- The alternative pathways of 17-hydroxyprogesterone leads to high levels of androgen and eventually testosterone biosynthesis, causing abnormal female genitalia.
- Lack of physical findings in male infants makes diagnosis more difficult in the newborn boys, causing a higher mortality (Figures A–C).

Treatment

- Newborn-screening has improved early diagnosis and timely treatment consisting of glucocorticoid and mineralocorticoid replacement.

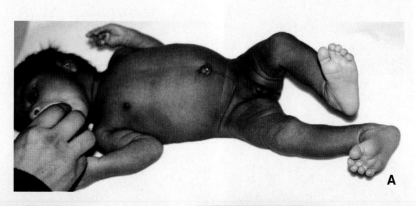

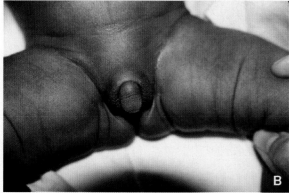
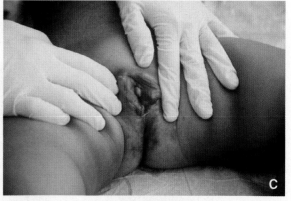

Figures A–C: A 14-month-old infant was seen for ambiguous genitalia. Hyperpigmentation and large clitoris were evident at birth. Her first hospital admission was at the age of 11 days for vomiting and weight loss. Her serum sodium at that time was 124 mmol/L, K 7.4 mmol/L, bicarbonate 16 mmol/L, testosterone 169 ng/dL, and 17-hydroxyprogesterone was >1,000 ng/dL. Ultrasound showed normal uterus and ovaries and no visible vagina. Karyotype was 46XX. Mutation panel; homozygous, salt wasting and simple virilizing, autosomal recessive. Her condition improved and she lost the hyperpigmentation in the skin, gingiva, and areola after treatment with hydrocortisone, flucortisone, and sodium chloride. **Figures A** and **B** before the clitorotomy and **Figure C** after the surgery.

CONGENITAL APLASIA OF DEPRESSOR ANGULARIS ORIS MUSCLE

Definition
- A congenital agenesis of the depressor angularis oris muscle.

Etiology
- Unknown.

Symptoms and Signs
- Congenital aplasia of depressor angularis oris muscle is best presented when a baby cries and the facial asymmetry becomes more obvious.
- The lower lip is pulled toward the healthy side (Figures A–C).
- The forehead, nasolabial, and eyelids are not involved and this differentiates it from facial palsy.
- There may be an associated cardiac anomaly.
- Moebius syndrome is mostly bilateral.

Treatment
- None. They improve with time.

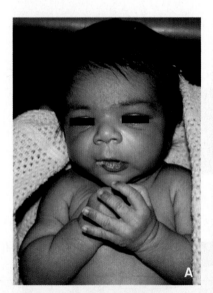
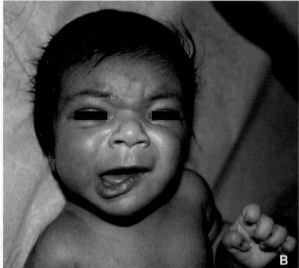
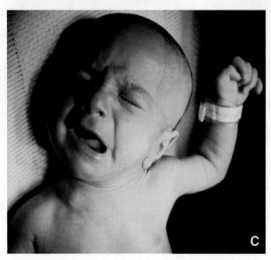

Figures A–C: Congenital aplasia of depressor angularis oris muscle in a 2-week-old infant **(Figure A)**, and then again at the age of 3 months **(Figure B)**, and in another newborn boy **(Figure C)**.

CONGENITAL EXTERNAL AUDITORY CANAL STENOSIS/ATRESIA

Definition
- Gross aplasia or hypoplasia of the auricle of the ear with a blind or absent external acoustic meatus.

Etiology
- Exposure to teratogens, hereditary factors, intrauterine positioning, or unknown cause.
- Mild ear canal stenosis is also occasionally seen in some syndromes such as Down's syndrome.
- Severe stenosis or atresia of the ear canal can be associated with other malformations of auricle and the middle ear (i.e., oculo-auriculo-vertebral dysplasia).

Symptoms and Signs
- Hearing loss and variability in the deformation of the auricle.

Treatment
- Hearing evaluation, computed tomography (CT), or magnetic resonance imaging (MRI) may be necessary to see the extent of the underlying deformity.
- Reconstructive surgery of the ear is normally done at the age of 5 years.

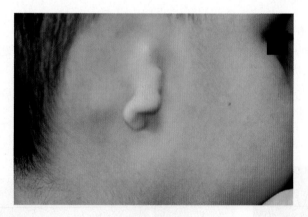

Hypoplasia and absent external acoustic meatus in a newborn.

CONJUNCTIVITIS

- Red or pink eye may be caused by a number of infectious or inflammatory causes, including bacterial, viral, and allergic.

CONJUNCTIVITIS, ALLERGIC
Etiology
- Allergens; for example, pollens, dust, and cat.

Symptoms and Signs
- Often seasonal and commonly bilateral with intense itching. History of allergy, itchy, watery eyes, chemosis, red edematous eyelids, and conjunctival papilla.
- Figures A–C.

Treatment
- Removal and elimination of the allergens, cold compresses, olopatadine, steroid eye drops, and oral antihistamines.

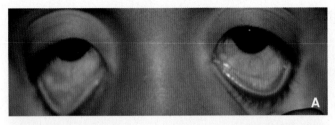

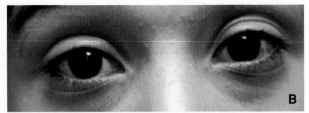

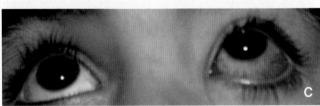

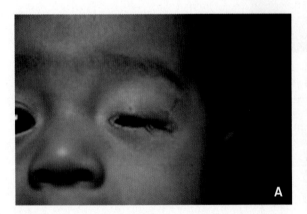

Figures A–C: These two teenagers presented on the same day with similar symptoms of itching and tearing of the eyes **(Figures A** and **B)**. They had bilateral injected watery eyes and slight edema of the eyelids. The child in **Figure C** had all of these symptoms in one eye (unilateral). They all had history of allergic diseases and no preauricular nodes or mucous in the eyes.

CONJUNCTIVITIS, INFECTIOUS

Etiology
- Many different bacteria, viruses, and chlamydia can cause eye infection (e.g., Haemophilus, gonorrhea, and herpes. The latter two can be devastating if not treated promptly and correctly).

Symptoms and Signs
- A feeling of a foreign body in the eye, redness, and discharge with some itching.

Treatment
- Antibiotics, in the form of eye drops or cream, can shorten the course of the disease and prevent the spread of infection.

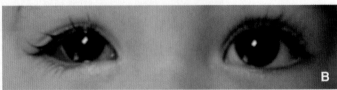

Figures A–C: These three children presented with the history of waking up one morning with glued eyes. Note swelling of the eyelids, injected conjunctivae, and the yellowish–greenish discharge.

CORNELIA DE LANGE SYNDROME

Definition
- Cornelia de Lange syndrome is a genetic disorder with severe mental retardation, short stature, and several other abnormalities.

C

Etiology
- It is caused by mutations with several genes involved (chromosome 5, 10, and X).

Symptoms and Signs
- Symptoms can be very mild and unrecognizable in some and may be severe in others.
- Developmental delay, short stature, and low birth weight.
- Hirsutism, coarse hair growing low on the forehead and neck, short neck, thick eyebrows, synophrys (thick eyebrows which meet in the middle), long eyelashes, microcephaly, brachycephaly, long philtrum, anteverted nostrils, low-pitched cry, thin lips turned down at angles, clinodactyly, single transverse palmar crease, heart defects, and cryptorchidism are some other findings in this syndrome (Figures A–E).

Treatment
- Management of the individual problems.

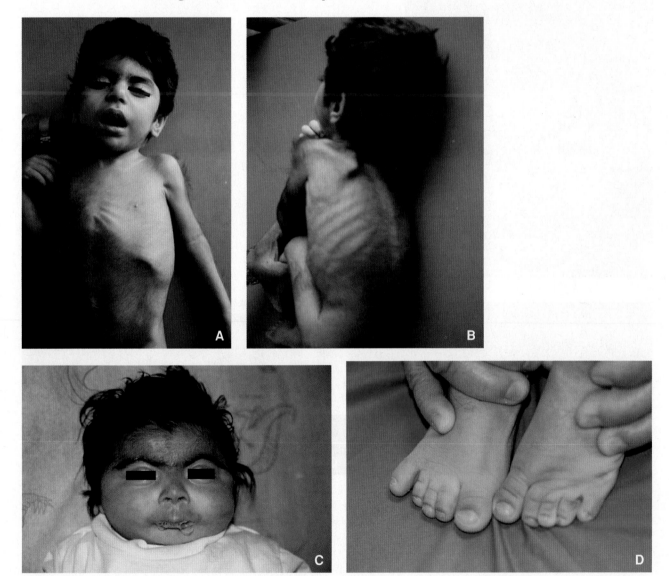

Figures A–G: The patient in **Figures A** and **B** had severe mental retardation, hirsutism, synophrys, thick long eyelashes, and pectus carinatum. The patient in **Figure C** is an 8-month-old male with typical facies of the syndrome. **Figure D** demonstrates macrodactyly of the right fifth toe. **Figures E** and **F** show bilateral macrodactyly of the second finger and hyperflexibility of the fingers. This boy in **Figure G** is now 8 years old, can sit without support, and can be fed, although he has some difficulty with fluids, and still has a gastric tube for fluids.

figures continues

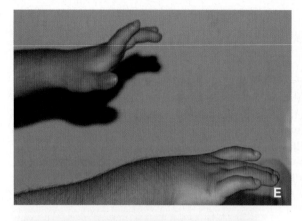

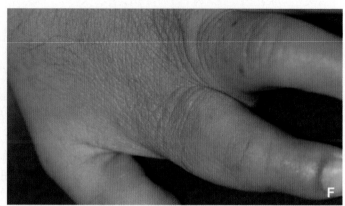

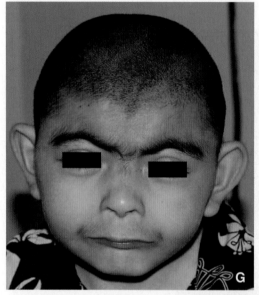

(figures cont.) **Figures E–G**

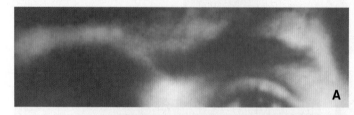

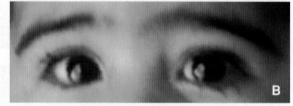

Figures A–C: Unibrow (synophrys) in isolation is common in some ethnicities and not necessarily syndromic.

CRANIOSYNOSTOSIS

Definition
- Premature closure of the cranial sutures.
- Craniosynostosis can be primary or secondary.
- Primary craniosynostosis is due to premature closure of one or more sutures due to abnormalities of skull.
- Secondary craniosynostosis is due to failure of proper brain growth.

Etiology
- Unknown. Some cases are syndromic.

Symptoms and Signs
- The skull deformity may be noticeable at birth.
- Clinical manifestations depend on the specific fused suture(s) as well as on the timing of closure. Anterior plagiocephaly is more common in girls and is due to the unilateral coronal synostosis. Features include widened skull, flattening of the forehead with an elevated eyebrow on the affected side, and asymmetrical features of the face.

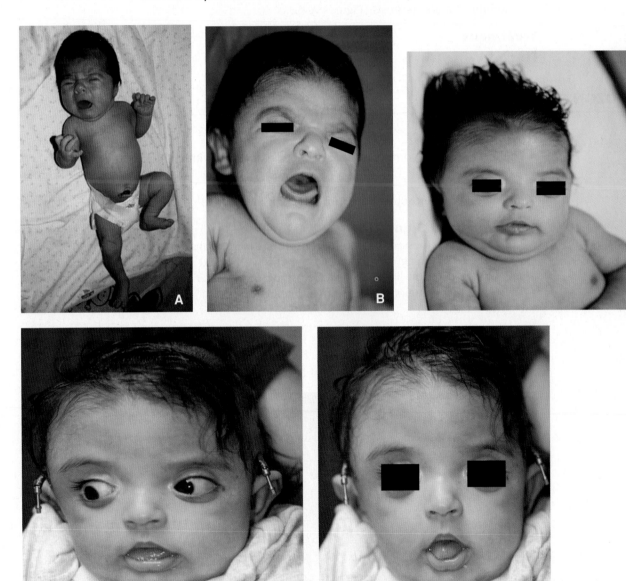

Figures A–B: This newborn had nonsyndromic, isolated craniosynostosis due to bilateral fusion of the coronal sutures or turricephaly (also known as oxycephaly, acrocephaly, tower head, and steeple head). She developed seizures at 8 months of age, without any signs of increased intracranial pressure. Head MRI, CT, and EEG were normal. She remained asymptomatic and lost to follow-up at 18 months of age.

Figures C–E: A 2-month-old female infant with microcephaly. The anterior and posterior fontanelles were closed at birth. She has exophthalmus, strabismus, anisometropia, midface hypoplasia, and low-set ears. Her cranial CT scan revealed synostosis of bilateral coronal, left lambdoid, left squamosal, and perhaps the sagittal sutures. **Figure C** is precraniotomy. **Figures D** and **E** are postcraniotomy.

- Posterior plagiocephaly: Results from unilateral lambdoid synostosis. The head appears skewed from the occipital view.
- Scaphocephaly (dolichocephaly): It is secondary to fusion of the sagittal suture and results in a narrow, long head. It is the most common type of craniosynostosis.
- Trigonocephaly: Secondary to metopic synostosis and it results in a triangular-shaped head.
- Turricephaly: There is premature fusion of bilateral coronal sutures that is inadequately treated. As a result, the head is cone shaped.
- Crouzon syndrome, Apert syndrome, and Chotzen syndrome are some other examples of syndromic craniosynostosis (Figures A–G).

Treatment
- Surgery.

CROUZON SYNDROME

Definition
- The most common form of genetic disorder associated with craniosynostosis.

Etiology
- Inherited as an autosomal dominant trait with incomplete penetrance.

Symptoms and Signs
- A deformed compressed back-to-front skull or brachycephaly. Strabismus, shallow orbits, wide-set eyes, bulging eyes, maxillary hypoplasia, beaked nose, under developed upper jaw, bifid uvula, cleft lip, and palate are some of the other possible abnormalities.
- These children commonly have normal intelligence.
- Figures F and G.

Treatment
- Surgery.

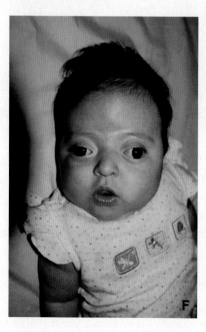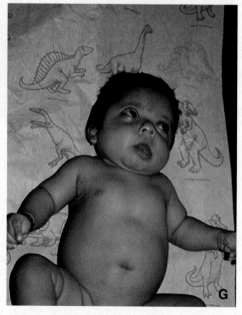

Figures F–G: A 10-week-old girl with Crouzon syndrome. Note brachycephaly, wide-set, bulging eyes, and strabismus.

C

CUTANEOUS LARVA MIGRANS (CREEPING ERUPTION)

Definition
- Cutaneous larva migrans is a self-limiting cutaneous parasitic infection seen mostly in tropical and subtropical parts of the world.

Etiology
- It is caused by the larva of several nematodes, the two major ones are Ancylostoma (Gr. Ankylos, bent or crooked) braziliense and *Ancylostoma caninum,* the infective larva of cats and dogs, which contaminate the soil.
- Individuals who are exposed to the soil contaminated with larva such as walking bare feet or laying on the sand are at risk.
- Larva can travel about 1 to 2 cm a day in the epidermis.

Symptoms and Signs
- Intense itching.

Treatment
- This is a self-limited disease. The larvae die without treatment and there is complete skin resolution.
- Oral albendazole can be administered orally, if necessary.

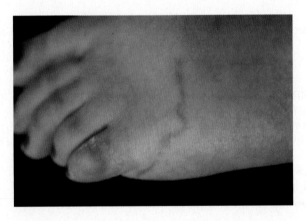

A 22-year-old girl was visiting Peru in the rain forest. She returned to Los Angeles with a rash on her foot. Had no fever or itching. Raised, erythematous, serpiginous track of cutaneous larva migrans.

CUTIS MARMORATA

Definition
- An uncommon disorder in pediatrics characterized by a reticulated, purplish-blue mottling of the skin.

Etiology
- Unknown.

Symptoms and Signs
- In most cases, it is present at birth, increases gradually and eventually fades away during childhood.
- This skin pattern may persist beyond infancy in certain conditions such as Down's syndrome, trisomy 18, and Cornelia de Lange syndrome.
- In the majority of the cases, the skin changes are distributed in a generalized, covering the trunk, and the extremities. The skin pattern can be segmental or localized in others.
- Figures A and B.

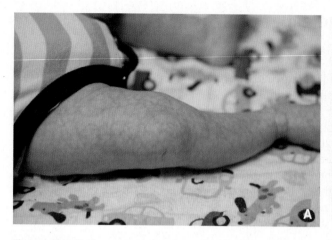
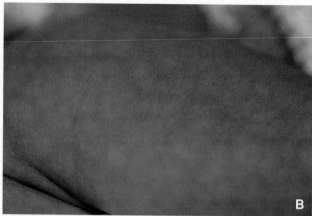

Figures A–B: Cutis marmorata in a 2-month-old otherwise healthy child (**Figure A** and close-up view in **Figure B**).

Treatment
- No treatment is needed.

CYST (Gr. Kystis, sac)

Definition
- An abnormal closed cavity containing a liquid or semisolid liquid and found anywhere in the body.

Etiology
- Epidermal cysts (epithelial, sebaceous, or pilar) most often arise from inflamed hair follicles and rarely from trauma to skin.
- They result from proliferation of surface epidermal cells within the dermis.
- The keratin made within the closed space is responsible for the creation of a cyst.

Symptoms and Signs
- Epithelial cysts are found mostly on the face, scalp, nape of the neck, and chest.
- They are slow-growing, round and raised 5 to 50 mm nodules.
- Figures A–E.

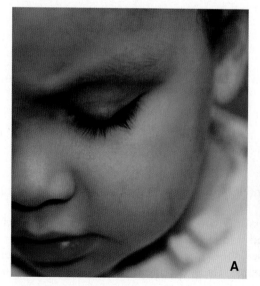

Figures A–C: Dermoid cysts of the upper eyelid and eyebrows.

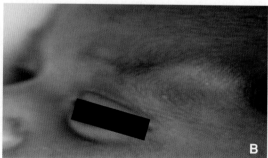

figures continues

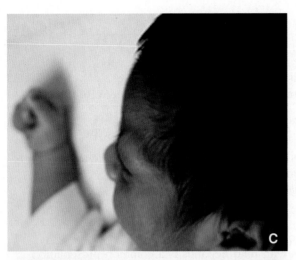

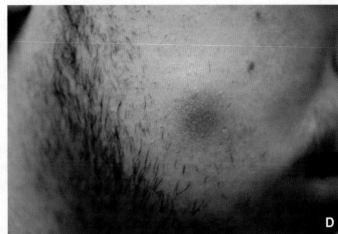

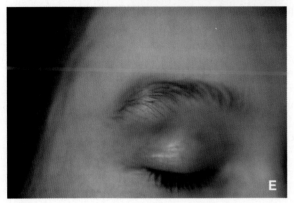

(*figures cont.*) **Figure D** is an infected cyst of the cheek.

Figure E: A cystic swelling over the right eyebrow appeared approximately a month after he was hit in the area by a ball. It has been drained twice and quickly spontaneously refilled every time. The cyst is nontender, firm, and mobile. It was eventually successfully removed surgically.

Treatment
- Incision and removal of the cystic sac.
- Malignant degeneration is rare.

CYST, RETROAURICULAR

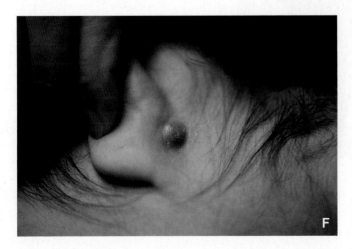

Figure F: This 13-year-old girl had noticed a painless growth behind her left ear for a few weeks. There was a brownish-gray, oval, nontender, soft, slightly movable cyst behind her left ear. She was offered surgery to remove it but her mother preferred to watchful observation. Meanwhile, it has remained asymptomatic and has not grown in size.

CYTOMEGALOVIRUS DISEASE (CMV)

Definition
- CMV is the most common congenital viral infection in the United States.
- Depending on the age and host resistance, this virus can cause a variety of different clinical syndromes.

Etiology
- Human CMV is a member of the herpes virus group, is highly host-specific and ubiquitous; causing disease in the human, monkey, and rodents.
- It is the most common nongenetic congenital cause of deafness.

Symptoms and Signs
- The disease in children is often asymptomatic.
- An infectious mononucleosis-like illness with mild hepatitis is a common presentation.
- Congenital form can present with intrauterine growth retardation (IUGR), hepatosplenomegaly, jaundice, retinitis, purpura, microcephaly, and intracerebral calcifications (Figure).
- Hearing loss and learning disability may be discovered later in childhood.
- CMV is much more severe in the immunocompromised.
- A fourfold antibody titer rise in the paired serum is considered diagnostic of CMV.
- There are some uniquely large cells bearing intranuclear inclusions, specific to CMV.
- Viral cultures from the nasopharynx, oropharynx, urine, stool, may be helpful.

Treatment
- Ganciclovir.

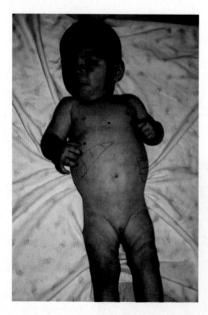

A 3-month-old female with congenital CMV infection. She failed her newborn hearing test, has hepatosplenomegaly, and several hemangiomas.

DACRYOCYSTOCELE (DACRYOCELE)

Definition
- Dacryocystocele, also called dacryocele or congenital nasolacrimal sac mucocele, is the enlargement of the lacrimal sac with fluid.

Etiology
- Obstruction of both the proximal and distal portions of the nasolacrimal duct.

Symptoms and Signs
- Usually noted during the newborn period. A bluish swelling of the skin overlying the lacrimal sac with superior displacement of the medial canthus.

Treatment
- High rate (90%) of spontaneous resolution by 6 months of age.
- Referral to ophthalmologist in cases of persistence beyond 6 months of life or the presence of infection (Figure).

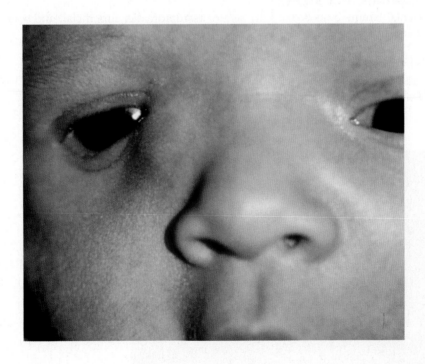

DACRYOSTENOSIS

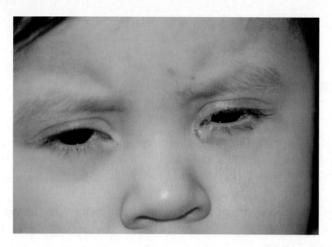

A 13-month-old girl with greenish yellow mucous discharge from bilateral eyes; left more than right. The discharge has been off and on since birth.

DENTAL LAMINA CYST

Definition
■ Congenital cysts on the alveolar ridge, AKA gingival cyst of the newborn.

Etiology
■ Cysts originating from remnants of dental lamina.

Symptoms and Signs
■ Dental lamina cysts are usually single, asymptomatic, superficial, and seen on the alveolar ridge (Figure).

Treatment
■ Transient in nature.
■ Exfoliate within a few weeks.

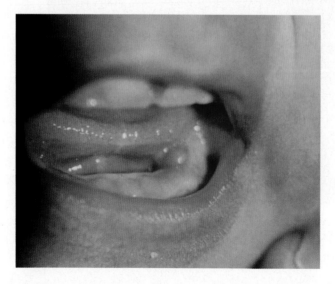

Dental laminal cyst in a 6-day-old.

D

DERMATITIS ARTEFACTA

(See Neurotic Excoriation).

DERMATOGRAPHISM

Definition
- Dermatographism is a form of physical urticaria with an exaggerated skin reaction to physical stimulus.

Etiology
- Unknown. Release of vasoactive mediators from mast cells is suspected.

Symptoms and Signs
A wheal-and-flare can be seen a few minutes after skin irritation, resulting in itching. Dermatographism can be divided into:
1. Simple: The most common form, wheal and erythema, is provoked following stroking or pressure on the skin. Wheals typically reach maximal size in 5 to 7 minutes and begin to fade by 15 minutes. They result in mild itching.
2. Symptomatic: More common in adults and only slightly different than the simple form. Lesions appear in less than 5 minutes and last up to 30 minutes. Reaction may be follicular, inflamed, and swollen (Figures A–D).

Treatment
- Avoidance of precipitating physical triggers. Use antihistamines for symptomatic relief.

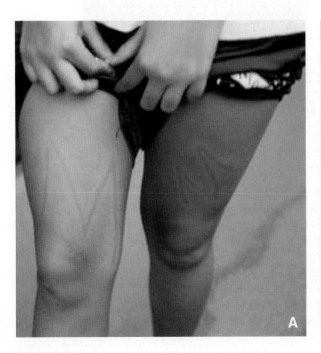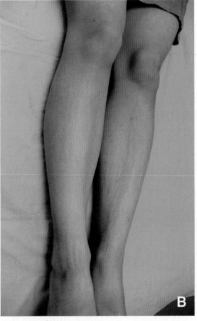

Figures A–B

figures continues

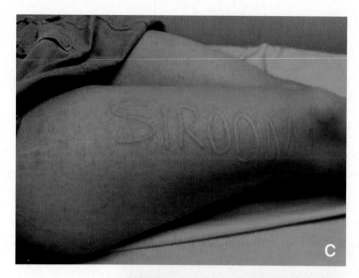

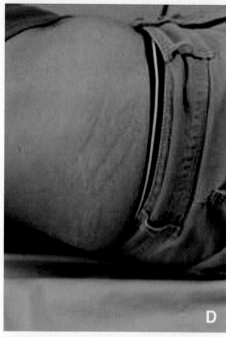

(figures cont.) **Figures C–D**

DIARRHEA

Definition
- Passage of frequent, loose, and watery stools.
- Diarrheal diseases are one of the leading causes of mortality and morbidity in children worldwide, particularly when superimposed on malnutrition in the developing world.

Etiology
- A wide variety of organisms including viruses, bacteria, and parasites can cause diarrhea.
- Acute infectious diarrhea is divided into:
  1. Noninflammatory: Caused by bacterial enterotoxins, viral destruction of intestinal villi, and parasitic infections (e.g., enterotoxigenic *Escherichia coli,* rotavirus, and *Vibrio cholerae*).
  2. Inflammatory diarrhea: Commonly caused by bacteria that directly attacks the intestinal villi (e.g., Aeromonas, *Campylobacter jejuni,* E. coli, *Plesiomonas shigelloides,* Salmonella, Shigella, *Clostridium difficile,* and *Yersinia enterocolitica*).

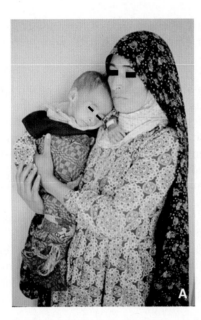 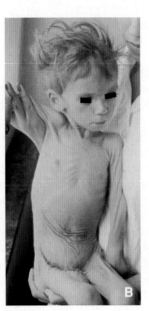

Figure A: Dehydration, malnutrition, and exhaustion following several bouts of diarrhea in an 11-month-old infant.

Figure B: A 22-month-old child with severe malnutrition (calorie–protein) following repeated bouts of diarrhea.

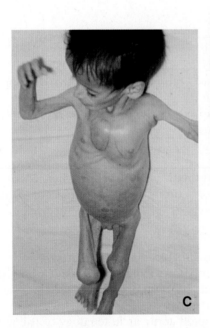 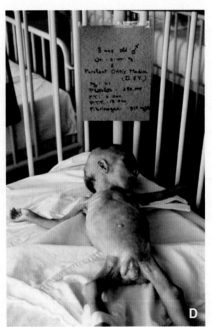

Figure C: Calorie malnutrition in an 11-month-old girl, following a prolonged period of diarrhea. Note the two abscesses on her chest. The weight of the pus drained from these two abscesses was equal to 20% of her body weight.

Figure D: Dehydration and malnutrition with a few purpuric spots on the abdominal wall in an 8-month-old boy, following poor nutrition, infections, and frequent diarrhea. He was brought to the hospital due to an "ear infection," with severe otorrhea. Culture of the ear discharge did not grow any pathogens, probably due to the oral antibiotics prescribed prior to his admission. His weight was 3.1 kg, hemoglobin 11.1 g/dL, platelet count 280,000/micro L, P.T. 11 seconds, P.T.T. 18 seconds, and fibrinogen 217 mgm/dL.

- Viral causes includes rotavirus, enteric adenovirus, and Norwalk-like virus.
- Diarrhea is classified as persistent or chronic when it lasts more than 14 days.

Symptoms and Signs
- Depends on the offending organism and the patient's overall health status.
- Rotavirus, the incidence of which has dropped appreciably since the use of rotavirus vaccines has a sudden onset with fever and vomiting, followed by watery diarrhea.
- In cholera, the majority of patients are asymptomatic but a small number have severe watery diarrhea that can cause a significant electrolytes loss, leading to rapid death.
- Helicobacter pylori can cause epigastric pain, nausea, vomiting, and bloody stool.
- Shigella infections begin with abdominal pain, cramps, tenesmus, and diarrhea with mucoid stool with or without blood.
- Nontyphoid Salmonella begins with fever, abdominal cramps, and diarrhea.
- Dehydration is the most common complication of diarrhea.
- Hemolytic uremic syndrome (*E. coli*), arthritis (Salmonella, Shigella, Yersinia, and Campylobacter), nephropathy and glomerulonephritis (Shigella, Yersinia, and glomerulonephritis) Guillain–Barré syndrome (Campylobacter) are some other and less frequent complications of diarrhea.

Treatment
- Rehydration (oral and intravenous) is the cornerstone of treatment.
- Proper and timely recognition of dehydration and its severity are essential for its management.

DIGEORGE SYNDROME

Definition
- A primary immunodeficiency diseases caused by the defective development of the pharyngeal pouch.
- It is manifested by hypoplasia or aplasia of the thymus and parathyroid gland, hypocalcemia, and cardiac defects.

Etiology
- Dysmorphogenesis of the third and fourth pharyngeal pouches.
- The majority have a small deletion of chromosome 22, at position 22q11.2 (the DiGeorge syndrome chromosome region).

Symptoms and Signs
- Phenotypic expression of disease is variable.
- Recurrent upper and lower respiratory tract infections. Hypertelorism, palatal abnormalities, micrognathia, low-set and posterior-rotated ears, and seizure due to hypocalcemia (hypoparathyroidism).
- A variety of cardiac defects (interrupted aortic arch, tetralogy of Fallot, truncus arteriosus, ASD, VSD, and vascular rings).
- Approximately 1% of patients have complete absence of thymus and severe combined immunodeficiency syndrome (SCID), speech delay, learning disability, and hyperactivity (Figures A–E).

Treatment
- Treatment must be personalized.
- Treatment of hypocalcemia. Correction of cardiac defects.
- Bone marrow transplantation.

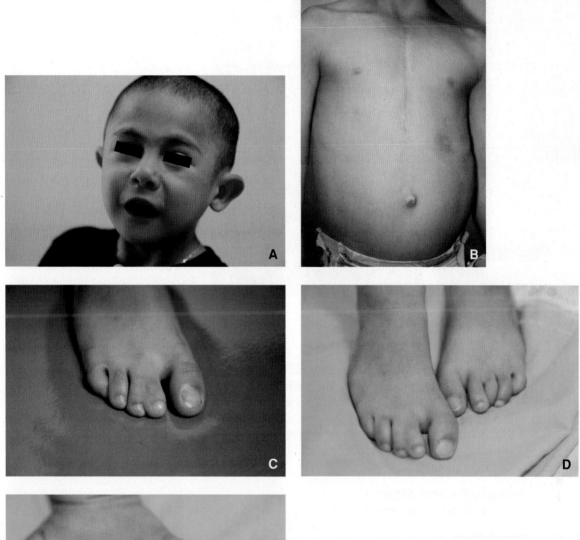

Figures A–E: A 38-week small-for-gestational-age infant with dysmorphic features, Tetralogy of Fallot, large patent ductus arteriosus, and chromosome 22q11 deletion, consistent with DiGeorge syndrome. He is now 4 years old. His weight is 11.3 kg, height is 81.5 cm, and head circumference is 45 cm, all of which are well below the 3rd percentile for his age. He has had numerous hospital admissions for upper and lower respiratory tract infections, two laryngoscopies, Nissen fundoplication for reflux, and a gastrostomy tube placement. He has clinodactyly of the left fifth finger, large gap between the first and second toe, bilateral clinodactyly of the fifth toes, and syndactyly of the second and third toe in the right foot.

DISSEMINATED INTRAVASCULAR COAGULATION (DIC)

CONSUMPTIVE COAGULOPATHY

Definition

- A heterogenous group of conditions that result in consumption of clotting factors, platelets, and anticoagulant proteins and intravascular deposition of fibrin leading to both thrombosis and hemorrhage.

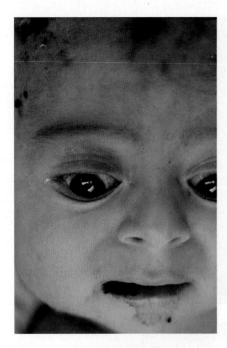
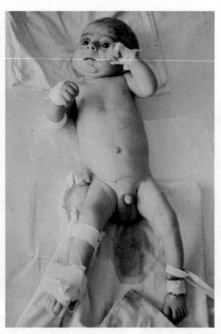

DIC in a 9-month-old boy who had protein–calorie malnutrition (marasmic kwashiorkor) and diarrhea. The stool cultures were negative but he was given antibiotic prior to his hospital admission. Note bloody stool, ecchymosis, purpura of the forehead, scalp, periorbital area, chin, left lower chest, and abdomen.

Etiology
- Meningococcemia, snake bite, rickettsial infections, malignancies, purpura fulminans, and giant hemangioma can be associated with DIC.
- Tissue necrosis, hypoxia, acidosis, shock, and endothelial damage are among the trigger factors.
- The deficiency of platelets; factor 2, factor 5, and factor 8; prothrombin and fibrinogen; consumption of physiologic anticoagulants and procoagulants can result in hemorrhage and thrombotic susceptibility.

Symptoms and Signs
- Bleeding, petechiae, and ecchymosis.

Treatment
- Treatment of the precipitating factor or factors is essential.
- Treatment of the consequences such as acidosis, hypoxia, and shock.
- Blood components. Protein C and heparin may be useful.

DOWN SYNDROME

Definition
- A chromosomal disorder with variable degrees of disability in mental and physical developments.

Etiology
- Down syndrome is caused by trisomy 21, the most common trisomy.
- Three types of cytogenetic abnormalities can result in trisomy 21.
  1. Presence of extra chromosome 21.
  2. Robertsonian translocation involving trisomy 21 (4%).
  3. Trisomy 21 mosaicism—normal population of cell line coexists with trisomy cell line (2%).
- The incidence of trisomy increases with advancing maternal age.

D

Symptoms and Signs

- Mental and growth retardation, hypotonia, flat face, up-slanted palpebral fissures, and epicanthic folds, speckled irises, short broad hands, hypoplasia of the middle phalanx of the fifth finger, simian creases, dysplasia of the pelvis, high-arched palate, intestinal atresia, and cardiac malformations.

Treatment

- The immediate problem is parental acceptance.
- Early management and correction of congenital abnormalities.
- The cardiac defects should be dealt with in a timely manner.
- Repeated infections, esotropia, refractory errors, hearing difficulties, cryptorchidism, and possible hypothyroidism should be attended to.
- Genetic counseling for the assessment of recurrence risk.
- Annual audiology evaluation during the first 3 years of life, annual thyroid screening.
- Their growth should be monitored on specific growth charts available for children with Down syndrome.

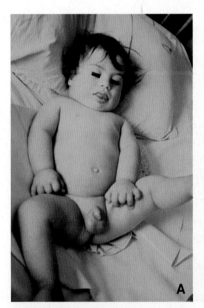
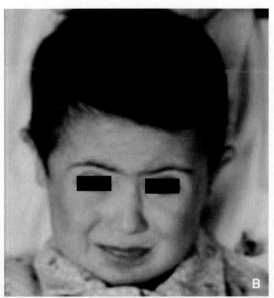
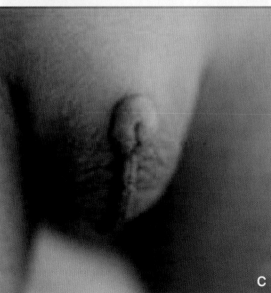
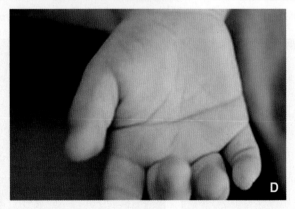

Figures A–C: Two boys with Down syndrome and typical facies. The boy in **Figure A** also has facial eczema. The boy in **Figure B** has micropenis and undescended right testicle **(Figure C)**.

Figure D: Simian crease.

figures continues

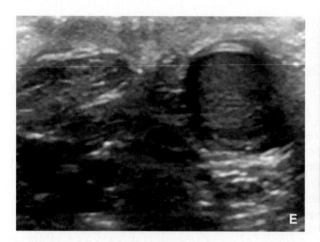

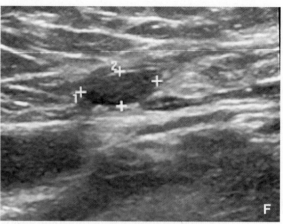

(figures cont.) **Figures E–F:** Transverse sonographic view of the scrotum demonstrates a normal left testicle within the scrotum **(Figure E)**. Targeted sonographic imaging of the right groin demonstrates a small atrophic right testicle within the inguinal canal compatible with an undescended right testicle **(Figure F)**.

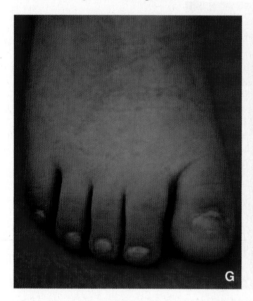

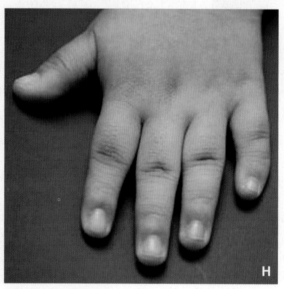

Figures G–H: Broad first toe and curly fifth finger (clinodactyly) in Down syndrome.

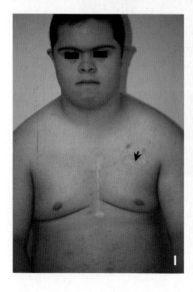

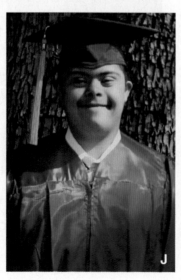

Figures I–K: An 18-year-old male with Down's syndrome **(Figure I)**. He had a large ventricular septal defect, which was repaired. He developed a complete heart block following the surgery **(Figure K)**, and required a pacemaker. He is doing well in special education and he recently graduated from high school **(Figure J)**. He is socially shy but can feed, dress, and bath himself. Plays Soccer, Hockey and Basketball. Note the pacemaker, arrow **(Figure I)**.

figures continues

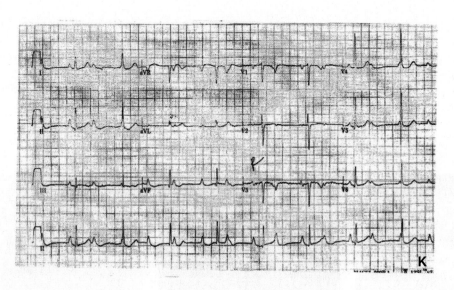

(figures cont.) **Figure K**

DRUG ERUPTIONS

Definition
- Drug allergies are common in children and present with a wide spectrum of signs and symptoms.

Etiology
- Hypersensitivity to a drug, which may or may not be IgE mediated.

Symptoms and Signs
- Drug reactions are the most common hypersensitivity reaction.
- Drug eruptions have a large range of presentation: Urticaria, angioedema, serum sickness–like reaction, fixed drug, lichenoid, drug hypersensitivity syndrome, pustular, acneiform, vasculitis, pseudoporphyria, drug-induced lupus, toxic epidermal necrolysis (TEN), and Stevens–Johnson syndrome (SJS).
- Acute type I hypersensitivity reaction is IgE mediated. Examples include hypersensitivity to penicillin and latex. These reactions generally occur within an hour of drug administration. Urticaria, angioedema, rhinitis, wheezing, shortness of breath, nausea, vomiting, diarrhea, and cardiovascular collapse may occur.
- Type II is cytotoxic reaction caused by antibody interacting with an antigen of the cell surface. Examples include hemolytic disease of the newborn, transfusion reactions, and pemphigus.
- Type III is toxic immune complex reaction; examples are glomerulonephritis, serum sickness, and Arthus-type reaction.
- Type IV is delayed-type hypersensitivity reaction; examples are tuberculin skin test and allergic contact dermatitis.
- An example of non-IgE mediated reaction is red man syndrome, which is related to the rate of vancomycin infusion.
- Delayed hypersensitivity occurs beyond the 1 hour of acute type I hypersensitivity and appears to be primarily T cell mediated. Maculopapular rash, erythema multiforme, urticaria, or more serious reactions such as blistering in SJS or TEN are some examples.
- The drug reaction seen mostly in pediatric population is a diffuse, small, red, or pink macula-papular rash with symmetrical distribution, pruritus and low-grade fever, presenting within 1 or 2 weeks of exposure (Figures A–H).

Treatment

- The offending antibiotic or chemical should be removed.
- Pretreatment with antihistamines and steroids can be effective in preventing type I hypersensitivity reactions.
- Treatment of delayed hypersensitivity drug reaction is mostly supportive. Includes oral antihistamines and bland emollients.

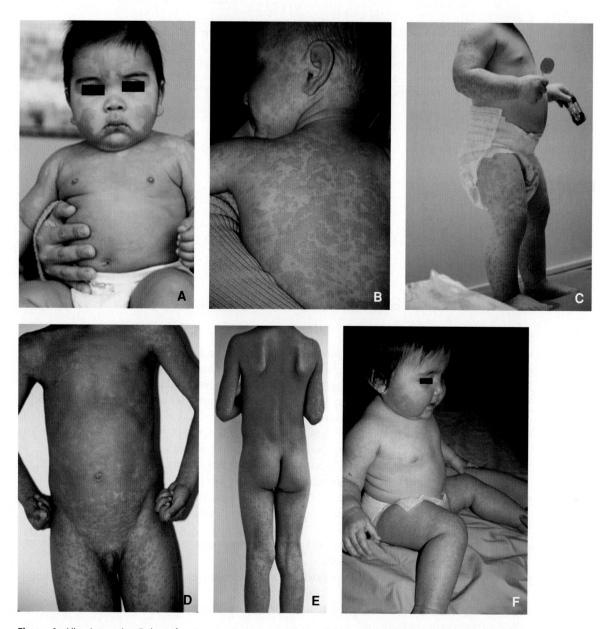

Figure A: Allergic reaction 5 days after Augmentin was prescribed to this 9-month-old boy for otitis media.

Figures B–C: Skin rash developed in this 1-year-old girl 9 days after the initiation of Amoxicillin **(Figure B)** and 1 week after Augmentin, in this 1-year-old boy **(Figure C)**.

Figures D–F: Cephalexin-induced morbilliform rash in a 14-year-old boy **(Figures D and E)** and in a 10-month-old girl **(Figure F)**.

figures continues

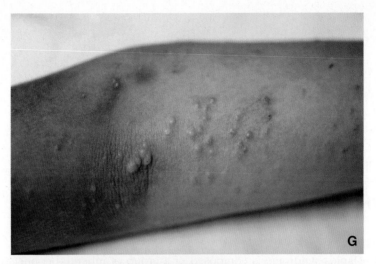

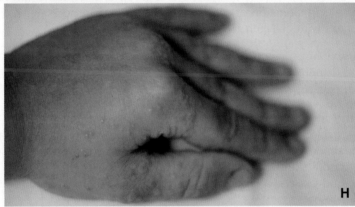

(figures cont.) **Figures G–H:** Drug hypersensitivity in a child who was put on Cephalexin and then on Azithromycin for "sore throat," without first obtaining a throat culture. He was subsequently diagnosed with infectious mononucleosis. There were numerous skin-colored papules on the dorsum of hands, extensors of the elbow and the knees.

ECZEMA (Gr. Ekzein, to boil over)

(See Atopic Dermatitis).

EHLERS–DANLOS SYNDROME (CUTIS ELASTICA)

Definition
- Ehlers–Danlos syndrome is composed of a group of inherited connective tissue disorders which results in alteration of structure, production, or processing of collagen or proteins that interacts with collagen.

Etiology
- Genetic mutation. The classical type Ehlers–Danlos syndrome is inherited in an autosomal dominant pattern.

Symptoms and Signs
- Loose, unstable joints resulting in dislocation, subluxation, or hyperextension, easy bruising, abnormal wound healing, and scar formation.
- Velvety-smooth skin which may be stretchy and translucent.
- Fragile blood vessels; complications may include abdominal aortic aneurism and valvular heart disease.
- Low muscle tone and weakness may be the presenting feature in the newborn.
- Other features of Ehlers–Danlos include kyphoscoliosis, club feet, premature rupture of membranes, periodontitis, platelet aggregation problems, and nerve compressions such as carpal tunnel syndrome.
- Figures A–F.

Treatment
- Supportive treatment.

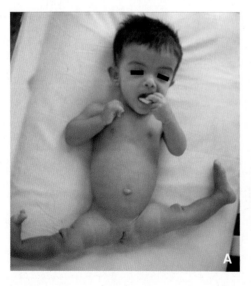

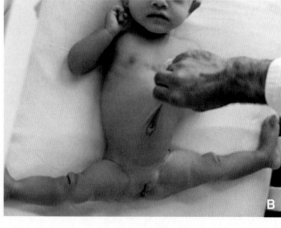

Figures A–B: Ehlers–Danlos in an 11-month-old baby.

figures continues

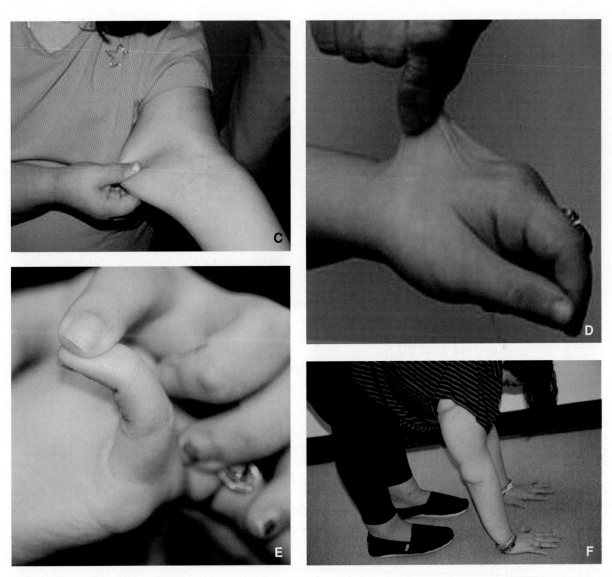

(figures cont.) **Figures C–F:** Ehlers–Danlos in a 12-year-old girl. Note stretchy skin, dorsiflexion of the fifth finger greater than 90 degrees and ability to touch palms to the floor.

EPSTEIN-BARR VIRUS INFECTION

(See Infectious Mononucleosis).

ERYSIPELAS (Gr. Erythros, red + pella, skin)

Definition
- Erysipelas is a relatively rare skin infection involving the upper dermis and the superficial lymphatics.

Etiology
- The majority of cases are caused by group A beta hemolytic streptococci. Either through a disruption of the skin barrier or by bacteremia.

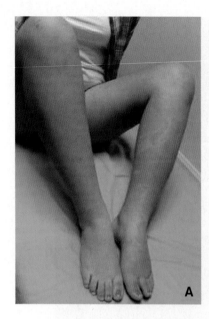 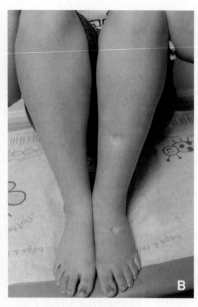

Figures A–B: This teenage girl presented with fever, shivering, abdominal pain, and rash. Note erythema on the legs, more prominent on the shins, and the pitting edema.

Symptoms and Signs
- It has an abrupt onset of symptoms including fever, chills, warm erythematous skin that is raised above the level of the surrounding skin. Has distinct and well-marginated borders.

Treatment
- IV antibiotic in case of systemic symptoms, ceftriaxone or cefazolin, penicillin in mild infections, erythromycin or clindamycin in cases of penicillin allergy. (Beware of antibiotic resistance.)

ERYTHEMA AB IGNE (Ab igne, L.; Redness from fire, hot water-bottle rash, fire stains, laptop leg)

Definition
- Erythema ab igne is a localized skin reaction to heat, presenting as an area of reticulated hyperpigmentation and erythema.

Etiology
- Chronic and repeated exposure to heat in the form of hot water bottle, heating pad, laptop batteries, open fire place, car heater, or space heater.
- It is believed to be due to the swelling of the medium veins in the skin.

Symptoms and Signs
- Erythema ab igne is characterized by mottled skin in areas exposed to the heat which turn into reticulated annular or gyrate erythema, and eventually progress to a pale pink and then to a purplish-dark brown color.

Treatment
- Removing the heat source.
- Mildly affected areas may self resolve within a few months.
- Topical tretinoin and laser therapy may improve the appearance of abnormally pigmented skin.
- Squamous cell carcinoma is a rare complication.

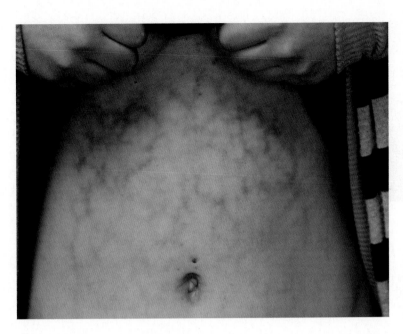

This 10-year-old girl had noticed this asymptomatic discoloration during the past 2 weeks. Hot water bottle was the culprit. She stopped the habit of going to bed with hot water bottle on her abdominal wall, and the reticulation gradually resolved.

ERYTHEMA INDURATUM (NODULAR VASCULITIS)

Definition
- Erythema induratum of Bazin is a vasculitis of large vessels and panniculitis that mainly manifests on the calves, thighs, or heels.

Etiology
- It was formerly believed to be a hematogenous dissemination of mycobacterium. But may also be secondary to other infections such as histoplasmosis or idiopathic.

Symptoms and Signs
- Symmetrical, tender subcutaneous nodules which may ulcerate.

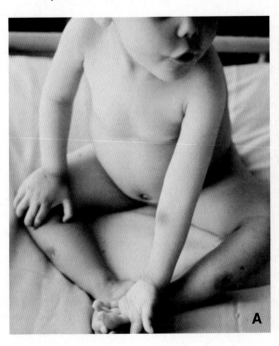

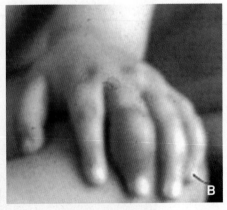

Figures A–C: This 2-year-old boy was brought in for sore on his shins and swelling of the left third finger. No fever or any other symptoms. He was a well-nourished boy with two tender, purplish, ulcers on his shins. His left third finger was tender and swollen in the middle phalanx and the spleen tip was palpable. He also had Vitamin D deficiency rickets. His chest x-ray was negative but his skin tuberculin test (PPD) was positive.

figures continues

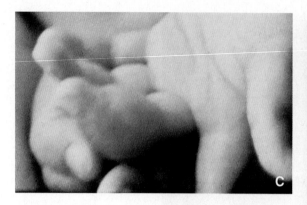

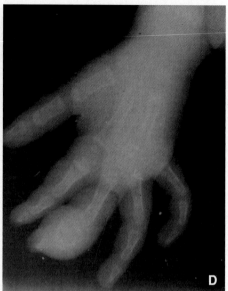

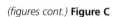
(figures cont.) **Figure C**

Figure D: Frontal view of the left hand demonstrates expansion with mixed destruction and sclerosis of the middle phalanx of the third digit with marked soft tissue swelling.

Treatment
- Treatment of the underlying infection.

ERYTHEMA INFECTIOSUM (FIFTH DISEASE)

Definition
- A contagious disease of childhood mostly affecting children between the ages of 3 to 12 years.

Etiology
- Human parvovirus B19.

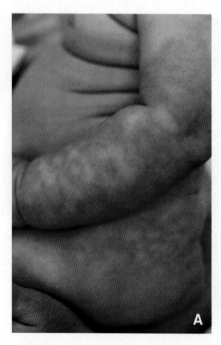

Figures A–C: The rash spreads rapidly to the trunk and proximal extremities. Macules turn into a lacy reticulated rash with central clearing. Palms and soles are spared.

figures continues

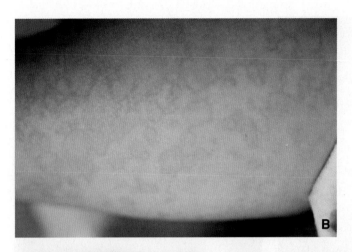

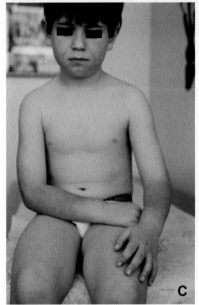

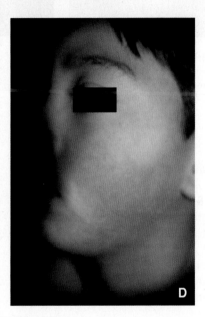

(figures cont.) **Figure D:** "Slapped-cheek" or "sunburned" in erythema infectiosum.

Symptoms and Signs

- Incubation period is 4 to 14 days.
- Only 20% of children have a mild fever.
- Classically begins with intense redness of both cheeks "slapped-cheek appearance."
- May then spread to the extremities, chest, and abdomen with a lacy, pink macular eruption, lasting 3 to 5 days (Figures A, B, and C).
- Symmetrical arthritis of hands, wrists, and knees may occur.
- Aplastic anemia can occur in children with underlying sickle cell disease or thalassemia.
- Erythema infectiosum in pregnant women may result in hydrops fetalis or fetal death.

Treatment

- Supportive care. Blood transfusion may be required to treat aplastic crisis or hydrops fetalis.

ERYTHEMA MULTIFORME

Definition

- Erythema multiforme is an acute immune-mediated condition.
- Distinctive target-like lesions on the skin are pathognomonic.

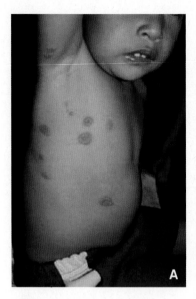
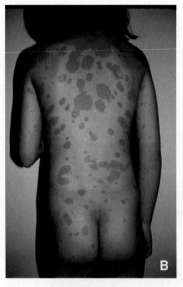
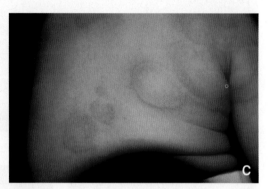

Figure A: Erythema multiforme in a toddler.

Figure B: A 6-year-old girl with 8 days of increasing rash, preceded by cold symptoms and a fever of 38.9-degrees celsius, 2 days prior to the rash.

Figure C: Bull's eye (iris, target-like, or doughnut-shaped) lesions in erythema multiforme.

Etiology
- Multifactorial.
- Infection: HSV is the most often implicated pathogen.

Symptoms and Signs
- Round erythematous papules that evolve into classic target lesions.
- Appear in symmetrical distribution on extensor surface of extremities and subsequently spread centrally.
- There may be some mucosal involvement.
- The skin lesions, unlike urticaria, may not disappear within hours.
- Usually symptomatic and rarely pruritic.
- Figures A–C.

Treatment
- Supportive care. Lesions fade within a few weeks.

ERYTHEMA NODOSUM (Gr. Nodosus, having nodes or projections)

Definition
- Erythema nodosum is an abrupt onset of symmetric, tender, erythematous nodules on extensor surface of extremities.

Etiology
- Erythema nodosum is considered a delayed hypersensitivity reaction to various drugs, infectious and inflammatory agents.
- Infectious: Streptococcal infections, tuberculosis, Yersinia, histoplasmosis, and coccidiomycosis.
- Inflammatory causes: Inflammatory bowel disease, sarcoidosis, and spondyloarthritis.
- Erythema nodosum can also be a reaction to certain drug such as oral contraceptives, sulfonamides, or phenytoin.

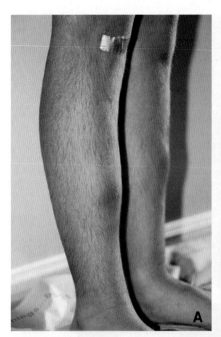

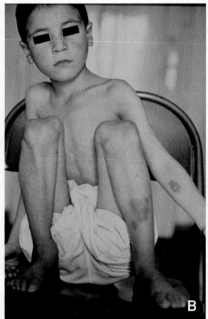

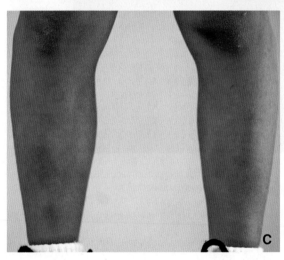

Figure A: A 9-year-old asymptomatic boy had this eruption on his legs for 3 weeks. His chest x-ray was suggestive of coccidiomycosis.

Figures B–C: Figure B is Erythema nodosum in a 12-year-old boy with spinal tuberculosis. Note the positive PPD on the left forearm. **Figure C** is Erythema nodosum in Juvenile Idiopathic Arthritis.

Symptoms and Signs
- Pretibial red, tender, nodular lesions in deep dermis and subcutaneous tissue.
- A high sedimentation rate (ESR) may be found in the majority of cases.

Treatment
- Treatment of the underlying condition.
- Figures A–C.

ERYTHEMA TOXICUM

Definition
- A benign cutaneous eruption in the neonatal period.

Etiology
- Unknown.

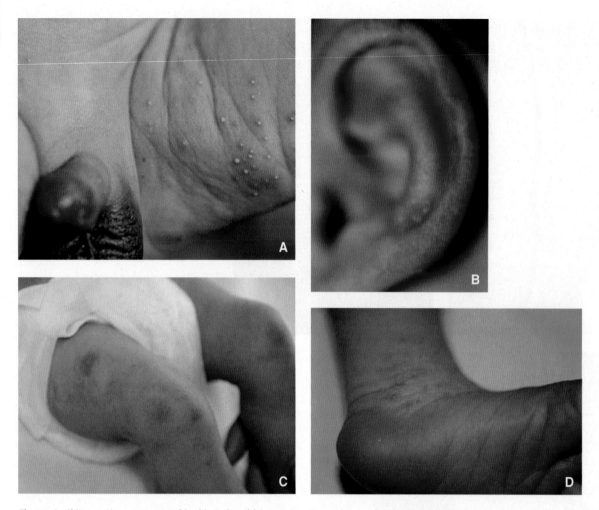

Figure A: Skin eruptions were noted in this 5-day-old asymptomatic newborn a few hours after birth. Numerous macules, papules, and vesicles on an erythematous base can be seen mostly on the anterior aspect of the thighs, axilla, abdomen, and back.

Figures B–D: A skin culture from some of these pustules were negative for staphylococcal infection. Erythema toxicum on the ear, thigh, and ankle of a 4-day-old.

Symptoms and Signs
- Asymptomatic and self limiting.
- Small, firm yellow-white, vesiculopustular papules on an erythematous base, which develop within the first 3 days of life.
- It can occur anywhere on the body and often sparing the palms and soles.

Treatment
- Unnecessary.
- The skin lesions disappear within 1 to 2 weeks.

ESOTROPIA

Definition
- Esotropia is a form of strabismus in which one or both eyes turn inward.

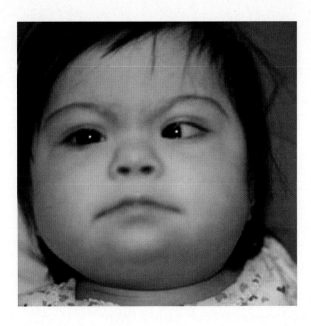

Esotropia in a 12-month-old girl with Down syndrome.

Etiology
- Unknown in the majority of cases.
- Congenital or infantile esotropia present at birth and up to 6 months of age.
- Weakness of one or more eye muscles.
- Cranial nerve palsy.
- Brain tumor.
- Eye injury.
- Retinopathy of prematurity.
- Accommodative esotropia due to hyperopia may present at 2 to 3 years of age.

Symptoms and Signs
- Crossed-eye appearance due to inward turning of one or both eyes (Figure).

Treatment
- Treat underlying medical condition.
- May require corrective surgery.

EXOSTOSIS

(See Multiple Hereditary Exostosis).

FACIAL PALSY

(See Bell's Palsy).

FANCONI ANEMIA

Definition
- Fanconi anemia is the best known constitutional pancytopenia.

Etiology
- Possible genetic predisposition to bone marrow failure.
- Autosomal recessive mode of inheritance.
- Can be associated with other genetic disorders such as Down syndrome.

Symptoms and Signs
- There is a spontaneous chromosome break, defective DNA repair, increased susceptibility of hematopoietic cells to oxidant stress, and decreased cell survival.
- Various physical abnormalities: Hyperpigmentation and café-au-lait spots.
- Skeletal abnormalities, especially absent or hypoplastic thumbs, and short stature.
- Organ abnormalities.
- Pancytopenia normally follows thrombocytopenia, leukopenia, lymphopenia, and anemia.
- Macrocytosis, poikilocytosis, and anisocytosis.
- Hypoplastic or aplastic bone marrow.

Treatment
- Steroids and androgens.
- Bone marrow transplantation.

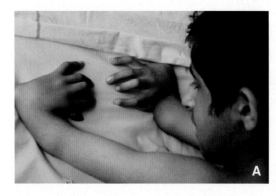

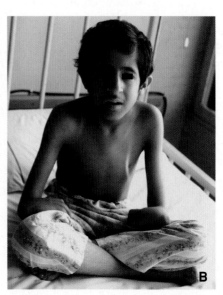

Figures A–D show a 14-year-old male with Fanconi anemia. Note the bilateral radial deviated hands due to absent radius and pectus carinatum.

figures continues

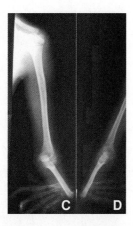

(figures cont.) **Figures C–D:** Absence of the radius and thumb aplasia.

FIBROMA, BENIGN NONOSSIFYING

Definition
- Nonossifying fibroma is, as the name implies, a benign, nonaggressive tumor consisting mostly of fibrous tissue. It is one of the more common benign tumors in children.

Etiology
- Unknown.

Symptoms and Signs
- Asymptomatic, unless it is large enough to cause pain or lead to a fracture.

Treatment
- Spontaneous regression can be expected after skeletal maturity.
- Bone grafting may be recommended when more than 50% of the bone is taken up by the lesion.
- Figures A–E.

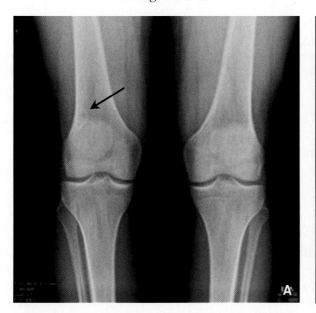

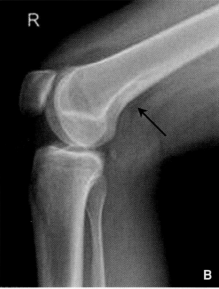

Figures A–E: A 12-year-old male with a 2-week history of pain in the right knee which was exacerbated by running and playing basketball. No associated swelling or deformity was present. However, the patient was slightly tender below the right patella. **Figures A** and **B:** Frontal and lateral x-rays of the right knee demonstrate an eccentric, cortical-based lucent lesion with a smooth sclerotic margin and narrow zone of transition. No matrix calcification is present.

figures continues

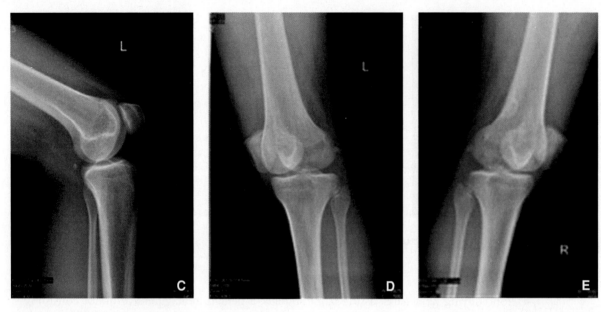

(figures cont.) **Figures C–E:** Over time, these lesions become increasingly sclerotic and eventually resolve. No further imaging or follow-up is necessary when this characteristic pattern is recognized.

FIFTH DISEASE

(See Erythema Infectiosum).

FINGER AND TOE CLUBBING (HIPPOCRATIC FINGERS)

Definition
- A deformity of distal phalanges of fingers or toes without constant osseous changes.

Etiology
- Bronchogenic carcinoma and other neoplasms.
- Lung abscess, emphysema, and bronchiectasis.
- Cystic fibrosis.
- Chronic obstructive lung disease.
- Sarcoidosis.
- Inflammatory bowel disease.
- Sprue.
- Neoplasms of the esophagus, liver, and bowel.
- Cyanotic congenital heart disease.
- Subacute bacterial endocarditis.
- Infected arterial graft.
- Aortic aneurysm.
- Patent ductus arteriosus.
- Arteriovenous fistula of major extremity vessel.
- Hyperthyroidism (Graves disease).

Symptoms and Signs
- Increased convexity of the nail fold.
- Fluctuation and softening of the nail bed.
- Loss of the normal angle between the nail bed and cuticula.
- Hypertrophy of the proximal end of the phalanx.

- Shiny and striation of the nail and skin.
- Schamroth's test (missing "diamond" between two opposing fingers. See the "diamond" in a healthy girl) (Figure C).
- Figures A–F.

Treatment
- Treatment of the underlying cause.

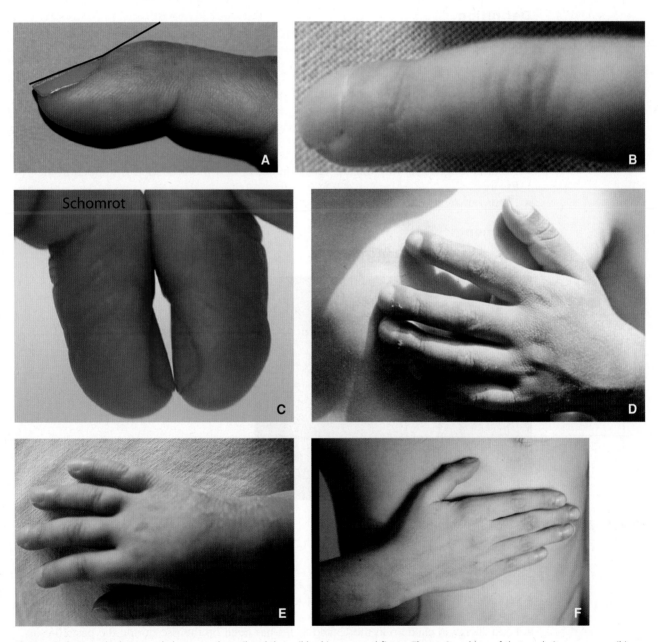

Figures A–B: Note the large angle between the nail and the nail bed in a normal finger, **Figure A** and loss of that angle in a convex nail in finger clubbing, **Figure B**.

Figure C: Schamroth's test. Note the "diamond" between two opposing fingers in a healthy young girl. This "diamond" is lost in finger clubbing due to the deformed nails.

Figures D–F: Finger clubbing in bronchiectasis **(Figure D)**. Finger clubbing in congenital cyanotic heart disease **(Figure E)**. Note nail changes in all and cyanosis in **Figure F**.

FINGER SUCKING

(See Acral Leak Dermatitis).

FISSURED TONGUE (SCROTAL TONGUE)

Definition
- Fissured tongue is a benign condition characterized by deep grooves in the dorsum of the tongue.

Etiology
- Congenital or inherited, also can be part of a syndrome like Down's syndrome caused by incomplete fusion of the two halves of the tongue.
- Infection, malnutrition, Vitamin A deficiency, and trauma.

Symptoms and Signs
- Fissured tongue is asymptomatic, unless infected, or a piece of food is trapped in the fissures.
- Fissures may also be interconnected.

Treatment
- Careful cleansing and rinsing.

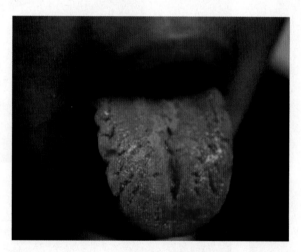

A 12-year-old male with fissured tongue since birth.

FOOD ALLERGY

Definition
- "An adverse health effect arising from a specific immune response that occurs reproducibly on exposure to a given food." National Institute of Allergy and Infectious Diseases (NIAID).
- Food allergy in children in the United States has been on the rise during the past 10-years.
- Distinguish from nonimmunogenic reaction to food, lactose intolerance.

Etiology
- Food allergy is the result of an adverse immune response to a food protein (IgE mediated).
- There is controversy about the role of food allergies in causing atopic dermatitis but more than 30% of children with moderate to severe atopic dermatitis have food allergies.
- A large number of children diagnosed with food allergy are not allergic to the suspected foods (using double blind placebo controlled challenge).

- It is unlikely that isolated asthma or allergic rhinitis is related to food allergy.
- Increasing quantities of food specific IgE are associated with increasing risks of clinical allergies.
- The incidence of respiratory allergies is two to four times higher in children who have food allergy.
- Over time, many children lose their sensitivity to food; especially to milk, eggs, soy, and wheat; therefore the prevalence of food allergy decreases with age.
- Food allergies that begin in adulthood may persist.
- Any food can cause an allergic reaction but the most common foods causing food allergy in children are milk, egg, peanut, wheat, soy, tree nut, shellfish, and fish.
- Food allergy should be distinguished from food intolerance.

Symptoms and Signs

- The most feared reaction of food allergy is *anaphylaxis, which is IgE mediated.*
- *Gastro intestinal food allergies* (e.g., eosinophilic esophagitis, eosinophilic gastro enteritis, food protein–induced allergic proctocolitis, and oral allergy syndrome, most common with fruits and vegetables with shared allergy with pollen).
- Swelling of the lips and tongue, oral pruritus, nausea, vomiting, reflux, colicky abdominal pain, and diarrhea.
- *Dermatologic manifestations* of food allergy (e.g., acute urticaria, contact urticaria, angioedema, allergic contact dermatitis, and exacerbation of atopic dermatitis).
- Pruritus, erythema, and morbilliform eruption.
- *Respiratory reactions* (e.g., allergic rhinitis and asthma).
- Sneezing, rhinorrhea, nasal congestion, pruritus, itching throat, hoarseness, dry staccato cough, chest tightness, dyspnea, and wheezing.
- *Primary pulmonary hemosiderosis with hypersensitivity to cow's milk* (Heiner syndrome).
- *Cardio vascular reactions* (e.g., tachycardia, bradycardia, hypotension, dizziness, fainting, and loss of consciousness).

Treatment

- Symptomatic treatment of reactions by epinephrine, other vasopressors, bronchodilators, antihistamines, oxygen, IV fluid, and corticosteroids.
- Avoidance of allergens.
- Auto injectable epinephrine for children at risk of anaphylaxis.
- Oral immunotherapy.
- Carry medal alert bracelet or necklace.

CASHEW ALLERGY

EGG ALLERGY

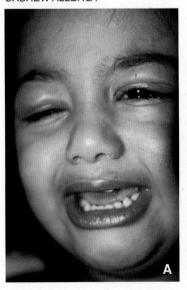

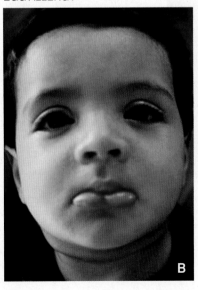

Figure A: This 2-year-old girls' eyelids and lips became swollen and developed urticaria on her chest 2 hours after eating some cashews. An epinephrine shot relieved her of her discomfort.

Figure B: This 1-year-old girl was given egg (yolk and white) at 9 a.m. She began to cough an hour later. Swelling of the lips, ears, and eyelids developed after 2 p.m. (5 hours later).

figures continues

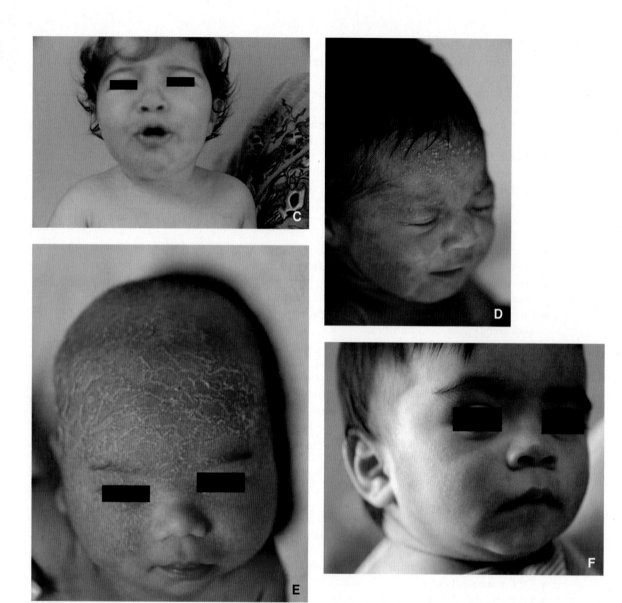

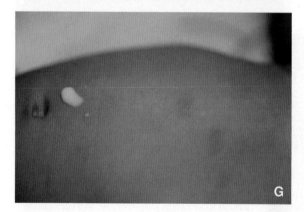

(figures cont.) **Figure C:** This 1-year-old baby was allergic to milk and was raised on soy formula. Her grandfather, unaware of this allergy, gave her a tea-spoon of ice cream on her birthday, which she soon vomited, her face became red, and her lips became swollen soon afterward.

Figure D: This 3-week-old girl developed this rash a few days after she was put on a cow's milk–based formula. A change to soy did not change the skin disorder. But, the rash resolved within 2 weeks on a hypoallergenic, casein hydrolyzed formula. This baby's karyotype is 44, triple X.

Figure E: This 4-week-old presented with these skin changes; erythema, scaling of the scalp, and generalized eczema. He was on a cow's milk–based formula. A trial of soy formula was unsuccessful. He was put on an amino acid based formula. He improved rapidly, and his skin was clear within 3 weeks.

Figure F: The mother of a successfully breast fed 9-month-old boy was told to stop breast feeding and give him formula. He developed facial erythema, some urticaria, and injected conjunctivae 20 minutes following a bottle of cow's milk–based formula. His reaction to cow's milk was more pronounced when he was given a bottle of formula at the age of 9 days; he vomited and his face turned red.

Figure G: A 5-month-old breast-fed infant boy who developed skin rash and hives 15 minutes following each bottle of cow-based formula. No diarrhea, vomiting, or coughing. A few drops of milk were placed on the abdomen to which he had an erythematous skin reacted within 10 minutes.

FRACTURE CLAVICLE

Definition
- Fracture of the clavicle, a bone well enveloped in a thick periosteum, is not an uncommon finding in the newborn.

Etiology
- Trauma as a result of a difficult vaginal or forceps delivery. In older children, a fall or direct impact on the clavicle.
- Fractures of the distal tip of clavicle, in infants and toddlers, can be the result of child abuse.

Symptoms and Signs
- Excessive crying in the newborn, and complain of pain in older children, and lack of or reduced movement of the affected arm.

Treatment
- A padded figure-of-eight for 2 to 3 weeks to reduce mobilization and pain. Addition of a sling in older children can be helpful.

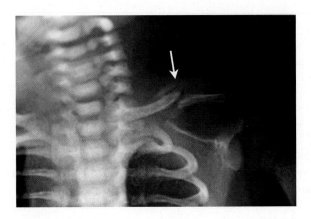

Eleven-day-old newborn who had an uncompli-cated and normal delivery. Baby cried excessively on dressing and undressing. Left clavicle x-ray: Mildly displaced fracture through the midportion of the clavicle (*arrow*). Surrounding periosteal reaction indicates the presence of healing.

FRENULUM (L., dim. of frenum bridle)

Definition
- Frenulum or frenum is a small tissue that restricts or secures movements of an organ.

Etiology
- A minor congenital anomaly.

Symptoms and Signs
- Frenulum or frenum of the lip is a thin mucosal tissue that connects the upper lip mucosa to the gingiva between the upper central incisors.
- When hyperplastic, it can cause diastema (midline gap). Lingual frenulum or ankyloglossia connects the inferior of the tongue to the floor of the mouth.
- Frenula, in the majority of cases, are an isolated finding, becoming less evident with age.

Treatment
- Surgery is rarely needed.

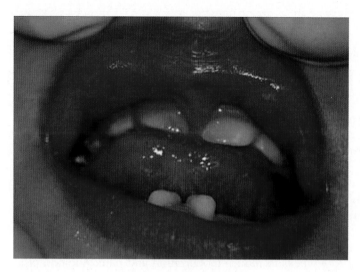

A labial frenulum in an asymptomatic 2-year-old boy.

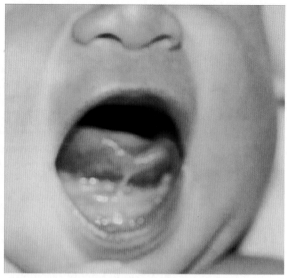

A lingual frenulum (ankyloglossia) in an asymptomatic infant.

FURONCULOSIS

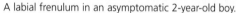

Definition
- The presence at any time of several furuncles or persistent recurrence of furuncles.

Etiology
- Infectious: *Staphylococcus aureus*.
- Predisposing factors are any skin injury, obesity, dermatitis, hyperhidrosis, diabetes mellitus, malnutrition, low serum iron, and HIV infection.
- Close contact with a carrier or carriage of *S. aureus* in the nares, axilla, or perineum can cause recurrent furunculosis.
- Figures A and B.

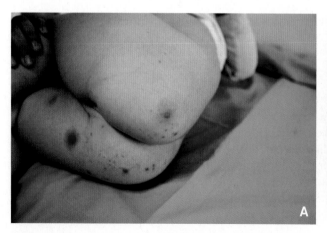

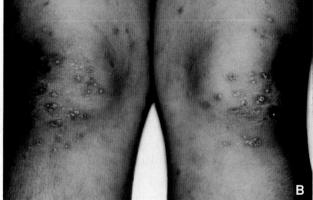

Figures A–B: Furunculosis in two children.

Symptoms and Signs

- Indurated lesions mainly on the face, neck, axilla, groins, and buttocks soon develop central necrosis and eventually rupture, leaving a scar.
- Furuncles on the upper lip or cheek can rarely lead to cavernous sinus thrombosis.

Treatment

- Hygiene, regular bathing, and antimicrobial soaps are very important first steps.
- Loose-fitting clothing, warm moist compress, and drainage if needed.
- Penicillin resistant antibiotics or in cases of penicillin allergy, clindamycin, cephalosporin, or erythromycin can be used.
- Application of mupirocin ointment in the nares may prevent further recurrences.

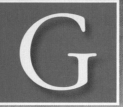

GANGLION CYST

Definition
- A ganglion cyst is a swelling found most commonly in the region of or on the joints and tendons of the hands and feet.

Etiology
- Unknown.

Symptoms and Signs
- Ganglia are typically found on the dorsum of the wrist and volar aspect of the radial wrist.
- They are usually asymptomatic, may disappear and reappear over time.
- Rarely, can compress the underlying radial or median nerves and cause loss of sensation or weakness.

Treatment
- Often self limited.
- Aspiration or surgical removal if painful or interference with function.

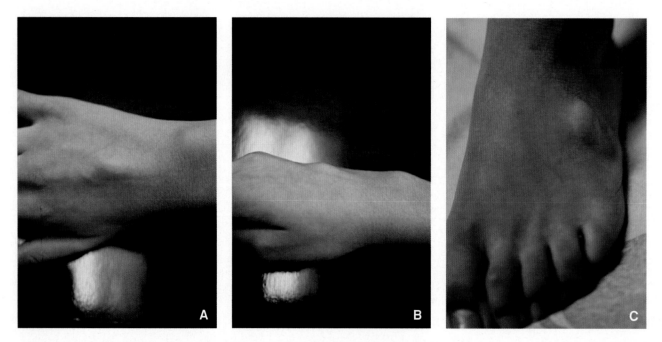

Figures A–C: Figures A and B, ganglion cyst of the hand; **Figure C**, ganglion cyst of the foot.

GANGRENE (L. gangraena, Gr. gangraina, putrefaction)

Definition
- Gangrene is a serious and potentially life-threatening condition, which may begin with a small sore, ending in putrefaction and necrosis of a large mass of tissue or that of an entire organ.

Etiology
- Infection (e.g., *Clostridium perfringens*).
- Ischemia: Often of the lower extremities as a result of peripheral vascular disease and diabetes.

Symptoms and Signs
- There are two main types of gangrene: dry and wet.
  1. Dry gangrene: Due to ischemia begins in the distal part of a limb. Minimal if any putrefaction.

     Pallor, dull ache, and cold feeling in the affected organ. The affected organ becomes dry, black, and smaller. The liberated hemoglobin, from the hemolyzed red blood cells, interacts with hydrogen sulfide released by bacteria forming iron sulfide which gives the black color to the affected tissues.
  2. Wet gangrene: Often develops in moist areas such as the lungs, mouth, and the bowel. Pressure ulcers in heels, sacrum, and buttocks are also categorized as wet gangrene. Multibacterial etiology associated with a very poor prognosis.
- Figure.

Treatment
- Debridement, surgery, amputation.

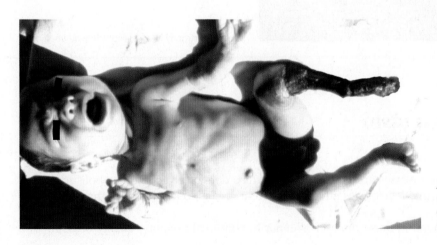

A skin infection in an 8-month-old was not managed timely and adequately. He had developed gangrene by the time he got to the Children's Hospital in Tehran.

GIANOTTI–CROSTI SYNDROME

(See Papular Acrodermatitis of Childhood).

GINGIVAL ENLARGEMENT (GINGIVAL OVER GROWTH, GUM HYPERTROPHY)

Definition
- Gum enlargement caused by a variety of factors.

Etiology
- Drug induced: Phenytoin, cyclosporine, and calcium channel blockers.
- Systemic factors: Scurvy, leukemia, granulomatous diseases (Wegener's disease, sarcoidosis).
- Infections: Viral or bacterial. Viral gingivostomatitis and poor oral hygiene.

Symptoms and Signs
- Erythema and swelling of the gingiva, gross enlargement of the gums, migration of teeth, secondary infections, and impaction of permanent teeth.

Treatment
- If possible, discontinuation of the drug causing gingival enlargement, oral hygiene, and gingivectomy.

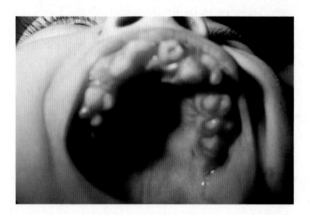

Gum hypertrophy in an epileptic boy on phenytoin.

GLYCOGEN STORAGE DISEASE (GSD)

Definition
- Glycogen storage diseases are characterized by disorders of glycogen metabolism due to liver enzyme deficiencies affecting different organs, but principally the liver.
- The glycogen found in these diseases is either in abnormal quantity, quality or both.

Etiology
- A rare autosomal recessive disorder due to the deficiency or absent activity of glucose-6-phosphatase enzyme in the liver, kidney, or/and intestinal mucosa.

Symptoms and Signs
- Inability to produce free glucose from glycogen leads to hypoglycemia and lactic acidosis in the neonatal period.

- Subsequent hyperuricemia, hyperlipidemia, seizures, and hepatomegaly.
- Fat cheeks, doll-like facies, short stature, thin extremities, large abdomen, and enlarged kidneys.
- Intermittent diarrhea, easy bruising, epistaxis, remarkably elevated triglycerides, cholesterol, and phospholipids.
- In older children; delayed puberty, multiorgan system involvement, polycystic ovaries, pancreatitis, atherosclerosis, reduced bone mineral content, renal disease (nephrolithiasis and nephrocalcinosis), and pulmonary hypertension.
- Diagnosis: Epinephrine or glucagon injections which fail to raise serum glucose levels. Liver biopsy.

Treatment
- Maintain euglycemia.
- Dietary supplements of vitamins and minerals, and treatment of hyperlipidemia.
- Liver transplantation.

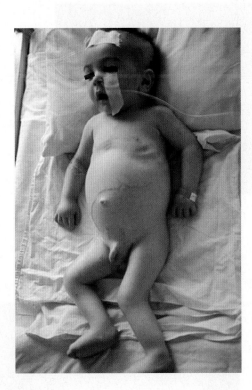

A 9-month-old boy was admitted with seizure and found to have hepatomegaly and hypoglycemia.

GRANULOMA ANNULARE (L. granuloma, a small particle or grain)

Definition
- A small nodular raised lesion forming a ring pattern consisting of an aggregation of mononuclear inflammatory cells surrounded by a rim of lymphocytes.

Etiology
- Granuloma formation represents a chronic inflammatory response caused by infectious or noninfectious agents.

Symptoms and Signs

- Often an asymptomatic, self-limited skin disease which is more common in females.
- Circular (annulare) or half circular (arciform).
- Skin colored, erythematous, or violaceous.
- Ring of small, firm papules 1 to 5 cm.
- Dorsum of hands, fingers, extensor aspects of arms and legs, and trunk are more prone to these lesions.
- Figures A–G.

Treatment

- Surgical or electrocautery (cauterization) for histologic diagnosis and treatment.

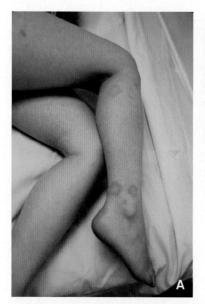

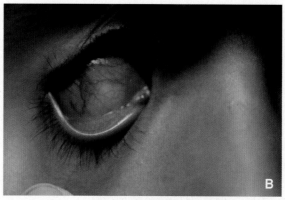

Figure A: Granuloma annulare in a 13-year-old girl.

Figure B: Granuloma of the eye.

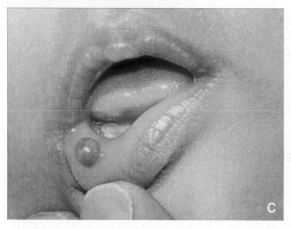

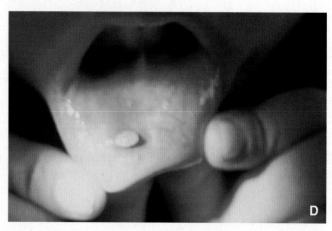

Figure C: Granuloma of the lip in a toddler.

Figure D: Granuloma of the oral mucosa.

figures continues

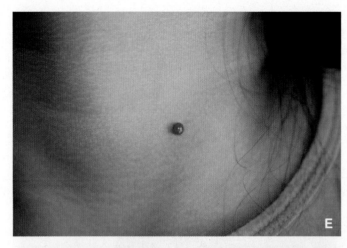

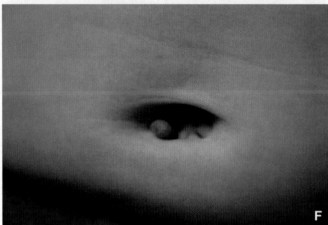

(figures cont.) **Figure E:** Granuloma, pyogenic. A growing papule on the neck of a 10-year-old girl. No associated pain or itching.

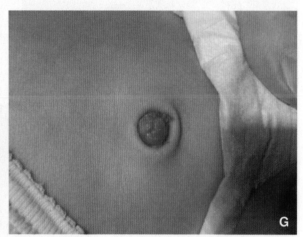

Figures F–G: Granuloma of the umbilicus in two newborns.

GYNECOMASTIA (Gr. gynec, woman + mastos, breast)

Definition
- Excessive growth of the male mammary gland(s).

Etiology
- Physiologic gynecomastia can be seen in both male and female newborns. The condition is due to circulating maternal estrogen, is self limited and resolves within a few weeks of life.
- Pubertal, secondary to hormonal changes.
- Drug induced: For example, estrogens, androgens, anabolic steroids, isoniazid, ketoconazole, cimetidine, ranitidine, omeprazole, Methotrexate, digitoxin, enalapril, methyldopa, spironolactone, diazepam, haloperidol, alcohol, amphetamines, marijuana, and phenytoin.
- Congenital disorders: For example, Klinefelter syndrome.

Symptoms and Signs
- Asymptomatic enlargement of the breast, mostly bilateral, without discoloration or tenderness. Nipples appear normal.
- Gynecomastia is in sharp contrast to mastitis, which is associated with fever, pain, tenderness, redness, and indrawn nipples.

Treatment

- Depends on the etiology. Often, reassurance, discontinuation of the medication causing the gynecomastia, and treatment of the underlying cause.
- Gynecomastia in older children, and particularly boys, may require surgical resection primarily for cosmetic and psychological reasons.
- Figures A–D.

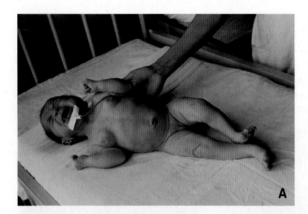

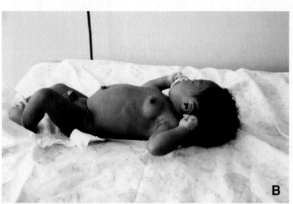

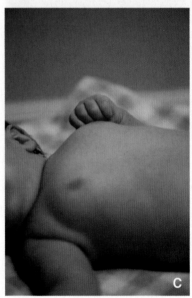

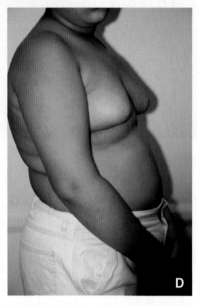

Figures A–B: Bilateral gynecomastia in a 1-month-old girl, a tetanus survivor **(Figure A)** and bilateral gynecomastia in a 2-week-old boy **(Figure B)**.

Figure C: A healthy 4-week-old girl with gynecomastia.

Figure D: Gynecomastia in an obese teenage boy.

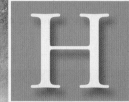

HAND-FOOT-AND-MOUTH DISEASE

Definition
- Hand-foot-and-mouth disease is an acute viral illness, characterized by a vesicular rash, on the oral mucosa and the extremities.

Etiology
- It is caused by nonpolio enteroviruses: Coxsackie virus A16 and enterovirus 71.
- The disease spreads by fecal–oral transmission or by direct contact with saliva. Vertical transmission to newborns may occur during late stages of pregnancy.

Symptoms and Signs
- The incubation period is 3 to 6 days.
- A low-grade fever may or may not accompany the maculopapular, vesicular, or pustular rash, which appears on the oropharynx, extremities, and the buttocks.
- Central nervous system or pulmonary complications may occur with certain viral serotypes (enterovirus 71).

Treatment
- Usually a self-limited disease. Treatment is symptomatic as patients improve within a week.
- In order to limit viral transmission, children with open lesions must avoid group activities.

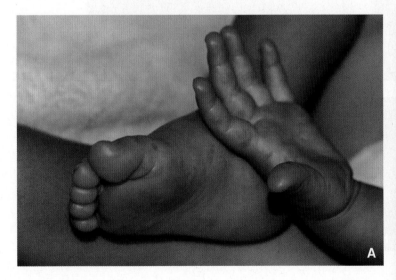
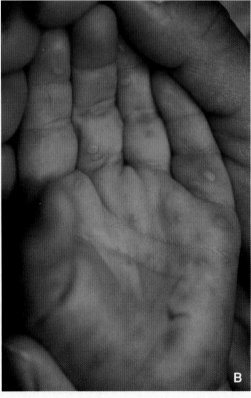

Figures A–H: Maculopapular and vesicular rashes on the hands, feet, buttocks, and groin of children with hand-foot-and-mouth disease. In **Figure G**, vesicles can be seen on the oral mucosa as well. **Figure H** is the close-up view of the lesions on the groin.

figures continues

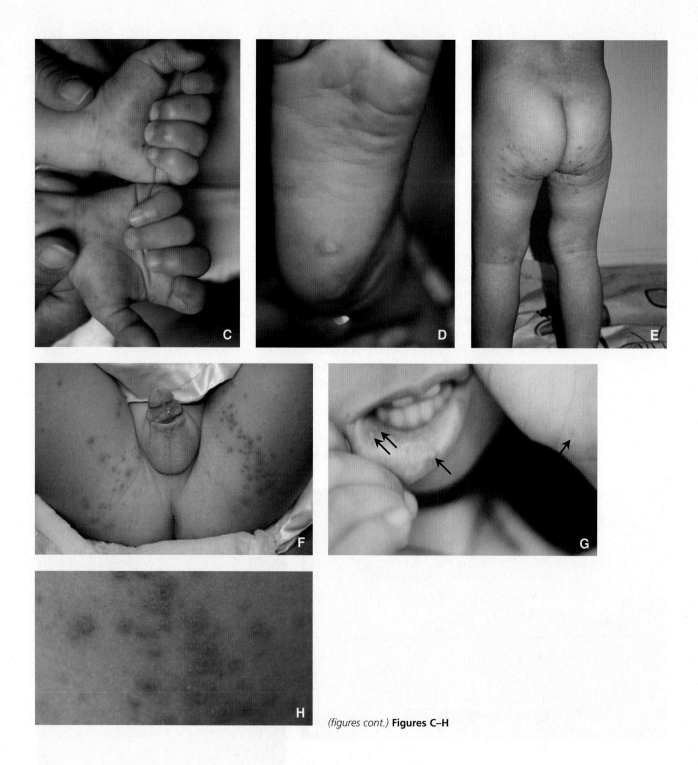

(figures cont.) **Figures C–H**

HEMANGIOMAS AND CAPILLARY VASCULAR MALFORMATIONS

HEMANGIOMAS

Definition

- Benign, congenital, vascular tumor of endothelial cells which are characterized by a growth phase and an involution phase.

Etiology

- Exact mechanisms remain unknown. However, there appears to be an abundance of positive vasculogenic factors expressed by the hemangioma during the growth phase. Apoptotic factors then counteract the vasculogenic factors during the involution phase.

Symptoms and Signs

- Most hemangiomas are not visible at birth. They present several weeks or months postnatally. The proliferative phase, which is characterized by rapid growth, occurs during the first year of life. This is followed by a slow involution phase which may take up to 5 years.
- They are more frequent in females, premature infants, and twins.
- Complications include ulceration and bleeding.
- Airway compromise and visual field deficits may occur with airway and periorbital hemangiomas.
- Hemangiomas located over the midline of lumbosacral area are associated with spinal dysraphism.
- The presence of five or more hemangiomas should raise concerns for the possibility of the existence of visceral hemangiomas.
- High output heart failure is a rare complication of hepatic and large cutaneous hemangiomas.
- Figures A–H.

Treatment

- Often a self-limited condition.
- Intralesional or systemic steroids, propranolol, interferon alpha, vincristine, laser therapy, and surgical resection have all been used with various success rates.
- Embolization of visceral hemangiomas in case of high output cardiac failure.

CAPILLARY VASCULAR MALFORMATIONS

Definition

- Malformed dilated blood vessels in the skin. In contrast to hemangiomas, they are nontumorous and have normal endothelial turnover (see Hemangiomas).

Etiology

- Congenital anomalies of capillary morphogenesis. Nevus simplex and nevus flammeus (port-wine stain) are the two most common examples.

Symptoms and Signs

- Nevus simplex (stork bite, angel kiss, salmon patch) occurs in approximately 40% of infants as pink to red blanchable patches. Lesions are most commonly located over the eyelid, glabella, and midline of the nape of the neck.
- Nevus flammeus (port-wine stain) are rare capillary malformation which occurs in approximately 0.3% of newborns. May occur on any part of the body, and typically presents as unilateral pink or red patch that enlarges proportionally as the child grows.

Treatment and Outcome

- Nevus simplex: Typically disappears within the first 2 years of life, with the exception of lesions on the nape of the neck. They may be associated with spinal dysraphism when located over the lumbosacral area, especially when another lumbosacral abnormality is present.
- Rarely, they are associated with genetic syndromes such as Beckwith–Wiedemann syndrome.
- Nevus flammeus, persist in the majority of cases through adulthood, progress to darker thickened nodules. Laser therapy has improved the outcome.

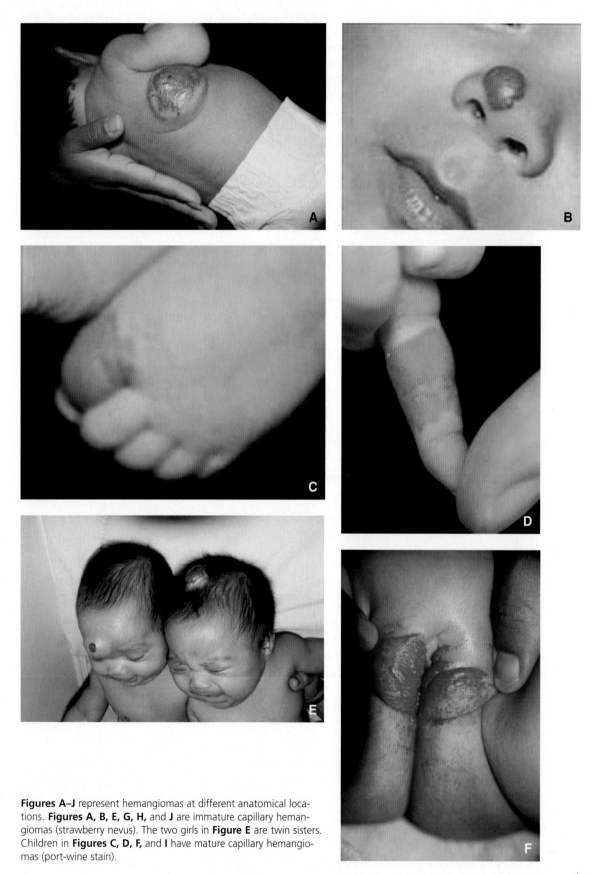

Figures A–J represent hemangiomas at different anatomical locations. Figures A, B, E, G, H, and J are immature capillary hemangiomas (strawberry nevus). The two girls in Figure E are twin sisters. Children in Figures C, D, F, and I have mature capillary hemangiomas (port-wine stain).

figures continues

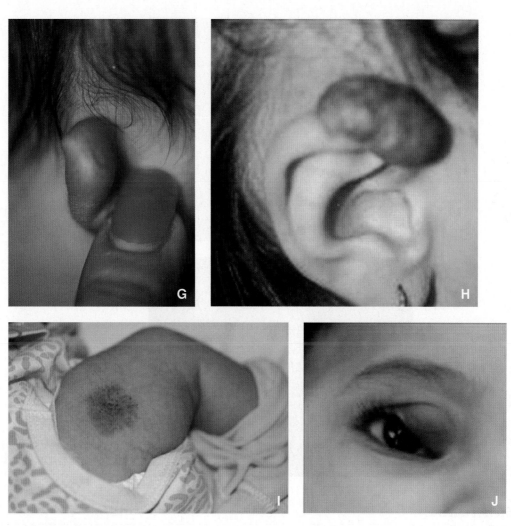

(figures cont.) **Figures G–J**

HEMANGIOMA OF THE NECK

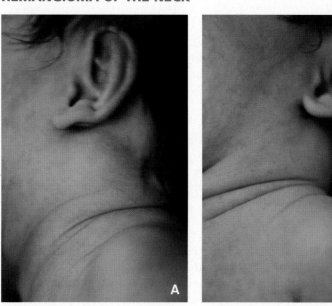

Figures A–B:
Hemangioma of the neck found incidentally in a 6-month-old child who presented with failure to thrive. There is also positional edema in the neck.

figures continues

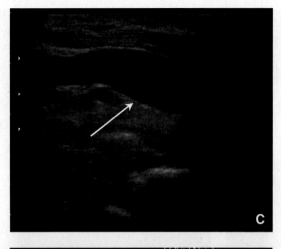

(figures cont.) **Figure C:** Doppler ultrasound image of the neck demonstrates a distended jugular vein with turbulent color flow pattern.

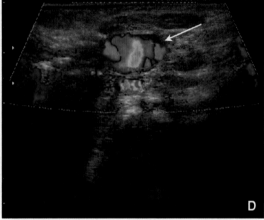

Figure D: Gray-scale sagittal ultrasound image of the neck demonstrates fusiform dilatation of the jugular vein.

HEMATOMA

Definition
- A localized collection of blood outside of the blood vessel.

Etiology
- It is caused by breakage of a blood vessel.
- Valsalva (coughing, sneezing, constipation, or other forms of straining), trauma, hypertension, bleeding disorders, antiplatelet or anticoagulant medications (aspirin or warfarin), and idiopathic causes.

Symptoms and Signs
- Asymptomatic in the majority of cases, but it depends mostly on the anatomical location of the hematoma.
- In subconjunctival hematoma, there is a collection of blood in the subconjunctival space along the sclera. It is a common and normal finding in newborn infants who are born via vaginal delivery.

Treatment
- Depends on the etiology and on the anatomic location of the hematoma.
- Consideration must be made regarding whether there is room for expansion of the hematoma, or bleeding is contained within a closed space such as the cranium.
- Most subconjunctival hematomas resolve spontaneously within 2 weeks.

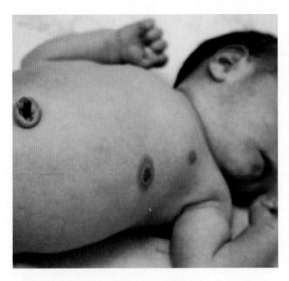

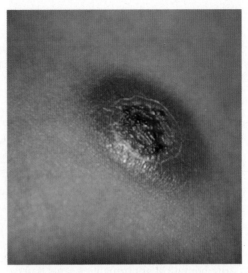

This asymptomatic 2-week-old baby was born with this hematoma on his abdominal wall.

Close-up view of the newborn's hematoma.

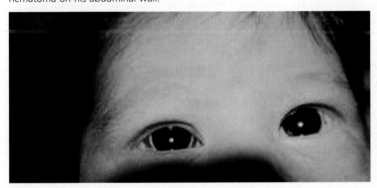

Bilateral subconjunctival hematomas in a 5-day-old otherwise healthy newborn and uncomplicated delivery.

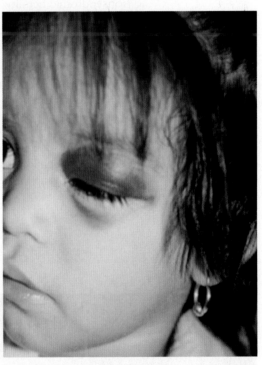

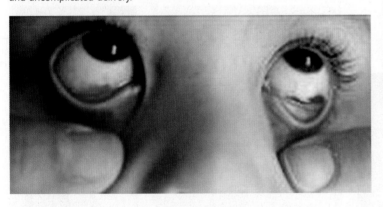

Hematoma of the left eyelids in a toddler following head trauma and fracture of the frontal bone.

Subconjunctival hematomas in a 15-year-old girl due to forceful coughing.

HEMIHYPERTROPHY

Definition

- Hemihypertrophy or hemihyperplasia is the enlargement of one side of the body or one part of the body.
- A 1.3-cm discrepancy in the lengths of the lower limbs at the age of 1 year, 2.3 cm at 5 years, 3.2 cm at 10 years, and 4.1 cm at 18 years is considered an abnormal finding.

Etiology

- Unknown.
- It can be syndromic as seen in certain diseases (Klippel–Trenaunay–Weber syndrome, Proteus syndrome, and Beckwith–Wiedemann syndrome) or nonsyndromic.
- It can also be classified as congenital or acquired (from radiation, infection, injury, or inflammation).

Symptoms and Signs

- It is not usually apparent at birth. Over the first few months of life, as one side of the face or extremity grows more than the contralateral side, hemihypertrophy becomes recognized.
- Hypertrophy (increase in the size of cells) or hyperplasia (increase in the number of normal size cells) is very difficult to differentiate from one another.
- Hemihypertrophy can be total, limited, or crossed (involving the contralateral upper and lower limbs).
- Hemihypertrophy may involve the eyes, ears, tongue, upper and lower extremities. The skin over the affected area may develop an increase in thickness, sweat glands, pigmentation abnormalities, and hair.
- Hemihypertrophy may also involve the internal organs, thorax, bones, and the cranium.
- Nonsyndromic hemihypertrophy can be associated with genitourinary abnormalities including cryptorchidism, inguinal hernia, renal cysts, sponge kidney, and horseshoe kidney.
- Cutaneous and vascular lesions are seen in syndromic hemihypertrophy.
- Increased risk of childhood cancers of the kidneys, adrenals, and liver has been documented in both syndromic and nonsyndromic hemihypertrophy.
- Figures A–E.

Treatment

- Depends on specific symptoms.
- Screening for childhood cancers by serial abdominal ultrasounds every 3 months until the age of 6 years, and every 6 months until puberty.

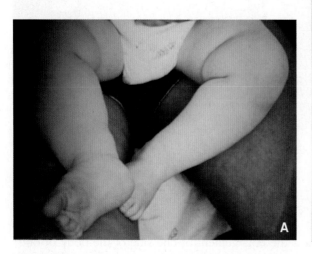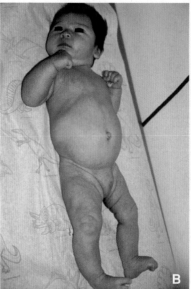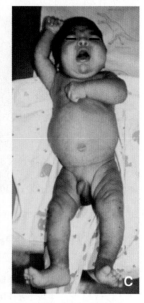

Figures A–C: Hemihypertrophy of the right leg in a 9-month-old **(Figure A)**, right hemihypertrophy in a 6-month-old **(Figure B)**, and a left hemihypertrophy in a 3-month-old **(Figure C)**.

figures continues

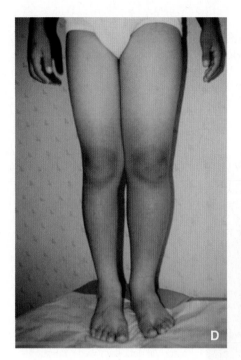
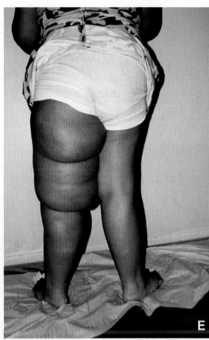

(figures cont.) **Figure D:** A 10-year-old girl with isolated hemihypertrophy of the left leg. She was otherwise healthy.

Figure E: A 13-year-old girl with hemihypertrophy of the left leg. She also has autism spectrum disorder, tuberous sclerosis, and obesity.

HEMOPHILIA

Definition
- A bleeding disorder due to defective, severe deficiency or absence of plasma coagulating factors VIII (hemophilia A) or IX (hemophilia B).
- May coexist with von Willebrand disease.

Etiology
- X-linked recessive condition which occurs almost exclusively in males. Combined incidence is 1 in 5,000 live male births.
- Hemophilia A is caused by numerous and diverse mutations in the factor VIII gene. These mutations include inversion in the tip of the long arm of chromosome X, nucleotide substitutions, and deletions.
- Hemophilia B (Christmas disease) also has a variety of specific gene defects affecting the factor IX gene.
- Hemophilia C refers to a rare bleeding disorder due to reduced levels of factor XI. The gene for factor XI is located on the distal arm of chromosome 4.

Symptoms and Signs
- Hemophilia A and hemophilia B are the most common and serious congenital coagulation factor deficiencies.
- Bleeding is the hallmark of this disease. It may occur anywhere but most frequently involves the joints (hemarthrosis) and muscles.
- May occur spontaneously or with slight trauma depending on specific factor levels.
- Deficiency of factors leads to an abnormal and delayed clot formation causing severe blood loss at the site of injury.
- Screening tests reveal prolonged activated partial thromboplastin time (PTT), but normal prothrombin time (PT) and platelet count.
- Figure.

Treatment
- Factor replacement therapy for prophylaxis and during active bleeding.
- Specific choice of factor (recombinant vs. plasma derived) will depend on the safety, purity, and cost.
- Complications (CNS bleed or hemarthrosis) require specific therapy in consultation with comprehensive hemophilia treatment center.

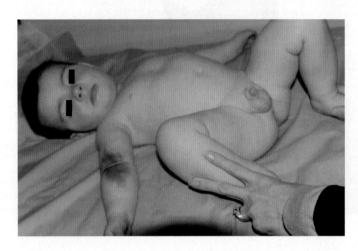

This asymptomatic 12-month-old boy bled extensively after routine phlebotomy. There was also a history of spontaneous hematoma in the right axilla. Hemophilia was suspected and factor VIII deficiency was confirmed by laboratory testing.

HENOCH–SCHÖNLEIN PURPURA (HSP, ANAPHYLACTOID PURPURA)

Definition
- Henoch–Schönlein purpura (HSP) is the most common form of systemic vasculitis in children.
- It is characterized by palpable purpura (without evidence of thrombocytopenia or coagulation defects), arthritis, abdominal pain, and kidney disease.

Etiology
- Unknown but immunologic, infectious, and environmental factors have been implicated.

Symptoms and Signs
- Many cases begin with an upper respiratory tract infection (streptococcus is often implicated).
- The purpura is the initial sign in 75% of cases.
- It may be preceded by urticaria.
- The rash is palpable, symmetrical in its distribution, and appears more frequently on the lower extremities. The buttocks, arms, trunk, and the face may also be affected, especially with nonambulatory toddlers.
- The abdominal pain is colicky in character, with or without nausea, vomiting, diarrhea, ileus, and bloody stools. Intussusception is a recognized complication.
- Nonpitting edema of the face, periorbital areas, scalp, hands, and feet.
- The arthritis is typically transient and migratory, more commonly involving the lower extremities. There is usually no joint effusion or associated long-term joint damage.
- Kidney involvement occurs in 20% to 50% of cases. The most common finding is hematuria and the majority of cases recover fully. However, those with associated hypertension, elevated creatinine levels, and proteinuria may develop progressive renal disease.
- Involvement of other organ systems is less common.
- Figures A–H.

Treatment

- There is a high spontaneous recovery rate.
- Symptomatic treatment includes pain management, rest, and appropriate hydration.
- Benefits of steroid therapy are inconclusive and their use is not recommended routinely.

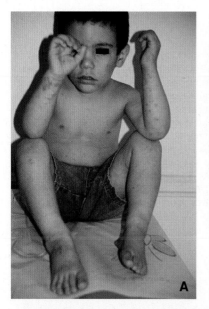
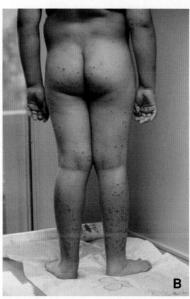
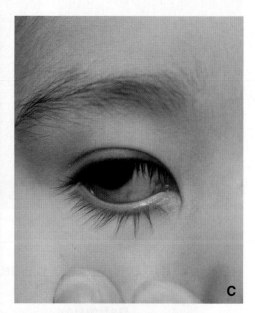
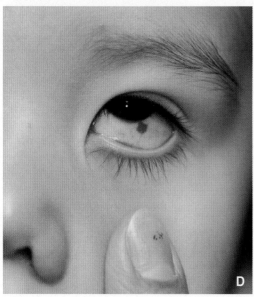
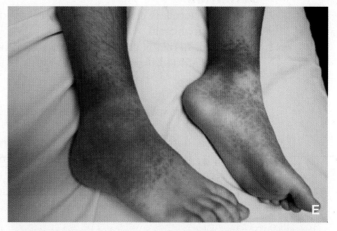
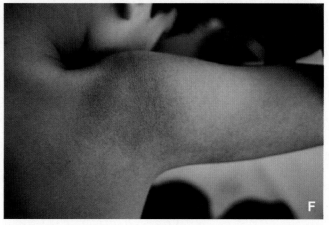

Figures A–F

figures continues

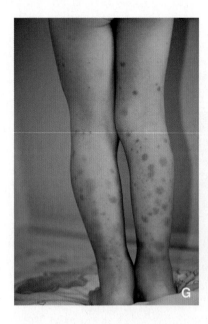
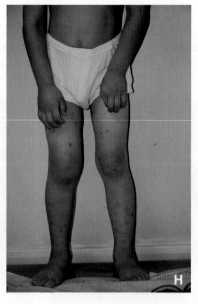

(figures cont.) **Figures A–H:** A 3–year-old boy presented with a bilateral, lower-extremity rash. The patient was afebrile and was not complaining of abdominal or joint pain. Laboratory evaluation including urinalysis, CBC, and ESR were all normal. Follow-up examination revealed pain and swelling on the right side of the lower thoracic spine, and an increase in purpuric and ecchymotic spots on his legs. He had pain and swelling of the right hand and knee. Short-lived abdominal pain was reported 8 days later. All symptoms resolved and there were no renal complications.

HERNIA (INGUINAL AND UMBILICAL)

Definition
- Inguinal hernia is characterized by protrusion of contents of abdominal cavity through the inguinal canal.
- Umbilical hernia is an outward protrusion of the abdominal organ or peritoneum through the area around the umbilicus.

Etiology
- Umbilical hernias are usually present at birth. They are caused by incomplete closure of the linea alba.
- Umbilical hernias may be acquired due to increase in the intra-abdominal pressure, for example, coughing, obesity, and heavy lifting.
- Indirect inguinal hernias are more frequent in premature infants. They result from failure of closure of the inguinal ring after the testicles descend into the scrotum.
- Direct inguinal hernias are due to weakness of the fascia of the abdominal wall.

Symptoms and Signs
- A bulge in the scrotum, groin, or umbilicus. It may appear more obvious while coughing and may fade when lying recumbent.
- Incarcerated hernia is defined by inability to reduce the hernia contents back into the abdominal cavity.
- Strangulated inguinal hernias (defined as vascular compromise of hernia contents) may present with sudden severe pain, fever, and tachycardia.

Treatment
- Umbilical hernias are common in newborns. The majority close spontaneously by the age of 3 years.
- Inguinal hernias should be treated surgically.
- Incarcerated hernias should be reduced manually or intraoperatively. Failure to do so may result in strangulation and subsequent peritonitis.
- Strangulated hernia is a surgical emergency.

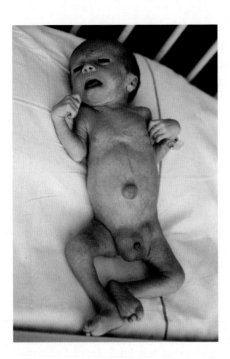

Bilateral inguinal and umbilical hernias and cutis marmorata in an asymptomatic 6-month-old.

HERPANGINA

Definition
■ A viral infection, characterized by fever, sore throat, and vesicles and on the posterior pharynx.

Etiology
■ Coxsackie A virus is the most frequent causative organism, but a variety of other enteroviruses can also cause herpangina.

Symptoms and Signs
■ Fever, sore throat, headache, backache, abdominal pain, and vomiting in older children.
■ Discrete lesions, typical of herpangina are 1 to 2 mm vesicles and ulcers that can grow up to 3 to 4 mm inside an erythematous ring, on the anterior tonsillar pillars, uvula, tonsils, soft palate, posterior buccal surfaces, and posterior pharyngeal wall.

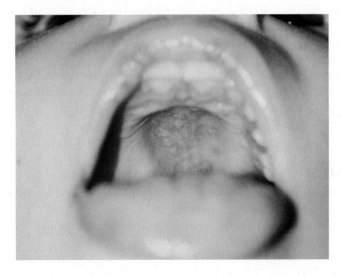

Herpangina in an 8-year-old girl.

Treatment
- Pain control.
- Maintain normal hydration status.
- Self-limited disease with expected recovery within a week.

HERPES (Gr., a spreading cutaneous eruption)

Definition
- Herpes simplex virus (HSV) 1 and HSV 2 are members of the Herpesviridae family of viruses. They possess biologic properties of latency and reactivation, which may cause recurrence of infection. They can cause a wide spectrum of illnesses; as mild as a herpes labialis and as serious as HSV encephalitis.

Etiology
- HSV 1 and HSV 2 are transmitted via direct contact with an infected area of skin or by secretions.
- Neonatal HSV infection may be acquired in the intrauterine, perinatal, or postnatal period.
- The possibility of sexual abuse should be considered in cases of genital or rectal herpes in a young prepubertal child.

Symptoms and Signs
- Incubation period is 2 to 12 days.
- Symptoms and signs depend on the age of the patient and the anatomic location.
- HSV establishes lifelong persistence in sensory ganglia neurons. Variety of stimuli, including fever, infection, or stress can cause reactivation.
- Neonatal infection:
  - Intrauterine infections may cause severe CNS findings (microphthalmia, retinal dysplasia, chorioretinitis, microcephaly, hydranencephaly, and calcifications).
  - Dermatologic findings include vesicles, ulcerations, and scarring.
  - Perinatally acquired HSV can cause three major types of infections in the neonate: (1) disseminated disease leading to hemorrhagic pneumonitis, liver failure, and meningoencephalitis; (2) localized CNS disease; and (3) localized disease of the skin, eyes, or mouth. The majority are acquired from mothers without a previous history of HSV.
  - Direct contact with active HSV lesions may lead to postnatally acquired HSV infection in a newborn.
  - Lesions appear as cluster of vesicles or bullae on an erythematous base. Any such appearing lesion in a newborn should be considered HSV until proven otherwise.
- Figures A–L.

GENITAL HERPES
- The most common manifestation of HSV 2 in adolescence and adults is genital herpes; however, HSV-1 infection rates have been on the rise.
- Fever, headache, pruritus, dysuria, inguinal lymphadenopathy, and vaginal or urethral discharge.
- Genital vesicles, which progress to ulcers, with subsequent crusting.

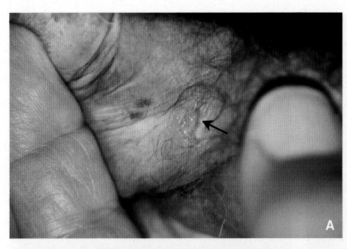

Figure A: *Herpes of the penis* in a 17-year-old boy who felt some itching and burning sensation of his penile skin for a few days and noted an ulcer.

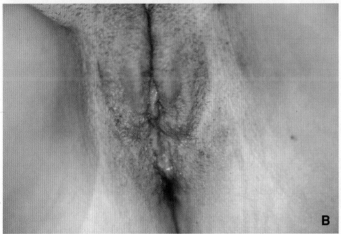

Figure B: *Herpetic vulvovaginitis* in a sexually active 16-year-old girl whose boyfriend had multiple partners. She was in a lot of pain and had several painful vesicles on the irritated labia major and labia minor.

- HSV persists in latent form for life; in trigeminal ganglion for HSV1 and sacral ganglion for HSV2, but any sensory ganglia may be involved.
- Recurrent lesions due to the latent virus are less painful.
- Figures A and B.

HERPES GINGIVOSTOMATITIS

- Most frequent manifestation of primary HSV 1 infection during childhood.
- Mostly found in children between 6 months and 5 years of age.
- Initial symptoms include fever, irritability, fetor oris, and refusal to eat or drink.
- Parents usually attribute these findings to teething.
- Subsequently clusters of vesicles may form on the tongue, lips, and palate. The gingiva appear red, inflamed, and may bleed at times.
- Symptoms resolve within 2 weeks. However, the latent virus can cause recurrent infections (Figures C–E).

Treatment

- Neonatal HSV, eczema herpeticum, and encephalitis should be treated aggressively with acyclovir.
- Recurrent genital HSV outbreaks may be prevented by oral antiviral therapy. Treatment strategies include episodic treatment and chronic suppressive therapy.

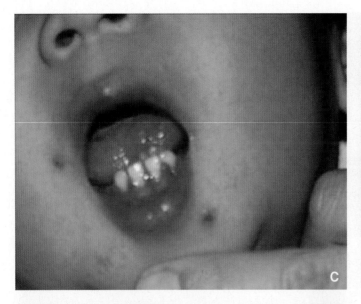

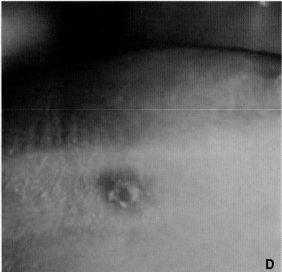

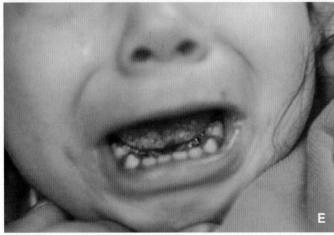

Figures C–D: An 18-month-old girl with swollen gums, numerous vesicles on the tongue, oral mucosa, and perioral area **(Figure C)**. A close-up view of a vesicle **(Figure D)**.

Figure E: *Herpetic gingivostomatitis.* This two-and-a-half-year-old girl's father, a physician, brought her to our house on a Sunday morning, for fever, crying, and refusing to eat or drink for 3 days. On examination she appeared irritable, was drooling, and had an inflamed oral mucosa with numerous vesicles on her tongue and perioral area.

HERPES SIMPLEX

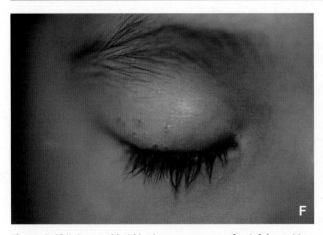

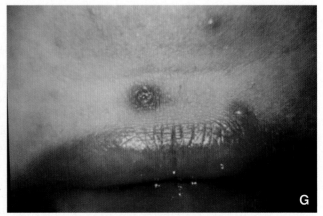

Figure F: This 6-year-old girl had an acute onset of painful, pruritic, vesicles over her swollen right eyelid. No fever or other vesicles noted elsewhere. There were no other family members with similar symptoms. Culture of the vesicles grew HSV 1.

Figure G: HSV reactivation following an upper respiratory tract infection.

figures continues

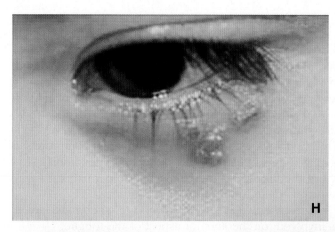

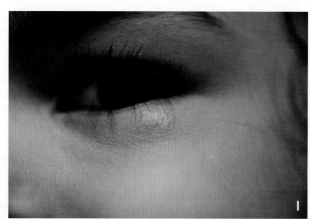

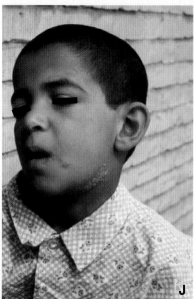

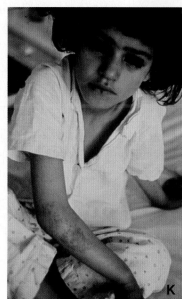

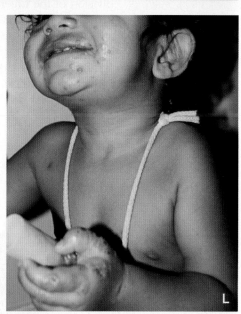

(figures cont.) **Figure H:** A 3-year-old girl with 1-day history of a rash below the left lower eyelid. Vesicular culture was positive for HSV 1.

Figure I: Recurrent herpes on the lower eyelid of a 9-year-old girl. HSV 1 grew from this lesion.

Figures J–K: HSV eruption noted on the face and right upper extremity of two young children who were being treated for meningococcal meningitis in Iran.

Figure L: Herpetic vesicles on the perioral area, oral mucosa, chest, and fingers (Whitlow) of a 14-month-old girl. Picture was taken on day 7 of her illness when her condition had improved and she was afebrile.

HERPES ZOSTER (Zoster Gr., a girdle; Zona L., a girdle shingles)

Definition
- Herpes zoster is characterized by an acute painful rash with vesicles in the dermatomal distribution.

Etiology
- Reactivation of a latent infection with varicella zoster virus (VZV) in the sensory ganglia.

Symptoms and Signs

- Most common in the elderly and the immunocompromised, rare in the neonates.
- Can be seen in children vaccinated with the varicella vaccine.
- Erythema and vesicles in a dermatomal distribution of one or more sensory nerves, but can be scattered beyond the dermatomes; unilateral, with rare contralateral involvement.
- Pain, hyperesthesia, and tenderness may be experienced before the skin manifestations.
- New lesions may appear up to 1 week after the appearance of the first lesion, and crusting and healing appears in the following 1 to 2 weeks.
- Herpes zoster is much more severe in patients with HIV and in the immunocompromised (possible complications of encephalitis, intravascular coagulopathy, and pneumonia).
- Infection of the ophthalmic branch of the fifth cranial nerve may cause permanent damage by the involvement of cornea, keratitis, and uveitis.
- Extracutaneous eruptions can be seen on the uvula, tonsils, and palate when maxillary division of the trigeminal nerve is involved; on the anterior aspect of the tongue, lips, buccal mucous membrane, and floor of the mouth when mandibular division is affected; and lesions on the ears, tongue, and auditory canal when geniculate ganglion is involved.
- Postherpetic neuralgia is rarely seen in children.
- Diagnosis is clinical but can be confirmed by viral culture from a vesicle.

Treatment

- Symptomatic.
- Antivirals given within 72 hours of eruption of the rash, shortens the course of the disease, and modifies the symptoms. Acyclovir; in children and adults; famciclovir, and valacyclovir can be used in adults.

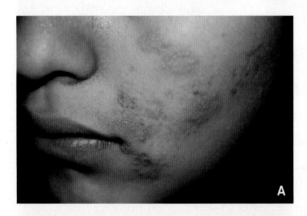

Figure A: Dermatomal distribution of herpes zoster in a teenage girl.

Figures B–C: A cluster of vesicles in herpes zoster **(Figure B)**, close-up view **(Figure C)**.

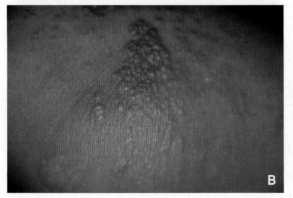

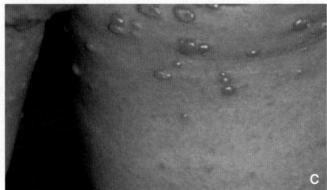

figures continues

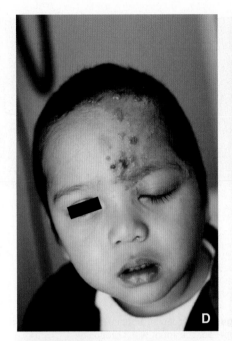

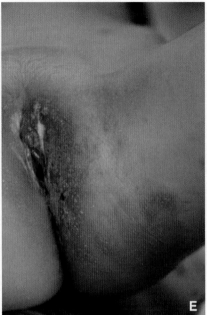

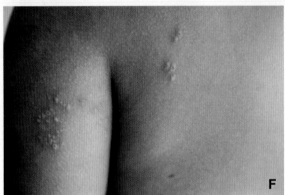

(figures cont.) **Figure D:** Day 4 in a 4-year-old boy with herpes zoster. The swelling of the left eyelid has diminished. Numerous vesicles are seen on the forehead on an erythematous base. His cornea remained intact.

Figure E: Herpes zoster vulvovaginitis in a 7-year-old girl. She had varicella at 1 month of age; 2 weeks after her older sister had severe varicella.

Figure F: Herpes zoster in a teenage boy. Dermatomas related to C5 and T1.

HISTIOCYTOSIS

(See Langerhans Cell Histiocytosis).

HORDEOLUM (L. barleycorn)

Definition
- Hordeolum, commonly known as "sty," is an acute inflammatory lesion of the eyelid.

Etiology
- Inflammation of the meibomian gland leads to internal hordeolum.
- Hordeolum externum is due to inflammation of the eyelash follicle or a lid margin tear gland.

Symptoms and Signs
- A hordeolum will present as an inflamed cystic lesion at the junction of the eyelid and the eyelashes (Figures A–C).

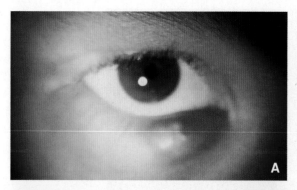
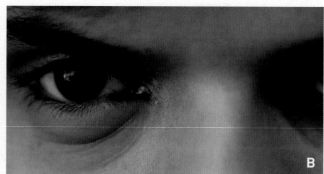
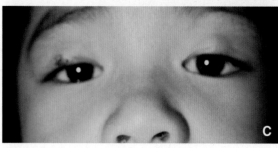

Figures A–C: demonstrate inflamed cystic lesions of the lower eyelid and upper lid, consistent with hordeolum.

Treatment
- Warm compresses with light massage.
- Trial of topical antibiotics and corticosteroids. However, clinical efficacy of topical treatments remains unproven.
- Incision and drainage (if lesion persists despite conservative medical management).

HYDROCELE

Definition
- A hydrocele is a pathologic accumulation of fluid around the testis.

Etiology
- Communicating hydrocele is usually caused by failure of processus vaginalis to close during development. Peritoneal fluid can move into the scrotum through a patent processus vaginalis and create a hydrocele.
- Noncommunicating hydrocele is secondary to production of fluid by mesothelial lining of tunica vaginalis, which is the covering of the testis.

Symptoms and Signs
- Hydroceles are smooth and nontender.
- Transillumination of scrotum confirms the diagnosis.
- Majority of hydroceles in newborns are noncommunicating.
- Communicating hydroceles may increase in size with the Valsalva maneuver.
- Hydrocele and inguinal hernia share the same etiology and may coexist.
- A noncommunicating hydrocele in older males can be the result of an inflammatory condition within the scrotum.
- Epididymitis, testicular tumor, torsion, or torsion of the appendix testis should be ruled-out (Figure).

Treatment
- The majority of noncommunicating hydroceles in newborns resolve by the first birthday.
- Surgery is indicated for communicating hydroceles persisting beyond 12 months of life.

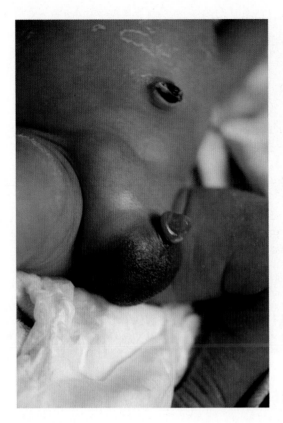

Coexisting hydrocele and inguinal hernia in a 5-day-old.

HYDROCEPHALOUS

Definition
- A diverse group of diseases resulting in abnormal accumulation of CSF within the ventricles.

Etiology
- Hydrocephalus may be caused by impaired CSF flow, reabsorption, and also by the excessive production of CSF. Impaired CSF flow (obstructive or noncommunicating hydrocephalus). Causes may include aqueductal stenosis, Chiari malformation, and Dandy–Walker malformation.
- Impaired CSF resorption (nonobstructive or communicating hydrocephalus). Causes may include subarachnoid hemorrhage, meningitis, and leukemic infiltrates.
- Excessive production of CSF is a rare cause of hydrocephalus. It may occur with a choroid plexus papilloma.

Symptoms and Signs
- Rapid increase in the head circumference of newborns, large bulging anterior fontanelle, dilated scalp veins, broad forehead, and downward deviation of the eyes (sunsetting sign).
- Pyramidal tract signs: Brisk tendon reflexes, spasticity (especially of lower extremities).
- Irritability, headache, lethargy, and papilledema.

Treatment
- Medical management of hydrocephalus includes serial lumbar punctures and diuretic therapy.
- Surgical management includes placement of ventricular shunts which drains CSF into the peritoneal cavity or into the right atria.

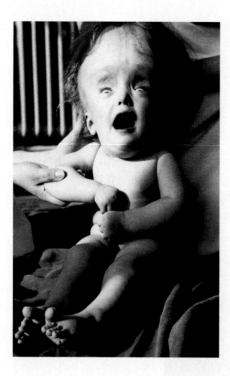

Large head, broad forehead, and sunsetting eyes in a patient with hydrocephalous.

HYPERCAROTENEMIA (CAROTENEMIA)

Definition
- Hypercarotenemia, which is a common finding in pediatrics, is the yellow discoloration of the skin due to raised serum beta-carotene levels.

Etiology
- The most common cause of hypercarotenemia is dietary. It is usually due to excessive intake of carrots or other vegetables that contain carotenoids.
- Carotenoids are absorbed by the GI tract and partially metabolized to vitamin A by the liver and intestinal mucosa.
- They are subsequently transported by lipoproteins to the peripheral tissue and contribute to the skin protection against the ultraviolet rays.
- Almost all reported cases of hypercarotenemia are from the Western world. Infection and intestinal diseases, all of which are more frequent in the developing countries, may impair the absorption of carotene.
- Human milk, particularly colostrum, contains a very high concentration of beta-carotene. As a result, hypercarotenemia is more common in breastfed infants.
- Hypothyroidism, anorexia nervosa, nephrotic syndrome, diabetes mellitus, advanced liver disease, and kidney disease can all cause secondary hypercarotenemia. This is secondary to hyperlipidemia and the inability to convert carotene to retinol.

Symptoms and Signs
- Well-appearing child without signs of systemic illness and normal physical examination (including no hepatosplenomegaly or lymphadenopathy).
- The first sign of hypercarotenemia is a yellow discoloration of the nose followed by the nasolabial folds, palms, soles, and gradually the entire body (Figures A–E).
- The yellow discoloration fades in the reverse order that it appears.
- The sclera and mucosa are *always* spared.
- Minor skin discolorations may not be as visible in darkly pigmented children.
- The distribution corresponds to areas where there are sebaceous glands which carotene is excreted from.

- Volume and size of beta-carotene–containing foods (carrots, sweet potato, and squash) are the most important factors in causation of hypercarotenemia. However, it appears that some children are more capable of handling carotene-loaded diets than others.

Treatment

- There is no need to treat hypercarotenemia in healthy children. Introduction of more variety in their diet will correct hypercarotenemia.

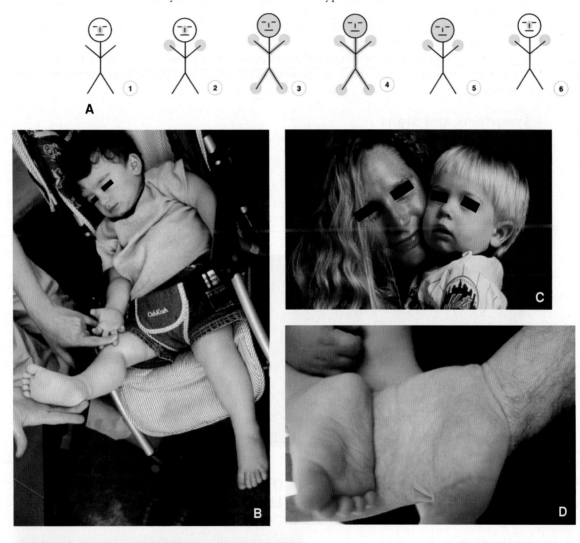

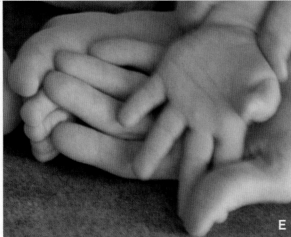

Figure A: The order-of-march of discoloration in hypercarotenemia.

Figure B: Yellow skin and clear sclera in an asymptomatic 2-year-old boy with hypercarotenemia. Note the color difference between him and his mother's hands.

Figures C–D: The yellow discoloration progresses very slowly. Parents rarely notice the change. The best way is to compare the baby's skin color with that of their own.

Figure E: Yellow hand and foot in an 11-month-old boy compared to his mother's hand with normal color.

HYPERHIDROSIS

Definition
- Hyperhidrosis is characterized by excess sweating (greater than what is physiologically required for body temperature regulation).

Etiology
- The causes of excessive sweating are numerous: Cortical (emotional and dysautonomia), hypothalamic (antipyretics and insulin), exercise, infection, metabolic (hyperthyroidism and diabetes mellitus), cardiovascular (shock and heart failure), vasomotor (Raynaud's phenomenon), neurologic (postencephalitic), and medullary (physiologic gustatory sweating).

Symptoms and Signs
- Wetness of the hands, axillae, and occasionally the entire body (Figure).

Treatment
- Emotional hyperhidrosis in the palms and soles may respond to aluminium chloride (Drysol), 10% glutaraldehyde soak, and 20% aluminium chloride in anhydrous ethanol.
- Aluminium chloride and anticholinergic agents may help in excessive sweating of the axillae.

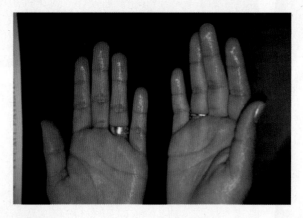

Emotional hyperhidrosis of palms in a teenage girl.

HYPERPHOSPHATEMIC TUMORAL CALCINOSIS (FAMILIAL TUMORAL CALCINOSIS WITH HYPERPHOSPHATEMIA)

Definition
- Hyperphosphatemic tumoral calcinosis is a rare metabolic disorder characterized by ectopic calcifications and hyperphosphatemia.

Etiology
- Autosomal recessive disorder with mutations in GALNT3 and FGF23 genes which lead to increased renal absorption of phosphate.

Symptoms and Signs
- Patients are usually otherwise healthy. They develop recurrent, firm, nontender masses around major joints including the shoulder, hips, and elbows.
- Normal serum calcium and high serum phosphorus levels.
- The signs normally appear during the first or second decade of life.
- Recurrence after a tumor has been resected is common.

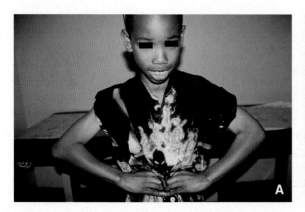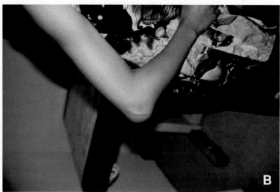

Figures A–B: Scar and keloid at the site of a previous surgery to remove a tumor from the distal humerus in this teenage boy with hyperphosphatemic tumoral calcinosis, before and after the removal of one of the tumors.

Figure B: This 8-year-old African American male has had pica and intermittent extremity and joint pain with swelling since the age of 2 years. His family history is significant for breast cancer which has affected both maternal and paternal aunts. The only abnormality on his physical examination was slight tenderness of the right elbow joint. Serum Ca level was 9.8 mg/dL, PO4 level was 8 mg/dL. Serum PO4 remained elevated on several subsequent tests. His CBC, serum lead level, and renal ultrasound were normal. Severe osteopenia of the lumbar spine and hips was noted on DEXA examination. CT scan of the elbow indicated periosteal thickening and a mass along the posterolateral aspect of the right elbow, primarily proximal to the elbow joint along the lateral aspect of the triceps. A repeat scan, 2 years later, revealed a 4-cm mass, in the left elbow joint which appeared to be extra articular. Nuclear medicine scan revealed focal pathology of the right elbow. MRI showed marrow edema within the midshaft of the left tibia. A tumor biopsy revealed histologic changes diagnostic of hyperphosphatemic tumoral calcinosis.

- Hyperphosphatemia is not the result of renal insufficiency or an abnormal parathyroid response.
- X-ray shows a round or oval well-demarcated mass of calcification in the periarticular soft-tissue.

Treatment
- Excision and re-excision of the recurring tumors.
- Normalization of serum phosphorus levels.

HYPERPIGMENTATION

Definition
- Abnormally darkened area of skin.

Etiology, Symptoms and Signs
- Hyperpigmentation may be categorized by endogenous or exogenous causes.
- Endogenous causes may be associated with the following disease conditions: Postinflammatory hyperpigmentation (postinflammatory melanosis) characterized by hyperpigmentation following cutaneous inflammation. Photodermatitis, pityriasis rosea, psoriasis, and eczematoid eruptions are among the factors causing this type of hyperpigmentation.
- Metabolic causes of hyperpigmentation:
  - Adrenal insufficiency (Addison's disease) is due to increased production of melanocyte-stimulating hormone by the pituitary gland. It causes hyperpigmentation of the skin (including areas not exposed to the sun) and mucous membranes. A similar pattern may be seen in patients with hyperpituitarism, Cushing's syndrome, and congenital adrenal hyperplasia.
  - Hyperpigmentation may be found in about 7% of children with hyperthyroidism.
  - Hyperpigmentation can also be seen in hemochromatosis, malnutrition, lymphoma, juvenile idiopathic arthritis, dermatomyositis, and chronic renal diseases.

- Hepatobiliary hyperpigmentation can be seen in the majority of patients with chronic liver disease.
- Familial progressive hyperpigmentation is a rare autosomal dominant condition which presents at birth as irregular hyperpigmented patches.

Exogenous factors
- Drug induced.
  - Chronic, high-dose, and long-term use of chlorpromazine. A bluish-gray discoloration more visible on the tip of the nose, the V of the neck, and cheeks.
  - Chronic use of antimalarial drugs such as chloroquine, quinacrine, or hydroxychloroquine. May cause a bluish-gray discoloration of the oral mucous membranes, face, neck, forearms, legs, nail beds, eyebrows, and eyelids.
  - Fixed drug eruption: Repeated exposure to a particular medication may lead to recurrence of a purplish-red, oval, round, or at times bullous circumscribed plaque. Barbiturates, antineoplastic agents, and phenolphthalein are a few of the medication under this category.
- Heavy metal toxicity.
  - Mercury poisoning: Slate-gray pigmentation best seen in areas of skin folds.
  - Silver poisoning (argyria) is a bluish-gray skin discoloration mainly found on the exposed parts of the body. May be caused by chronic use of eye/nose drops containing silver.
  - Gold poisoning (chrysiasis) is rare and similar to skin discoloration in silver poisoning.

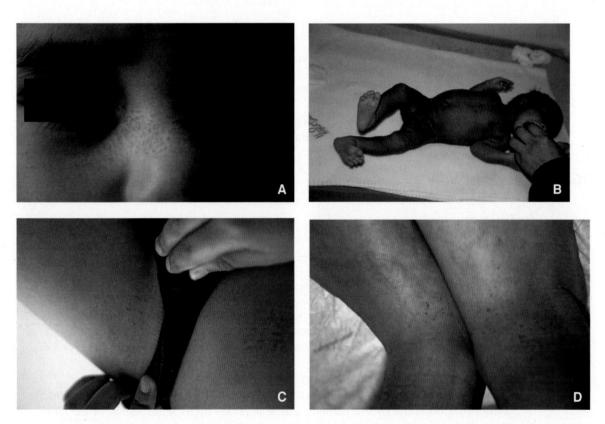

Figure A: Hyperpigmentation during recovery from protein malnutrition. Note the lighter color skin growing under the pealing old darker skin.

Figure B: Hyperpigmentation in congenital adrenal hyperplasia. Significant improvement was noted after the initiation of medical therapy.

Figures C–D: This healthy teenage girl returned from a vacation in Brazil with these hyperpigmented spots on her legs, for unknown reason. No family history of skin discoloration.

figures continues

Treatment
- Treatment of the underlying disease or removal of offending agent will lead to normalization of skin color.

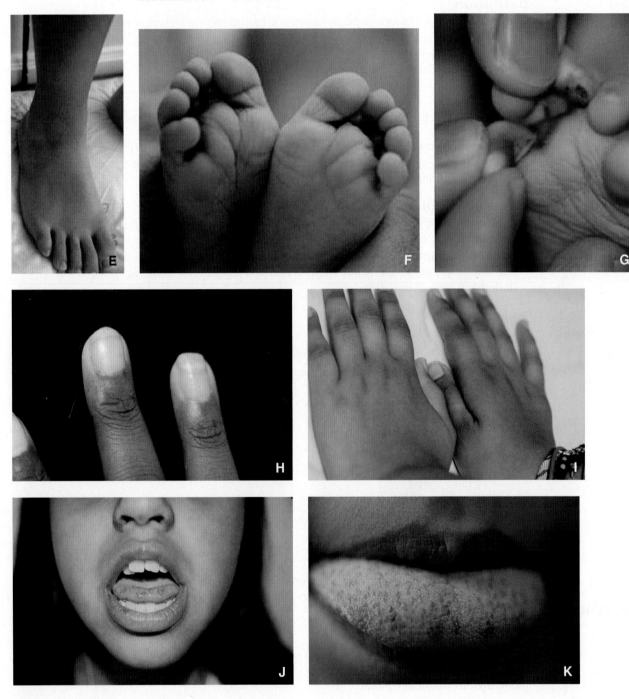

(figures cont.) **Figure E**

Figures F–G: This healthy 8-day-old baby boy presented with congenital hyperpigmentation between his toes. Skin cultures were negative for bacteria and fungus. The skin discoloration disappeared spontaneously within 2 months.

Figures H–I: This healthy 8-year-old Hispanic female presented with recent asymptomatic hyperpigmentation of the knuckles. The cause was not identified.

Figures J–K: This healthy 15-year-old has noted some asymptomatic hyperpigmented spots on the tip of her tongue for the past few months. The cause was not identified.

HYPERTRICHOSIS

Definition
- Hypertrichosis is characterized by excessive hair growth which is abnormal for race, sex, and age of an individual.
- It may be congenital or acquired.
- It may be confined to small area of the body or generalized.

Etiology
- The congenital forms of hypertrichosis are present at birth and are caused by genetic mutations.
- The acquired forms appear after birth. They may result from side-effects of particular medications (e.g., minoxidil and phenytoin), internal malignancy, or metabolic disorders (porphyria, anorexia nervosa, and hyperthyroidism).

Symptoms and Signs
- Excessive growth of hair, generalized or localized, with the exception of androgen-dependent hair of the face, axilla, and pubic area.
- A nevoid hypertrichosis is a solitary area of terminal hair growth with well-defined borders. If located in the lower back, it is called a "faun-tail" and may indicate an underlying spina bifida (Figure).

Treatment
- Hair removal by laser or electrolysis.
- Treatment of the underlying factors in acquired hypertrichosis.

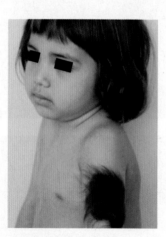

Localized hypertrichosis in an otherwise healthy toddler.

HYPOPARATHYROIDISM

Definition
- Hypoparathyroidism is a rare disorder characterized by the abnormally low secretion of parathyroid hormone (PTH).

Etiology
- Congenital hypoparathyroidism: Aplasia or hypoplasia of the parathyroid gland associated with DiGeorge/velocardiofacial syndrome (see DiGeorge syndrome).
- X-linked recessive hypoparathyroidism (hypocalcemic seizures in affected males secondary to a defect in development of parathyroid gland).
- Autosomal recessive hypoparathyroidism with dysmorphic features (microcephaly, micrognathia, deep set eyes, beaked nose, large floppy ears, mental and growth retardation).

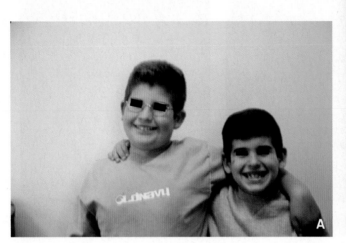
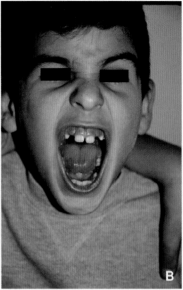

Figures A–B: Hypoparathyroidism in two brothers. The older brother was diagnosed, following weeks of pain in his calves and abdomen. He had abnormal teeth, low serum calcium, and high serum phosphorous levels. His younger brother, who had similar symptoms and also the same biologic markers, was diagnosed earlier.

- Autosomal dominant HDR syndrome (hypoparathyroidism, deafness, and renal abnormalities).
- Transient hypoparathyroidism due to suppression of parathyroid gland caused by maternal hyperparathyroidism.
- Autoimmune disorders. Immunologic destruction of the parathyroid gland as well as other endocrine organs.
- Acquired hypoparathyroidism following a surgery or infection.
- Hypomagnesemia may lead to suppression of the PTH secretion.

Symptoms and Signs
- Symptoms associated with chronic hypocalcemia: Movement disorders secondary to basal ganglia calcifications, cataracts, dental abnormalities, skeletal and craniofacial abnormalities, patchy alopecia, and brittle nails.
- Low PTH, hypocalcemia, high serum phosphorus level, and low 1,25[OH]2 D3 levels.
- Radiographic findings include increased bone density in the metaphyses.

Treatment
- Calcium and Vitamin D2 supplementation.

HYPOPIGMENTATION, POSTINFLAMMATORY

Definition
- The loss or removal of pigmentation of skin following any inflammatory skin disease.

Etiology
- Inflammatory injury to melanocytes results in decreased pigment production.
- Hypopigmentation is
  1. either genetic or developmentally controlled, like tuberous sclerosis and hypomelanosis of Ito or

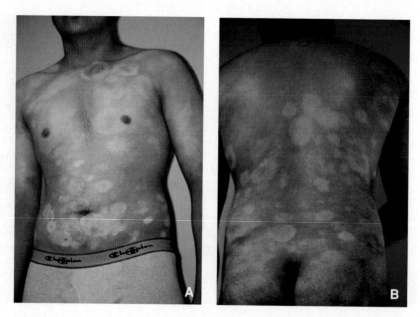

Figures A–B: A 15-year-old boy with extensive hypopigmentation following tinea versicolor.

2. a previously healthy skin which has now lost its pigmentation such as pityriasis alba, vitiligo, leprosy, and postinflammatory depigmentation, the best example of that is tinea versicolor.

Symptoms and Signs
- Asymptomatic loss of pigmentation in previously healthy skin following any inflammatory skin disease such as pityriasis alba, tinea versicolor, and vitiligo. Figures A and B.

Treatment
- Treatment is not necessary, as the lesions resolve several months after the inflammatory disorder.

HYPOTHYROIDISM

Definition
- Hypothyroidism is a condition in which the thyroid gland does not produce adequate amounts of the thyroid hormone. Congenital hypothyroidism is one of the most common preventable causes of mental retardation.

Etiology
- Iodine deficiency is the most common cause of hypothyroidism worldwide.
- Congenital (cretinism).
  - Occurrence rate is 1/2,000 to 1/4,000 newborns.
  - Majority of cases (85%) are caused by thyroid dysgenesis which includes thyroid agenesis, ectopy, or hypoplasia.
  - Ten percent are due to an inborn error of thyroxine synthesis and transport. They are usually inherited in an autosomal recessive pattern. A palpable goiter may be found on physical examination of these infants.
  - Five percent are due to transplacental maternal thyrotropin-receptor blocking antibodies.

- Radioactive iodine for treatment of Graves' disease or thyroid cancer during pregnancy may cause congenital hypothyroidism.
  - Fetal exposure to excessive iodine.
- Acquired.
  - Autoimmune destruction of the thyroid gland (children with celiac disease, Down's syndrome, Klinefelter syndrome, and Turner syndrome are at great risk).
  - Thyroid injury: Head and neck radiation, drug induced (iodides, lithium), thyroidectomy and systemic diseases (cystinosis, histiocytosis X, and hemangiomas of the liver).
- Central hypothyroidism.
  - May be caused by congenital or acquired diseases of pituitary gland or hypothalamus.

Symptoms and Signs

- As a result of national and widespread and routine newborn screening program in the United States, the incidence of symptomatic congenital hypothyroidism has dropped dramatically.
- More common in girls and Hispanics. Lower incidence in Caucasians and African Americans.
- Asymptomatic at birth due to the presence of maternal thyroid hormone which crosses the placenta and also residual thyroid function in the newborn.
- Newborns may develop the following symptoms: Macroglossia, umbilical hernia, constipation, hypotonia, large fontanelle, prolonged physiologic jaundice, hypothermia, and coarse hair.
- Older children may develop deceleration of growth rate leading to short stature, delayed puberty, hypothermia, myxedema, somnolence, and constipation.
- High TSH and low serum T4 or free T4 in congenital or acquired hypothyroidism.
- Low to normal TSH and low serum T4 in central hypothyroidism.

Treatment

- Levothyroxine, 10 to 15 µg/kg/day, is the starting dose in the newborns. Goal is to keep the serum free T4 in the upper half of the normal range.
- Hypothyroid children may need up to 4 µg/kg/day of levothyroxine.

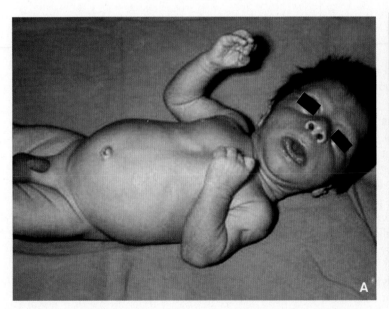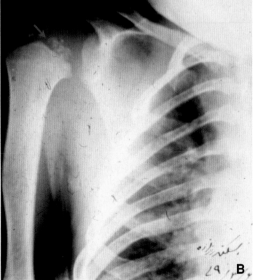

Figure A: An infant with congenital hypothyroidism. Note the large abdomen, large tongue, and coarse hair.

Figure B: Frontal view of the right humerus demonstrates stippling of the humeral epiphysis, which is characteristic of hypothyroidism.

I

ICHTHYOSIS

Definition
- Ichthyosis, also known as fish-scale disease or fish-skin disease, refers to a heterogeneous group of Mendelian disorders of cornification characterized by dry, scaly skin with erythroderma.

ICHTHYOSIS VULGARIS
- Accounts for more than 95% of the cases of ichthyosis.

Etiology
- Abnormal formation of filaggrin due to an autosomal dominant genetic mutation. Filaggrin plays an important role in the regulation of epidermal homeostasis.

Symptoms and Signs
- Incidence = 0.5 to 4 per 1,000 and male = female.
- Diagnosed mostly at 3 to 12 months of age. It is not apparent in the newborn period.
- White scales on extensor surface of extremities, hyperlinear palmar markings, atopic disorders (asthma, eczema, and allergies), and keratosis pilaris.
- Dry skin leads to bloody, painful cracks in the palms and soles.

Treatment
- Liberal use of topical emollients for exfoliation of scales is helpful.

X-LINKED ICHTHYOSIS
Etiology
- Inherited as an X-linked recessive disorder which leads to mutations of the gene for steroid sulfatase and leads to hyperkeratosis.

Symptoms and Signs
- Incidence 1/6,000 males.
- Majority of cases present during the first few months of life.
- Can be prenatally detected by amniocentesis.
- Large, dark, adherent scales cover the extensors, preauricular area, and posterior neck.
- Spares the flexors, face, palms, and soles.
- Asymptomatic corneal opacities.
- The placental steroid sulfatase deficiency may interfere with progression of labor and lead to cesarean delivery.
- Bilateral cryptorchidism.
- Generalized, brown polygonal scales seen in older adults and children.
- Temporary improvement over time.

Treatment
- Topical emollients including keratolytic agents and isotretinoin.

CONGENITAL ICHTHYOSIFORM ERYTHRODERMA

Etiology
- Autosomal recessive with the incidence of 1/180,000. Mutation may be caused by several genes.

Symptoms and Signs
- Presents as collodion baby at birth. Erythroderma with fine and lighter scaling. Less common findings include persistent ectropion (outward turning of lower eyelid) and scarring alopecia.

Treatment
- Emollients in the newborns. Topical retinoids and keratolytics in older children. Figures B–D.

LAMELLAR ICHTHYOSIS (L. lamella, a thin layer)

Etiology
- Autosomal recessive with the incidence of 1/300,000. Caused by defective gene encoding for transglutaminase 1.

Symptoms and Signs
- Collodion baby with translucent membrane encasing the body with generalized erythroderma. Ectropion and turning outward of the lip. Membrane generally dries out and sheds.
- Risk of hypernatremic dehydration and sepsis.
- Generalized, brown polygonal scales seen in older adults and children.

Treatment
- Emollients and systemic retinoids.
- Normal life span.

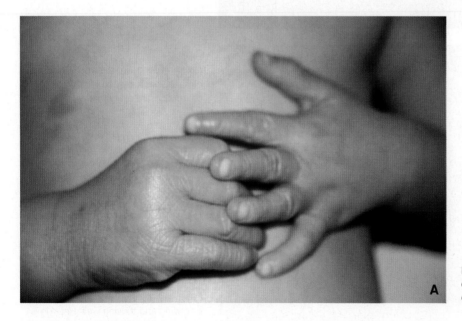

Figure A: A 2-year-old boy born with extremely dry skin. Ichthyosis vulgaris was confirmed by skin biopsy.

figures continues

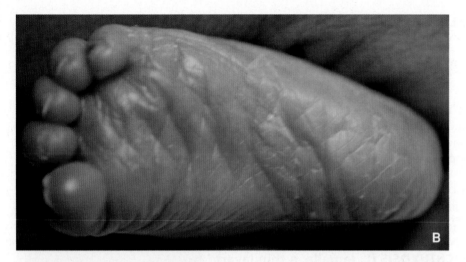

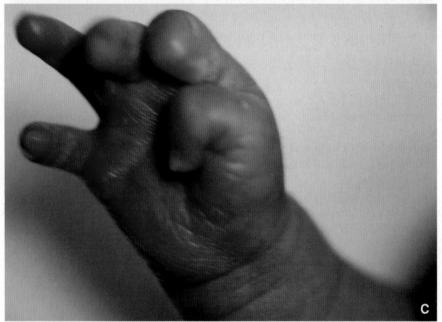

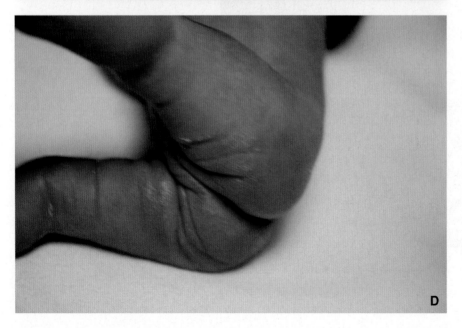

(figures cont.) **Figures B–D:** This 4-week-old baby girl is the product of a second-cousin consanguinity marriage. Delivered by C-section secondary to low amniotic fluid volume and breech presentation. Apgars were 9 and 9. Birth weight was 3,310 g. On physical examination, the skin was dry and cracks were noted on the abdominal wall, chest, and the extremities. Contractures of the extremities due to thick, dry skin were noted. The infant was diagnosed as a collodion baby. Mother has a family history of two cousins born with similar skin disorder. Her CBC, ESR, CRP, and electrolytes were normal and her Na = 142 mm/L. She was placed in 80% Giraffe humidification and covered with emollients. She is feeding and thriving well. Her skin is now dry and erythematous, worst in the diaper area.

IMPETIGO

Definition
- Impetigo is a highly contagious superficial skin infection which mainly affects children.

Etiology
- *Staphylococcus aureus* and *Streptococcus pyogenes* are the principal organisms responsible for impetigo.
- Bacteria enter the skin through a bite, injury, or after an upper respiratory tract infection.

Symptoms and Signs
- Localized lesions that begin as papules and subsequently progress to pustules that are filled with honey-colored fluid. The pustules subsequently break and form a characteristic golden crust.
- Lesions start in a single spot but may spread to other areas with scratching.
- Lesions involve the face, arms, and the legs.

Treatment
- Topical antibiotics (mupirocin) when lesions are few and are without bullae.
- Oral antibiotics for extensive lesions and also for the treatment of bullae. Local bacterial resistance patterns should be considered.
- Postinfectious sequelae include rheumatic fever and poststreptococcal glomerulonephritis.

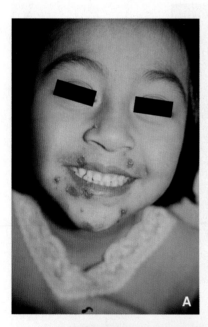

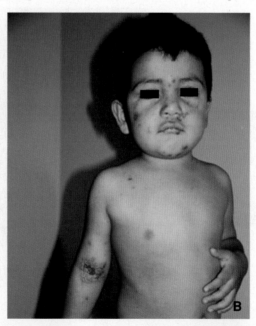

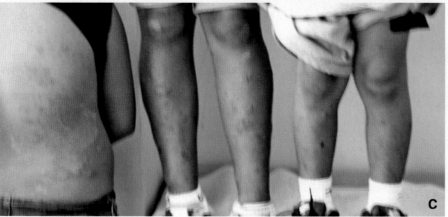

Figure A: Impetigo in a 5-year-old girl. Initial lesion was a pustule on the upper lip, which ruptured and spread to other parts of her face.

Figure B: An insect bite on the right elbow became infected and spread to the arms, face, and chest of this 2-year-old boy.

Figure C: This family went back home to a developing country for vacation. They returned with numerous insect bites which progressed to impetigo.

IMPETIGO OF THE NEWBORN (IMPETIGO NEONATORUM)

Definition
- This acute contagious disease of the skin is characterized by vesicles and bullae on an erythematous base.

Etiology
- It is caused by toxin-producing *S. aureus*.
- Parents and the hospital nursery staff are often the main source of infection.

Symptoms and Signs
- It manifests within the first and second weeks after birth.
- Impetigo of the newborn may present as bullae on any part of the body. More commonly occurs on covered areas that are exposed to moisture (diaper, axilla, neck fold).
- The bullae rupture easily with shallow erosion that is similar to a second-degree burn.
- The condition may remain localized or become widespread (Figures A–D).

Treatment
- Treatment is with appropriate, systemic, and antistaphylococcal antibiotics. Oral and topical antibiotics are not an appropriate therapy.

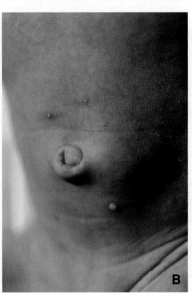

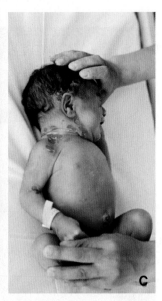

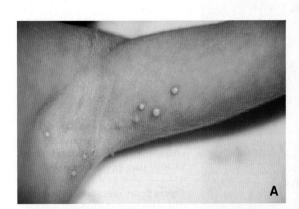

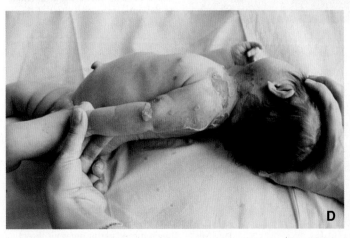

Figures A–D: Note the bullae in the axilla, neck fold, and periumbilical area. The newborns in **Figures A** and **B** were born in an American hospital, where an outbreak was reported. Their parents brought them to a pediatrician soon after the pustules were noted. The newborn in **Figure C** was born in an Iranian hospital and **Figure D** was a home birth in Iran. Note, in **Figures C** and **D**, the infection has spread widely by the time these children were brought to medical attention. Note the fairly limited, small bullae present in babies in **Figures A** and **B**, in comparison to the extensive, larger bullae (some ruptured) present in **Figures C** and **D**. *S. aureus* was cultured in all. This organism was also cultured from a "pimple" on the nose of a nurse working in the hospital nursery where the baby in **Figure C** was born.

I

INCONTINENTIA PIGMENTI

Definition
- Incontinentia pigmenti is a skin pigmentation disorder associated with abnormalities of the eyes, teeth, skeletal system, and the central nervous system.

Etiology
- An X-linked dominant disorder. It is usually lethal to the male fetus.

Symptoms and Signs
- There are four characteristic stages:
  - Stage 1: Vesicular. The first stage is noted in the newborns with blisters which are often preceded or accompanied by erythema. These may involve different regions of the body. The lesions appear as linear marks over the limbs and circumferentially around the trunk along the Lines of Blaschko. During stage one, peripheral eosinophilia may also be noted.
  - Stage 2: Verrucous. Wart-like or pustular lesions. Is characterized by hyperkeratosis or verrucous changes.
  - Stage 3: Hyperpigmented. Hyperpigmentation which typically appears as streaks or whorls. It may be present throughout childhood.
  - Stage 4: Atrophic/ hypopigmented. Seen in teenagers or adults is that of pale or atrophic streaks.
- Associated abnormalities include strabismus, cataracts, seizures, spastic paralysis, mental retardation, scarring alopecia, anodontia, or dystrophic nail changes. Figures A–D.

Treatment
- The cutaneous lesions usually do not require treatment; however, topical tacrolimus and corticosteroids have been used in an attempt to hasten the resolution of the inflammatory stage.
- Regular ophthalmologic evaluation is required to prevent complications.

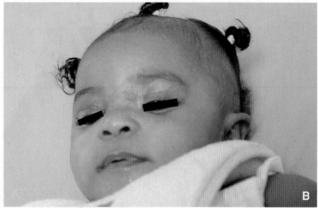

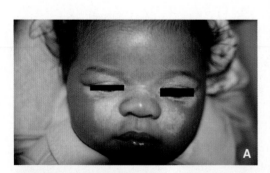

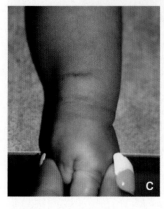

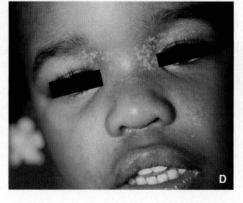

Figure A–D: A 1-month-old girl born with hypopigmentation. There are no male cousins in the family. Her mother has a history of one miscarriage and this is her only child. **Figures A–D** display incontinentia pigmenti at various stages. Hypopigmentation, hyperpigmentation, and streaks around her wrists. She has otherwise remained asymptomatic.

Figure D: The same patient at 4 years of age. Note the periorbital hypopigmentation.

INFECTIOUS MONONUCLEOSIS

Definition
- Infectious mononucleosis (IM), aka "kissing disease," mono and glandular fever, is an infectious, widespread viral disease to which 90% of adults have been exposed.

Etiology
- It is caused by the Epstein-Barr virus, which is a member of the herpes virus family, and spreads from person to person via saliva contact.

Symptoms and Signs
- Triad of fever, pharyngitis, and lymphadenopathy.
- Tonsils may be large and covered with exudate. Pharyngitis typically lasts longer in mono than in those caused by other organisms.
- Lymphadenopathy may be limited to cervical region or be diffuse.
- Hepatosplenomegaly and laboratory evidence of hepatitis are common.
- Large tonsils and the grossly enlarged lymph nodes can cause breathing difficulty.
- Constitutional symptoms include fever, malaise, anorexia, and weight loss.
- The infection is more often diagnosed in adolescents, but often unrecognized in younger or in less symptomatic children.
- A positive heterophil antibody test (monospot) which becomes positive during the second week of infection and the presence of atypical lymphocytes (greater than 10% of total lymphocytes) are diagnostic of acute infection.

Treatment
- Treatment is symptomatic, steroids may be used for severe tonsillar inflammation and impending airway obstruction.
- The use of ampicillin or amoxicillin can cause a maculopapular rash.
- Due to the risk of splenic rupture, it is advised to avoid contact sports during the initial 3 weeks of infection.

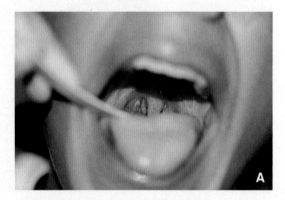

Figure A: Exudative pharyngitis in a 17 year old boy with infectious mononucleosis.

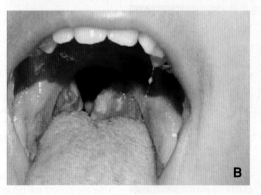

Figure B: A 14-year-old girl with fever, sore throat, loss of appetite and energy of 7 days duration. Her mother noted swelling of her neck 3 days prior to the office visit. She received Azithromycin for 3 days prior to the visit and without improvement. She had difficulty breathing the night before. She was afebrile with periorbital edema, visible glands on both sides of her neck, palpable anterior cervical lymph nodes, palpable spleen tip, and exudative pharyngitis. Her initial monospot was negative. However, repeat testing performed 10 days later was positive for infectious mononucleosis.

figures continues

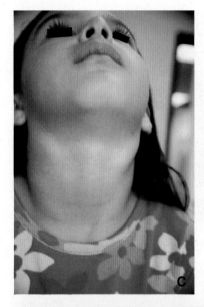

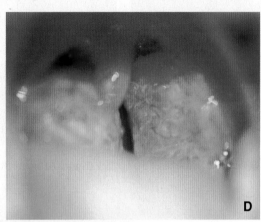

(figures cont.) **Figures C–D:** Teenager with infectious mononucleosis. Note cervical lymphadenopathy and exudative tonsillitis.

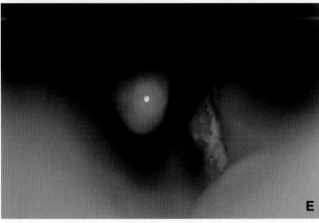

Figure E: This 17-year-old sexually active girl has had a severe sore throat for 10 days. She has anorexia, low-grade fever, cervical lymphadenopathy, and exudative pharyngitis. The liver and spleen tip were not palpable and there was no evidence of generalized lymphadenopathy. She had two negative throat cultures for group A streptococcus. Her monospot test was positive.

INGROWN TOENAIL (ONYCHOCRYPTOSIS, Onyx Gr., nail)

Definition
■ When one or both sides of toenails grow into the surrounding soft tissue of the nail bed.

Etiology
■ Infection causes granuloma in the nail bed, the growth of the nail in this tissue, or the healthy nail bed causes the symptoms.
■ Unsuitable tight foot-wear; shoes and socks.
■ Sweating in the socks and shoes creates a favorable environment for the bacteria to grow.
■ Trauma and sharp nail corners due to improper nail cutting may contribute to this problem.

Symptoms and Signs
■ Ingrown toenail is a common nail problem and much more common than ingrown finger nail and present with pain, erythema, and swelling of the toe.
■ Infection of the affected tissues is part of the disease (Figures A and B).

Treatment
■ Wedge resection.

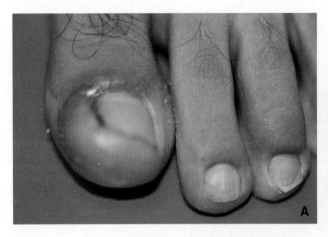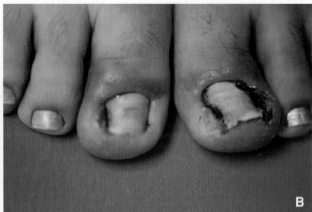

Figures A–B: Swelling and erythema of the first toe **(Figure A)** and severe, bilateral swelling and exudate in the nail bed **(Figure B)**.

IRITIS, TRAUMATIC

Definition
- Iritis is an inflammation of the iris or a form of anterior uveitis.

Etiology
- Trauma.
- Other factors such as infections (a variety of conditions ranging from herpes simplex virus to toxocariasis), autoimmune diseases, and cancer.

Symptoms and Signs
- Dull or throbbing pain, photophobia, and tearing.
- Asymmetrical pupils.
- White blood cells and proteins in the anterior chamber of the eye.

Treatment
- Cycloplegic agents, steroids.

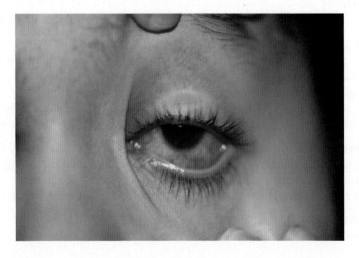

This 10-year-old's eye was sprayed with a water-gun while swimming. He developed photophobia, pain, blurry vision, and redness of his left eye for 8 days. He was afebrile, in pain with severe conjunctival injection, and cellular reaction in the left eye. He was diagnosed with anterior iritis and treated with steroid eye drops.

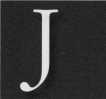

JUVENILE DERMATOMYOSITIS

Definition
- A rare, idiopathic, autoimmune myopathy of childhood.

Etiology
- Unknown, but may be an autoimmune response in genetically susceptible children in response to environmental triggers, including various infections. The peak incidence is between 5 and 10 years of age, and girls are twice as likely to be affected as boys.

Symptoms and Signs
- Symmetrical, proximal muscle weakness. Swollen eyelids, with reddish rash on upper eyelids. Scaly, red rash on the knuckles (Gottron's papules), skin ulceration, soft tissue calcifications, arthralgia, fever, weight loss, and fatigue.
- Complications include: Photosensitivity, osteoporosis (mainly from the steroids), GI perforation, and rarely, cardiac muscle involvement.
- Figures A–E.

Treatment
- Immunosuppressive therapy including corticosteroids, cyclosporine, and methotrexate.
- Sunscreen use for photosensitivity.
- Vitamin D and calcium supplementation for prevention of osteoporosis.

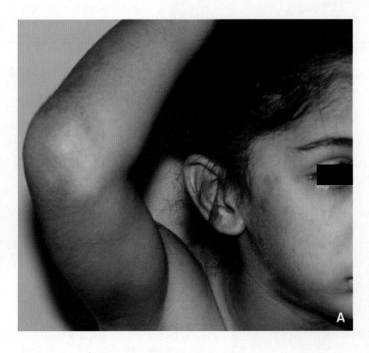

Figures A: Erythematous rash on the cheeks, elbows, and around the eyes.

figures continues

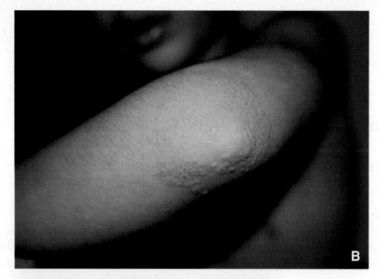

(figures cont.) **Figure B**

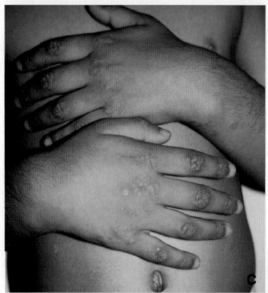

Figure C: We have been following this now 11-year-old boy since birth. He has asymptomatic dextrocardia. At 4 years of age he became symptomatic with fatigue, weakness, and a newly developed rash on his face, elbows, and knees. He was a well-nourished boy with an erythematous rash on his cheeks, forehead, around the eyes (heliotropic), elbow joints, knuckles, knees, and abdomen. Weakness of his flexor muscles were also noted at that time. The skin over the metacarpals were reddish-pink and hypertrophic (Gottron papules). CBC, sedimentation rate and urinalysis were normal. ANA was 4.5 (positive). He was diagnosed with juvenile dermatomyositis and treated with oral prednisolone and pimecrolimus cream. He has responded well to this therapeutic regimen.

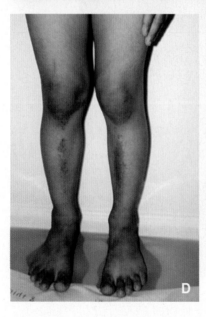

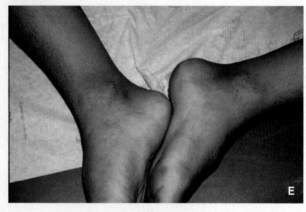

Figures D–E: A pinkish rash with some fine papules on the shins, ankles, and the feet.

JUVENILE IDIOPATHIC ARTHRITIS (JIA) (JUVENILE RHEUMATOID ARTHRITIS)

Definition

- Juvenile idiopathic arthritis is a broad term that describes a clinically heterogeneous group of inflammatory arthritides, which can be self-limited or chronic. It typically occurs in children under 16 years of age.

Etiology

- Unknown. Combination of genetic and immune-related factors. Environmental exposures may be at play.

Symptoms and Signs

- Depends on the subtype, but typically presents with painful, swollen joints which are not erythematous.
- There are three subgroups for JIA.

PAUCIARTICULAR JIA

- Affects less than five joints after 6 months of illness. Typically presents in children younger than 5 years of age, with a nontender, but swollen joint. It is more common in females.
- Diagnosis is based on the clinical findings and not based on any specific laboratory tests. ANA is positive in 80% of cases and correlates with the development of uveitis.
- Leg-length discrepancy is a well-known complication of pauciarticular arthritis.

POLYARTICULAR JIA

- Involves four or more joints after 6 months of illness and has a bimodal distribution of age at onset (first peak between 2 and 5 years, second peak between 10 and 14 years).
- Diagnosis is made upon clinical findings.
- Laboratory findings may include an elevated ESR and mild anemia.
- ANA is positive in 40% and is used as a marker for the development of uveitis. Internal organ involvement is otherwise rare.

SYSTEMIC ONSET JIA

- High-spiking daily fever, salmon-colored macular rash that appears with the fever, and arthritis (mono, oligo, or poly).
- Systemic signs and symptoms may include: Lymphadenopathy, hepatosplenomegaly, pericarditis, and pleuritis.
- There are no specific diagnostic tests. ANA is rarely positive. Elevated ESR, mild anemia, leukocytosis, and thrombocytosis are common findings.

Treatment

- Varies depending on the specific subgroup type.
- Nonsteroidal anti-inflammatory drugs (NSAIDs) are the first line of therapy for pain relief.
- Glucocorticoid intra-articular injections or other disease modifying antirheumatic drugs for control of inflammatory process (methotrexate, hydroxychloroquine, sulfasalazine) and antitumor necrosis factor have all been used with varying degrees of success (Figures A and B).

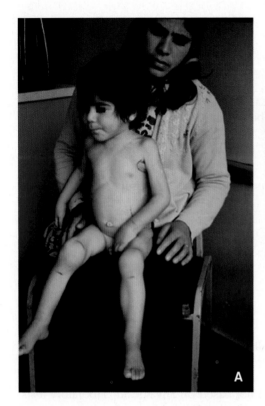

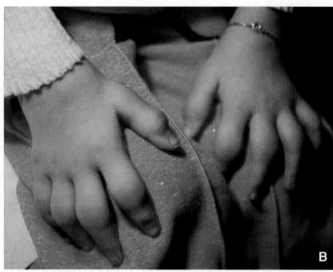

Figure A: Juvenile idiopathic arthritis in a 3-year-old boy. Note the swelling of the knees and of the left wrist, splenomegaly, and lymphadenopathy.

Figure B: Interphalangeal joint deformities in a 2-year-old girl with JIA. She presented with a history of 1-month-long fever, anorexia, and excessive crying. No other joints were involved.

JUVENILE XANTHOGRANULOMA

Definition
■ Juvenile xanthogranuloma (JXG) is a benign, self-limited disorder of non-Langerhans cell histiocytosis in infants and children.

Etiology
■ Unknown.

Symptoms and Signs
■ They present as solitary or multiple, yellow to reddish brown, cutaneous 0.5 to 2 cm papules or nodules that regress within a few months or sometimes a few years.
■ JXG is 10 times more common in Caucasians than in African Americans, male/female ratio is 1.4/1.
■ 35% are present at birth and 71% occur in the first year of life.
■ JXG is mostly confined to the cutaneous tissue in the head and neck area.
■ Systemic lesions are rare but may involve the eyes, liver, lungs, spleen, bones, and lymph nodes.
■ Ocular JXG may lead to hyphema, uveitis, iridis, secondary glaucoma, and blindness.
■ Ophthalmologic referral should be considered in children younger than 2 years who present with multiple lesions.

Treatment
■ Majority of cases resolves spontaneously.
■ Systemic lesions may cause symptoms of mass-effect. Treatment options include surgical removal, radiotherapy, or chemotherapy.

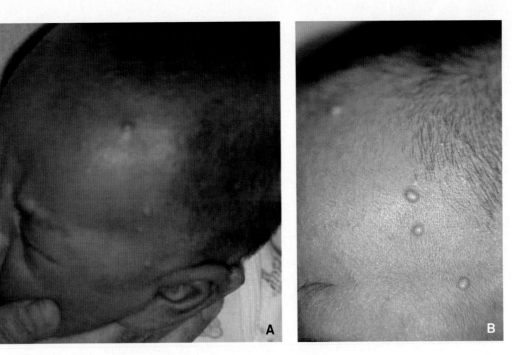

Figure A–B: This newborn male developed papules on his head and neck by 3 weeks of age. The papules were firm, dome-shaped, and orange yellow in color. The papules grew in numbers by 6 weeks of age. He was diagnosed with JXG with subsequent regression of nodules by the age of 3 years.

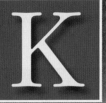

KALA-AZAR

(See Leishmaniasis).

KAWASAKI DISEASE (KD)

Definition
- Kawasaki disease is a multisystem, childhood disease of unknown etiology, characterized by vasculitis of the small and medium-sized blood vessels.

Etiology
- Unknown, possibly infectious, may be autoimmune.

Symptoms and Signs
- KD is characterized by 5 days or more of high fever, irritability, conjunctivitis, and generalized skin pealing. The rash can present as a maculopapular rash, erythema multiforme, or scarlatiniform, often more prominent in the groins, and can be full body.
- Lymphadenopathy, erythema and swelling of the hands and feet, strawberry-red tongue, and dry cracked lips due to necrotizing microvasculitis.
- Other manifestations of KD include hydrops of the gall bladder, diarrhea, mild hepatitis, urethritis, sterile pyuria, and thrombocytosis.
- Children can develop cardiovascular sequelae ranging from asymptomatic coronary artery ectasis (dilatation) or aneurysm formation to giant coronary artery aneurysms with thrombosis.
- Diagnosis is based on:
  - Five days or more of fever together with any four of the following:
    - Bilateral nonsuppurative conjunctivitis.
    - Polymorphous, nonvesicular rash.
    - Mucus membrane changes of the upper respiratory tract that may include erythema, fissures of the lips, crusting of the lips and mouth, strawberry-red tongue, exudative pharyngitis, and discrete oral lesions.
    - Peripheral edema or erythema of the hands and feet.
  - Cervical lymphadenopathy of at least 1.5 cm in diameter, which is mostly unilateral.
- Atypical KD, which is more common in children younger than 1 year of age, may present with less than four of the five criteria, and can yet progress to developing coronary artery aneurism.

Treatment
- Treatment is with IV gamma globulin, 2 g/kg, high-dose aspirin, 80 to 100 mg/kg/day, in divided doses, and corticosteroids.
- Figures A–H.

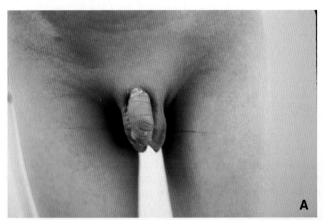

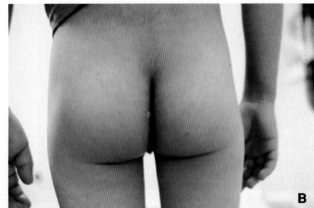

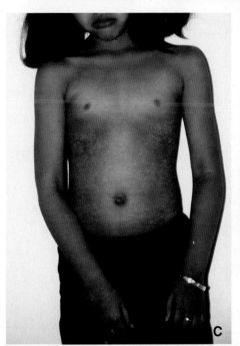

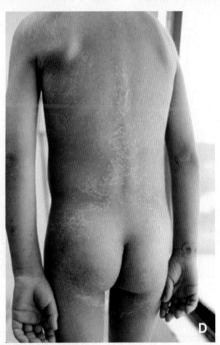

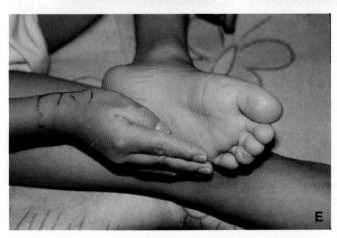

Figures A–B: This 6-year-old boy with a 4-day history of fever, loss of appetite, headache, sore throat, and rash. On examination, he had a temperature of 39.8°C, strawberry tongue, erythema of the lower abdomen, buttocks, legs, and pealing of the penis and perianal area. Erythema and slight swelling of the hands. Lips looked normal. His throat culture was negative for group A streptococci. He was admitted and treated with IV gamma globulin and aspirin.

Figure C: A 7-year-old girl presented with some pealing of the skin, following 16 days of high fever. She had severe hematuria and skin desquamation. No cardiac involvement. Her ESR was 100 and CRP 8.4.

Figures D–E: Desquamation of the skin in a 7-year-old boy with Kawasaki disease.

figures continues

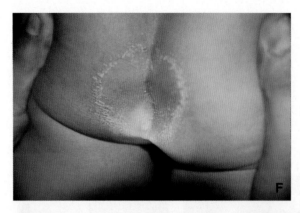

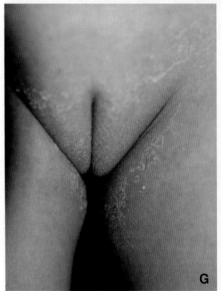

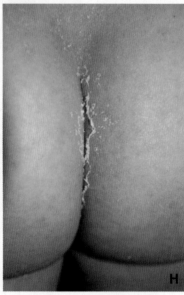

(figures cont.) **Figure F:** Skin desquamation in a 5-year-old boy, following 7 days of fever and stomach ache prior to admission, with cracked dry lips and strawberry tongue. He also had some coronary artery involvement.

Figures G–H: Skin desquamation in Kawasaki disease.

KEARNS–SAYRE SYNDROME (OCULOCRANIOSOMATIC DISEASE)

Definition
- Kearns–Sayer syndrome is a rare mitochondrial disorder.

Etiology
- Kearns–Sayre syndrome is inherited as a mitochondrial autosomal recessive or dominant or can be sporadic.

Symptoms and Signs
- Characterized by a triad of (1) progressive external ophthalmoplegia, (2) pigmentary retinopathy, and (3) onset before 20 years of age.
- Other features of this disease include heart block, increasing muscular weakness, ataxia, sensorineural hearing loss, multiple endocrine disorders, short stature, syncope, night blindness, and cerebrospinal fluid protein greater than 100 mg/dL.
- Prognosis is poor.

Treatment
- Supportive.

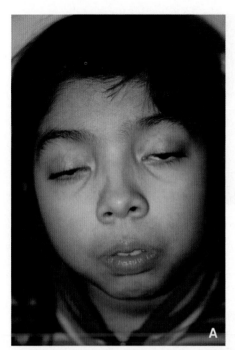

Figure A: This girl was adopted when she was 10 years old and we have no access to her past history other than knowing that her mother had used drugs. She was brought in at that age by her foster mother for learning disability, increasing fatigability, most noticeable when "asked to run at school," "sleeping-a-lot," and "her eye going outward all the time." Her weight was in the third percentile, and her height was well below the third percentile. Her pulse rate was 59 per minute. She had bilateral ptosis and esotropia of the right eye. Her vision was 20/50 in the right eye and 20/70 in the left eye, and she failed the hearing test. She was seen again 2 months later with the history that she had "fainted in the classroom," one day at 9 a.m., while sharpening her pencil, and vomiting a few days later. The only striking change at this time was a heart rate of 41 and a systolic murmur of 2/6 in the left midsternal border. Heart block was suspected and confirmed by EKG. She now has a dual-chamber pacemaker for a third-degree heart block. She is short, has chorioretinal atrophy with slight bilateral optic nerve atrophy, bilateral ptosis, severely impaired hearing, poor muscle strength, more noticeable in her legs (she gets tired after 5 to 10 minutes of walking), and has a tremor. Her head CT scan showed a small pituitary, minor calcification of the left intracranial vertebral artery, and slightly thin extra ocular muscles bilaterally. Normal female karyotype and normal renal ultrasound. Mitochondrial DNA analysis showed a large mitochondrial deletion. She has bilateral ptosis and chronic progressive external ophthalmoplegia (CPEO).

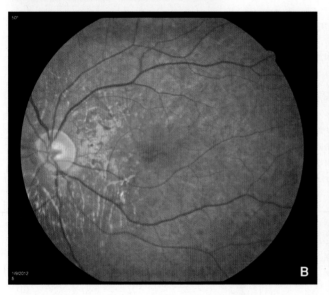

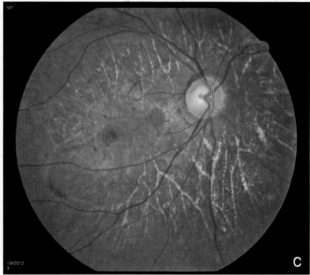

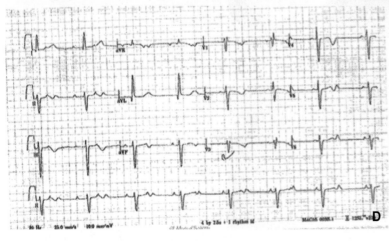

Figures B and C:
1. Chorioretinal atrophy.
2. Retinal pigment epithelium (RPE) changes.
3. Optic atrophy.

Figure D: Complete (third-degree) heart block and an atrial rate of approximately 84 per minute and ventricular rate of 44 per minute. There is no relationship between the P waves and the QRS complexes (P waves are "marching through" the QRS and the former is faster than the latter). The QTc is also prolonged which can also be seen in complete heart block.

figures continues

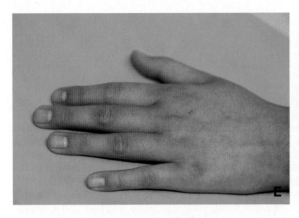

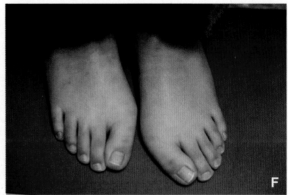

(figures cont.) **Figures E–F:** Arachnodactyly, slender and long fingers, and bunion worse in the left foot and in the same child.

KERATOSIS PILARIS (Kerato, any horny + osis) (KP)

Definition
- Keratosis pilaris, or follicular hyperkeratosis, is a common follicular skin condition in which keratin forms plugs within the hair follicles causing rough patches on the skin.

Etiology
- The excess keratin produced entraps the hair follicles forming hard plugs, a process known as hyperkeratinization.
- It is inherited in an autosomal dominant fashion.

Symptoms and Signs
- It is more common in the females and approximately 50% to 80% of adolescents are affected.
- In keratosis the skin is like chicken-skin or goose-flesh. The lesions are mostly on the upper extensor arms, thighs, cheeks, trunk, and buttocks and worse when dry. This cornification and contraction of erector pili muscles gives the skin its look.
- Worse during winter when the air is dry.
- Figures A–D.

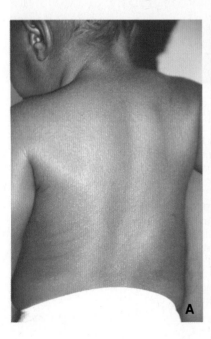

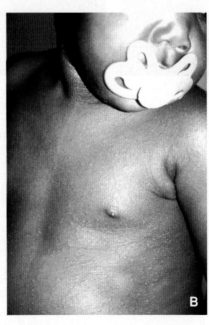

Figures A–B: Keratosis pilaris in a 9-month-old boy. Fine keratotic papules seen on the chest.

figures continues

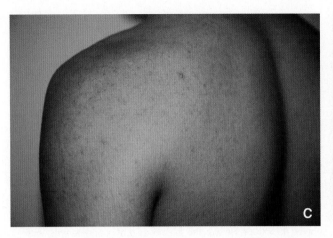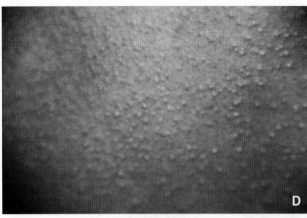

(figures cont.) **Figures C–D:** Keratotic pilaris in a teenage boy **(Figure C).** Magnified keratosis pilaris papules **(Figure D).**

Treatment
- Benign skin condition.
- Daily use of 10% to 25% urea cream or lactic acid in an emollient, steroid cream, or topical retinoic acid are helpful.
- The skin improves with age and the majority recover by the age of 30 years.

KLINEFELTER VARIANT

Definition
- A rare form of Klinefelter's syndrome with more anomalies.

Etiology
- A chromosomal aberration, mostly due to meiotic sequential nondisjunction during parental gametogenesis.
- The most common pattern in Klinefelter syndrome is 47,XXY.
- Mosaic patterns of 46,XXY/47,XXY or other combinations can be seen.
- The presence of more than two X-chromosomes is rare and is called Klinefelter variant.
- The Y-chromosome always determines a male phenotype.

Symptoms and Signs
- Mental retardation and other manifestations of Klinefelter are more severe with the increasing number of sex chromosomes.
- Mental retardation is severe in 49,XXXXY variant.
- Other features include short neck, epicanthus, strabismus, large mouth, flat upturned nose, deformed ears, small penis, hypoplastic testes, and cubitus valgus.

Treatment
- Testosterone replacement therapy.

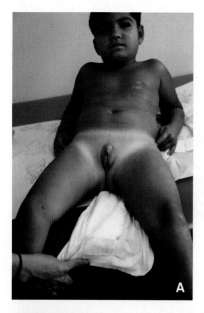

Figure A: A karyotype was performed soon after birth, due to his coarse features, short hair line, and abnormal ears, which showed 49,XXXXY. He was the second child of young parents, with adequate prenatal care, normal delivery, and a birth weight of 2.8 kg. He was delayed in his milestones and never talked. He was brought in for seizure at the age of 2 years. He had brachycephaly, hypertelorism, coloboma of the left iris, epicanthal folds, low nasal bridge, restricted carrying angle of the elbow, clinodactyly of the fifth fingers, flat feet, small penis, and hypoplastic testes. He was not short and did not have microcephaly.

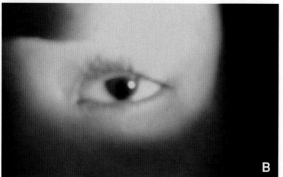

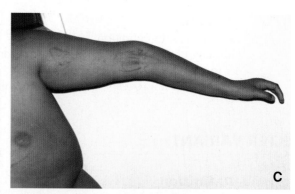

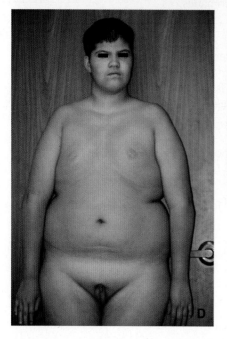

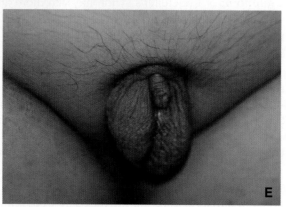

Figures B–C: Colobomata of the left eye **(Figure B)** and cubitus valgus of the left arm **(Figure C)** in Klinefelter variant.

Figures D–E: At age 14, he is obese, tall, has bilateral gynecomastia and clinodactyly of the fifth fingers, micropenis, hypoplastic testes, wide hip, and no speech.

KLIPPEL–FEIL SYNDROME

Definition
- Klippel–Feil syndrome is a rare congenital deformity characterized by fusion of any two of the seven cervical vertebrae.

Etiology
- Possibly hereditary.

Symptoms and Signs
- Low hair line, short neck, restricted neck movement, reduction of the cervical vertebrae, and hemi- or fused vertebrae signify this syndrome.
- Affected children may have many other problems such as Sprengel anomaly, scoliosis, congenital heart disease, syndactyly and hypoplastic thumb, deafness, webbed neck, torticollis, and renal abnormalities (Figure).

Treatment
- Symptomatic and at times surgery.

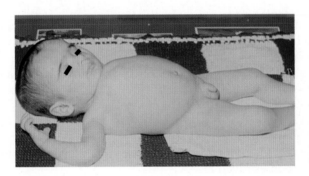

This 9-month-old boy was brought in for his inability to move his neck. He had a short hair line and three of his cervical vertebras were fused together. He had no other visible abnormality at that time.

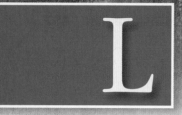

LABIAL ADHESION

Definition
- Labial adhesion occurs when the labia minora adhere together. It ranges in severity from partial to complete fusion.

Etiology
- Exact etiology remains unknown. It may be secondary to a combination of low estrogen levels and a local inflammatory process such as fecal soiling, vulvovaginitis, or eczema.

Symptoms and Signs
- Labial adhesion is more frequently seen in children between 3 months and 6 years of age.
- They are often asymptomatic and discovered during a routine physical examination.
- They appear as thin, pale, semitranslucent membranes that cover the vaginal entrance between the labia minora.
- Complications may include urinary dribbling, frequent urinary tract infections, and vaginal irritation.
- Figures A and B.

Treatment
- No treatment necessary for asymptomatic children. Adhesions usually resolve during puberty with increase in estrogen levels.
- Adhesions should be treated with an estrogen cream, if there is evidence of urinary symptoms.
- Possible side effects of treatment include breast-bud formation and vaginal bleeding.
- Surgery is recommended if adhesions and urinary symptoms persist despite estrogen therapy.

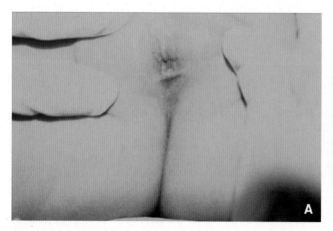
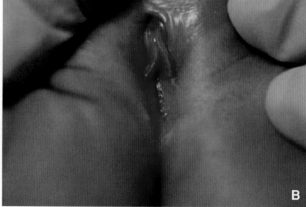

Figures A–B: Labial adhesions in a 5-year-old girl who was seen for recurrent urinary tract infections **(Figure A)** and an incidental finding in a 6-month-old **(Figure B)**.

LANGERHANS CELL HISTIOCYTOSIS (LCH)

Histiocytosis X, eosinophilic granuloma, Hand–Schuller–Christian syndrome, Letterer–Siwe disease.

Definition
- LCH is part of a group of clinical syndromes called histiocytosis. They involve an increase in number of immune cells called histiocytes which are part of the mononuclear phagocyte system. There are three major classes of LCH:
  - Unifocal disease: Historically known as eosinophilic granuloma. There is proliferation of Langerhans cells in a single or multiple bones without extraskeletal involvement.
  - Multifocal unisystem: Fever, bone lesions, and diffuse eruptions (most commonly involving the scalp and ear canals). May also involve the pituitary stalk, leading to diabetes insipidus. Hand–Schuller–Christian syndrome is the triad of lytic bone lesions, exophthalmos, and diabetes insipidus.
  - Multifocal multisystem: Also known as Letterer–Siwe disease. It is characterized by the proliferation of Langerhans cells in many tissues.

Etiology
- Unknown. May be an autoimmune phenomenon.

Symptoms and Signs
- Incidence is 1 in 200,000 people per year. Mainly affects children between the ages of 1 and 15 years. Peak incidence occurs in children 5 to 10 years of age.
- Painful bone swelling is the most common finding. Involves the skull, long bones, and the flat bones.
- Osteolytic lesions may lead to pathologic fractures.
- Bone marrow involvement and pancytopenia.
- Dermatologic findings include a variety of rashes: Seborrheic dermatitis of the scalp, red papules, and scaly erythematous lesions.
- Lymph node involvement: Lymphadenopathy and hepatosplenomegaly.
- Endocrine: Diabetes insipidus is most common. Hypothalamic–pituitary axis may also be involved.
- Lungs: Chronic cough or shortness of breath. An incidental nodule may be found on a chest radiograph.
- Diagnosis is confirmed by tissue biopsy. Birbeck granules on electron microscopy ("tennis racket" cytoplasmic organelles of unknown significance).
- Figures A–E.

Treatment
- Depends on the type of the lesion, severity, and the number of organs involved.
- Multifocal multisystem has a very poor prognosis, despite aggressive systemic chemotherapy.
- Solitary bone lesions may be treated via excision and limited radiation.
- Systemic disease requires chemotherapy.
- Hormonal supplementation for endocrine disorders.

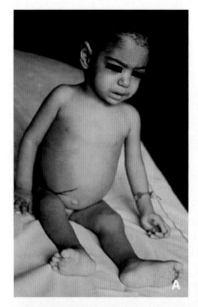

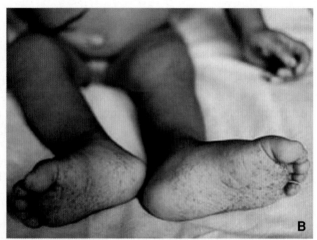

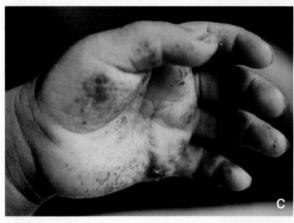

Figures A–C: This male toddler was brought in for evaluation of a "rash" on his hands and feet. Physical examination revealed bilateral perforated tympanic membranes with otitis media, hepatosplenomegaly, ascites, and petechia without fever or lymphadenopathy. The liver biopsy confirmed the clinical diagnosis of Langerhans cell histiocytosis.

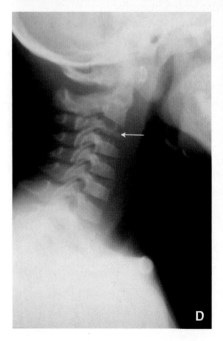

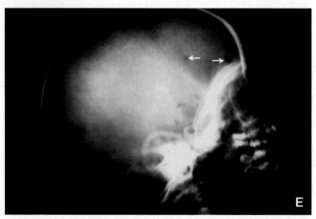

Figure D: Cervical spine x-ray, lateral view: There is complete flattening of the third cervical vertebral body (vertebra plana). This is a typical presentation of Langerhans cell histiocytosis.

Figure E: Lateral skull x-ray: Multiple well-defined lytic lesions (*arrows*) of the skull. The most commonly involved bony site is the calvarium, particularly within the frontal and parietal bones.

LEISHMANIASIS

Definition
- A tropical disease caused by protozoan parasites that belong to the genus Leishmania. It is most commonly seen in tropical and subtropical parts of the world with the exception of Australia and islands of the tropical Pacific Ocean.

Etiology
- It is transmitted by the bite of the phlebotomine sand flies. The leishmania invade and multiply within host macrophages and affect different host tissues (different leishmania species affect different tissues causing different clinical manifestations).
- Most forms are transmitted by rodents and dogs but some can be spread between humans.

Symptoms and Signs
- Many infections are asymptomatic. This may be secondary to genetic virulence of the parasite, human genetic predisposition, the immunologic and nutritional status of the host.
- Symptomatic leishmaniasis may be divided into four different types: Visceral, cutaneous, diffuse cutaneous, and mucocutaneous.
- Visceral leishmaniasis (kala-azar, Hindi for "black fever"): Marked by replication of parasites in the reticuloendothelial system (liver, spleen, and bone marrow). There is a subacute progression of fatigue, fever, weight loss, and splenomegaly. Anemia, thrombocytopenia, hepatic dysfunction, edema, and significant cachexia are common in later stages of the illness.
- Cutaneous leishmaniasis: Most common form. An ulcer is formed at the bite site. It may heal over within a few months to a year, or progress to the other forms of leishmaniasis.
- Diffuse cutaneous: Widespread skin lesions which physically resemble leprosy (without nerve involvement).
- Mucocutaneous: Skin ulcers which spread to the nose and the mouth causing significant tissue damage.
- Diagnosis is made by histopathologic studies of the affected organs by needle aspiration or biopsy. Visualization of amastigotes (form that leishmania parasites take in the host) within or outside of macrophages is required for diagnosis. Culture studies may take up to 2 to 4 weeks. Various serologic tests such as enzyme-linked immunosorbent assay (ELISA) are also available.

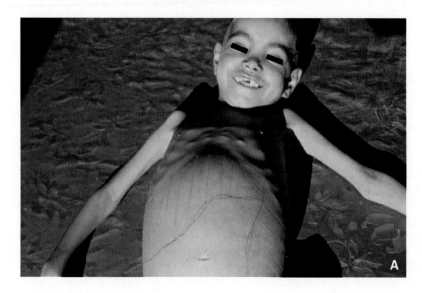

Figure A: Hepatosplenomegaly and cachexia in a child with leishmaniasis. This picture was taken weeks after treatment was initiated. Significant nutritional improvement was noted.

figures continues

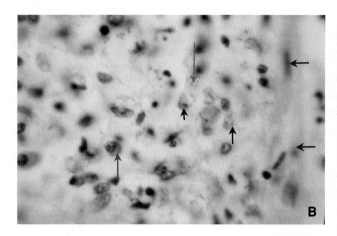

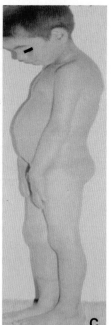

(figures cont.) **Figure B:** Liver biopsy of a patient with visceral leishmaniasis. *Red arrow:* Smooth muscle cells. *Blue arrow:* Presence of amastigotes within macrophages.

Figure C: A toddler with visceral leishmaniasis. He presented with fever and hepatosplenomegaly.

Treatment
- Treatment differs upon the type of leishmaniasis. Difficult to make universal recommendations, given different resistant patterns of the organism as well as differences in the genetic background and immune status of the patients.
- Cutaneous form has a high rate of spontaneous cure.
- Untreated visceral leishmaniasis has a 90% mortality rate.
- Therapeutic drugs include amphotericin and pentavalent antimonial drugs.
- Figures A–C.

LEUKEMIA

Definition
- A malignant disease of blood forming organs, which is progressive and characterized by abnormal proliferation and development of leucocytes and their precursors in the bone marrow.

Etiology
- Most of the childhood leukemias are acquired genetic diseases.
- Children with certain genetic syndromes are predisposed to childhood leukemias. For instance, the risk of developing acute lymphocytic leukemia (ALL) is 10 to 20-fold higher in children with trisomy 21.
- With the exception of specific genetic mutations, there is very limited knowledge about the causes of childhood leukemias. Other possible causes include environmental factors such as chemicals, radiation, and certain viral infections.
- The leukemias constitute approximately one-third of childhood cancers, and acute lymphoblastic leukemia is the most common type of childhood malignancy.
- The order of frequency for other types of leukemia in children is acute myelogenous leukemia, chronic myelogenous leukemia, and juvenile chronic myelogenous leukemia.

Symptoms and Signs
- The peak incidence is between 2 and 6 years of age. Leukemias are slightly more frequent in males.

- Children may present with nonspecific symptoms such as anorexia, fatigue, bone and joint pain, and low-grade fevers.
- Abnormal bleeding, purpura, and ecchymosis are common presentations of leukemia.
- Physical examination findings vary and may include petechia, lymphadenopathy, and hepatosplenomegaly.
- Retinal changes are common with central nervous system involvement.
- Diagnosis is made by the examination of peripheral blood. There is an increase in immature white blood cells (blasts) as well as anemia and thrombocytopenia.
- Bone marrow biopsy is confirmatory.

Treatment

- Depends on type and stage of leukemia.
- Patients should be referred to the appropriate tertiary care centers, where experts follow clinical protocols established by national or international cooperative groups.
- Figures A and B.

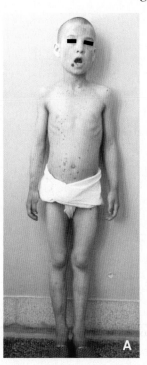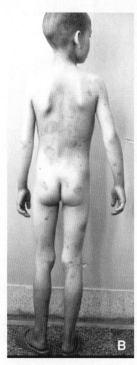

Figures A–B: This 12-year-old boy was brought in for evaluation of a rash. He had nonspecific joint pain which was diagnosed as rheumatic fever and he was treated with aspirin and penicillin. He started to bleed at the site of an IV insertion, which was controlled with pressure. On physical examination, he appeared pale with generalized purpura, ecchymosis, gingival bleeding, and splenomegaly. His peripheral blood smear indicated severe anemia, thrombocytopenia, and many "atypical lymphocytes." His bone marrow aspiration confirmed the clinical diagnosis of acute lymphoblastic leukemia.

LIPOATROPHY, ACQUIRED

Definition

- A dent due to localized fat loss at site of injection.

Etiology

- Commonly seen at site of corticosteroid and insulin injections.
- Has been reported with growth hormone, vitamin K, as well as other childhood vaccinations.
- May be avoided by making sure injection is within muscle tissue and not within the subcutaneous fat.

Treatment

- Purely cosmetic, may include fat transfers, injectable fillers, and implants (Figures A and B).

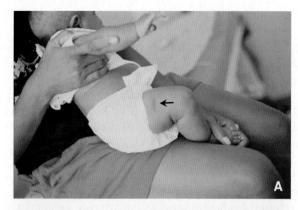

Figure A: Dent noted on the right thigh of a 3-month-old at the site of neonatal vitamin K injection.

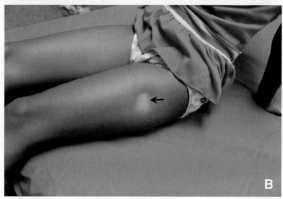

Figure B: A dent and depigmentation on the thigh of a teenager who had received several shots in that spot.

LIVEDO RETICULARIS (Livedo L., a discolored spot or patch on the skin)

Definition
■ Livedo reticularis refers to mottled or reticulated, purplish discoloration of the skin. It occurs most often on the lower extremities and the trunk.

Etiology
■ Unknown. It may be caused by vasospasm of the arterioles in response to cold, leading to hypoxemia, and dilation of capillaries and venules. Blood then stagnates within these vessels, giving it a characteristic appearance.

Symptoms and Signs
■ Lace-like, purplish discoloration of the legs, trunk, and arms. It often becomes aggravated in cold weather.
■ The condition may be benign (cutis marmorata) or may be a sign of serious pathology.
■ Development in a blotchy or interrupted asymmetrical distribution may herald the beginning of an autoimmune disease; idiopathic thrombocytopenia, rheumatoid arthritis, systemic lupus erythematosus, dermatomyositis, thrombotic thrombocytopenia, polyarteritis nodosa, or rheumatic fever.
■ Other potential causes include leukemia, cryoglobulinemia, cerebrovascular accidents, lymphoma, tuberculosis, and streptococcal infections.
■ Figures A–G.

L

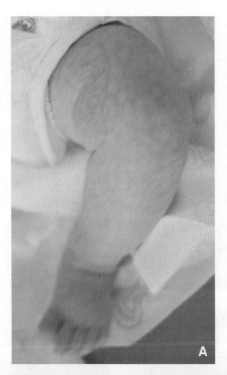

Figure A: Cutis marmorata in a 2-month-old baby.

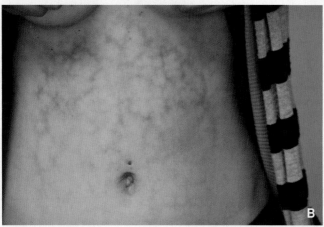

Figure B: This 14-year-old girl presented with this rash on her abdominal wall for 2 months. No pain, itching, or fever. She had a habit of taking a hot water bottle to bed and place it on her abdomen. The rash slowly resolved, once she gave up use of the bottle.

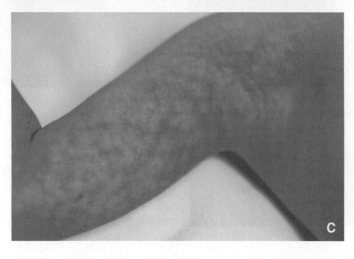

Figure C: This otherwise healthy 3-year-old girl's response to cold has always been this reticulation and discoloration since birth.

figures continues

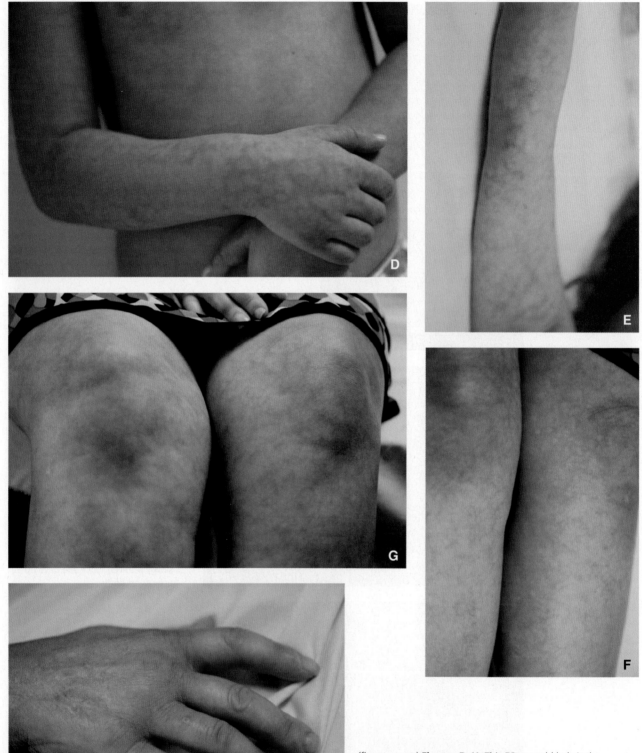

(figures cont.) **Figures D–H:** This 58-year-old lady is the maternal grandmother of the previous 3-year-old girl. She has scleroderma and Raynaud's phenomenon of her hands. Note the edema, erythema, and contracture flexion of her hand. Also note skin reticulation in the lower extremities.

Treatment
- Warming the body improves the discoloration in benign cases.
- Treatment of the underlying cause in pathologic cases.

LYMPHADENOPATHY

Definition
- Disease of the lymph nodes.

Etiology
- Lymph nodes may enlarge secondary to an infection, malignancy, or autoimmune disease.
- Depending on the cause, lymphadenopathy may be localized to one region of the body or generalized to multiple noncontiguous regions.
- Supraclavicular lymphadenopathy is associated with a high rate of neoplasm in children.
- Axillary lymphadenopathy is associated with a variety of infections including cat scratch disease.
- Epitrochlear lymphadenopathy may be secondary to a localized infection, mycobacteria, or malignancy.
- Inguinal lymphadenopathy is rarely associated with any particular illness, unless it is larger than 3 cm.
- Generalized lymphadenopathy may be secondary to systemic infection or illness, including influenza, EBV, measles, miliary TB, HIV, or systemic lupus.

Symptoms and Signs
- An enlarged lymph node may be palpable, visible, or detectable by different imaging techniques.
- Rubbery, mobile, minimally tender, and "shotty" lymph nodes are called "reactive" nodes. They are usually in response to a localized viral or bacterial infection.
- Acutely enlarged, erythematous, tender lymph nodes are suggestive of an infected lymph node.
- Fluctuance may suggest an abscess. *Staphylococcus aureus* and streptococcus are the two main causative organisms.
- Chronic, nontender, matted lymphadenopathy with surrounding indurated skin is suggestive of tuberculosis and nontuberculous mycobacteria.
- A firm, fixed, and matted node should raise concern for malignancy (leukemia and neuroblastoma in younger children, lymphoma in adolescents).
- Laboratory studies depend on the type of adenopathy (localized vs. generalized) as well as history and physical examination findings. A complete blood count, EBV titers, CMV titers, toxoplasma, cat scratch disease titers, ASO, anti-DNAse serologies, PPD skin test, HIV test, and chest x-ray are typically considered for diagnostic purposes.
- If cause remains unknown, a biopsy may be performed.

Treatment
- Treatment of the underlying cause. Some cases may need surgical debridement.
- Figures A–D.

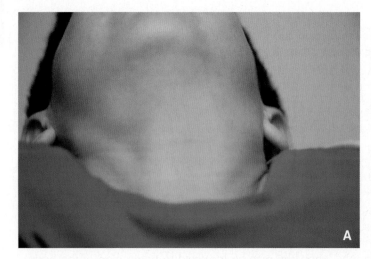

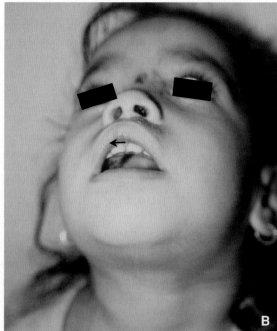

Figures A–B: Anterior cervical lymphadenopathy in streptococcal tonsillitis **(Figure A)**. Jugulodigastric lymphadenopathy in reaction to facial impetigo **(Figure B)**.

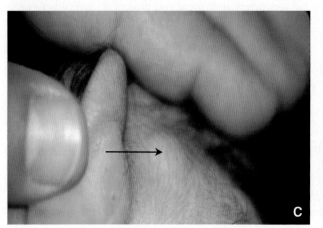

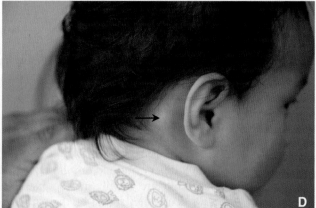

Figures C–D: Pre- or retroauricular lymphadenopathy can be pathologic, but also not uncommon to see in healthy children. Preauricular lymphadenopathy as a reaction to the preauricular dermatitis in a 1-year-old male **(Figure C)**. Preauricular lymphadenopathy in a healthy 3-year-old boy. It was noted by his mother 3 months ago **(Figure D)**.

LYMPHANGITIS

Definition
- Lymphangitis is the inflammation of a lymphatic vessel.

Etiology
- Lymphangitis is usually a complication of a bacterial infection at a location distal to the vessel.
- The most common pathogenic organisms in immunocompetent hosts are *Staphylococcus aureus* and *Streptococcus pyogenes*.

Symptoms and Signs
- Tender, red streak extending from the original infection site toward regional lymph nodes.
- There may be systemic symptoms including fever, chills, and regional lymphadenopathy.

Treatment

- Treatment of the causative organism.
- *Streptococcus pyogenes* infections have a significant risk for morbidity and mortality.
- Figures A–C.

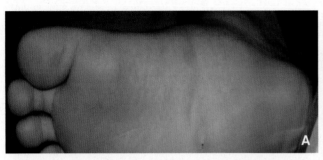

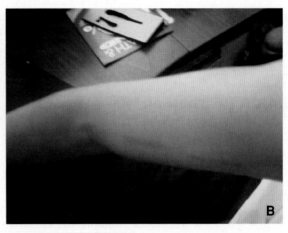

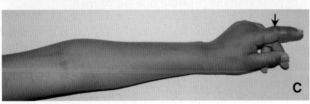

Figure A: This 10-year-old boy stepped on a zipper. He developed this rash the following day accompanied with pain and itching. A puncture wound is visible on the foot along with an erythematous streak which is extending proximally.

Figure B: A suspected arthropod bite in this 14-year-old girl was followed by swelling, redness, and itching the next day. A red, proximally extending streak was noted 2 days later.

Figure C: A 7-year-old boy was bitten by an arthropod. The left second finger was swollen and tender the following morning. Multiple, rapidly expanding streaks were noted on his left arm. There was no fever or other constitutional symptoms.

LYSOSOMAL STORAGE DISEASE

(See Mucopolysaccharidosis).

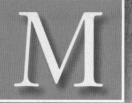

MACRODACTILY

(See Cornelia de Lange syndrome).

MALARIA (It. "bad air")

Definition
- Malaria is the most common and the most important parasitic disease of man.

Etiology
- Malaria is caused by protozoa and is transmitted by the bite of anopheles mosquitoes.
- Worldwide, millions of people are affected each year, and approximately 1 million individuals, most of whom are children, die from complications of the disease.

Symptoms and Signs
- Malaria can present with vague symptoms suggesting a viral infection. But in most cases, it begins with rigor (L. a chill) followed by high fever, headache, then profuse sweating.
- Patient may feel weak after the cycle, but can go back to school or work.
- Vomiting, diarrhea, and arthralgia may be present.
- This cycle is normally repeated every 2 or 3 days depending on the infecting species.
- These paroxysms are so regular that patients in the endemic areas know when to expect them, leave their job, go home, have the rigor, fever, and sweating, and go back to work.
- The rigor is one of the most severe chills seen in any disease.

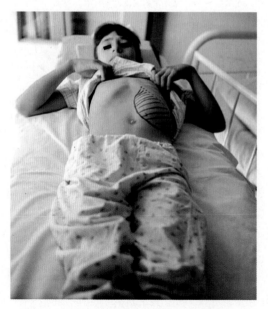

This 14-year-old girl had suffered several attacks of malaria (the first episode was at the age of 8 years). She could vividly visualize and describe the first episode of rigor which shook her, her bed, and her blankets as well as describe her severe sweating which soaked her mattress and its awful odor.

- A rare observation in this disease was a young woman with alternating days of fever and urticaria. The malaria parasite was seen in her blood smear. We treated the malaria and the urticaria (her reaction to the released malaria parasite, the merozoites into the blood) resolved.

Treatment
- The possibility of resistance, severity of the disease, and the infecting species determines the choice of drug therapy.
- Mefloquine, doxycycline, primaquine, chloroquine phosphate plus proguanil are some of the choices.

MALNUTRITION

Definition
- According to the World Health Organization, "The cellular imbalance between supply of nutrients and energy and the body's demand for them to ensure growth, maintenance, and specific functions." And, "a condition resulting from long-term inadequate intake of protein and energy that can lead to wasting of body tissues and increased susceptibility to infections."
- According to the United Nations, "Malnutrition kills 10 children every minute."

Etiology
- Inadequate nutrients, improper utilization, lack of health and education of parents and that of care takers, and infections.
- Inappropriate weaning practices, poor hygiene, and insufficient knowledge of food preparation causes repeated bouts of diarrhea which is the precipitating factor in many cases of malnutrition. Other infections such as measles, ear and skin infections further compromise the child's immune system causing loss of appetite, increased metabolism, increased loss of nitrogen, and depletion of the minimal nutrients available.
- There was a general belief that protein deficiency caused kwashiorkor and insufficient calorie ended in marasmus. But, this is an oversimplification of a complex problem.
- Protein, sodium, and potassium deficiencies, and possibly, other factors cause the edema in malnutrition (kwashiorkor).
- Marasmus may be due to the body's adaptation to starvation and kwashiorkor, dysadaptation.

Classification
- The following is perhaps the simplest classification of malnutrition:
  - Wasting. Acute, current short-duration malnutrition where weight for age and weight for height are low, but height for age is normal.

Wt/age	Wt/ht	Ht/age
↓	↓	Normal

  - Stunting. Past chronic malnutrition where weight for age and height for age are low, but weight for height is normal.

Wt/age	Wt/ht	Ht/age
↓	Normal	↓

- Wasting and stunting. Acute and chronic, or current long-duration malnutrition, where weight for age, height for age, and weight for height are low.

Wt/age	Wt/ht	Ht/age
↓	↓	↓

- *Welcome classification of protein–energy malnutrition*

Percentage of standard weight for age	EDEMA present	EDEMA absent
60–80	Kwashiorkor	Undernutrition
<60	Marasmic kwashiorkor	Nutritional marasmus

KWASHIORKOR (Ghana, abandoned or displaced)

Definition
- Kwashiorkor is a serious form of malnutrition more common in children younger than 3 years, with bulky, but insufficient food and particularly protein-poor as well as in many other nutrients.
- The role of infection in this pathology cannot be over emphasized. Diarrhea in particular, plays a major role in precipitating the clinical picture of kwashiorkor.

Etiology
- As discussed in malnutrition.

Symptoms and Signs
- Failure to grow adequately is the first and most important manifestation of protein–energy malnutrition. Poor appetite, muscular wasting, edema, skin changes, mental status changes (apathy), and hair changes both in color (reddish-brown) as well as bands of discoloration (flag sign).
- Hepatomegaly and purpura may be found. Both predict a poor prognosis.
- The increase and decrease in the amount of purpura has a prognostic value.
- Author believes purpura in malnutrition is caused by essential fatty acid deficiency although this hypothesis needs further investigation.
- Fatty infiltration of the liver, low serum protein, particularly albumin, and anemia are commonly found.

Treatment
- Hospitalization, treatment of possible infection (if any), and proper diet.
- In the developing world, every attempt at intravenous fluid management carries a significant risk of introducing an infection. Therefore, injections in general and intravenous therapy in particular must be avoided. In addition, many of these malnourished children lack any appreciable muscle mass and contaminated needles may carry organism directly into the underlying bony structures.
- The food provided to the child, who would often have a very poor appetite, must be complete in needed nutrients, be pleasant visually and palatable in needed nutrients.
- Parents and particularly mothers should participate in the preparation of food and feeding.
- Figures A–C.

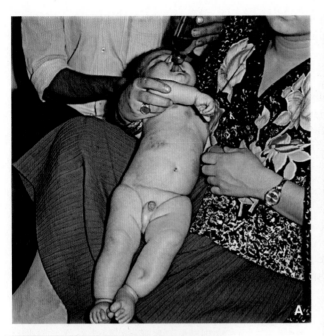

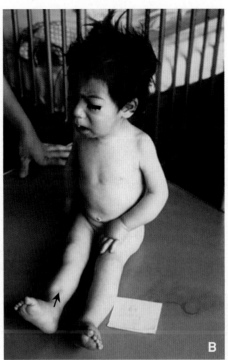

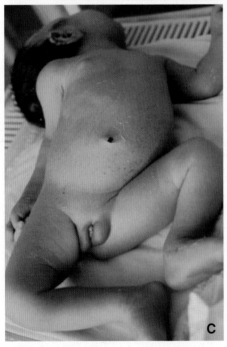

Figure A: Kwashiorkor in a 12-month-old boy, the only child of a young middle class family, and breastfed for 8 months. Cow's milk and solids were introduced at that time without any expert instructions. The infant then had many bouts of on-and-off diarrhea. Note that infant does not look thin or wasted. Note the pitting edema on his legs, purpura and ecchymosis on his lower chest and on his abdominal wall. Also, the mother appears to be financially well-off. Note the gold watch, ring, and bracelets on the mother's wrist; and yet, the baby is not being fed from a proper baby bottle, but instead, was fed using a medicine vial. The improper feeding is not due to the lack of financial resources, but rather due to the lack of proper training of the parents.

Figure B: 1-year-old boy with protein malnutrition. Weight of 6.7 kg. Edema of the face, eyelids, hands and legs.

Figure C: Edema, abdominal distention, and purpura on the abdominal wall of infant with protein malnutrition.

MARASMUS (Gr., Marasmus, a dying away)

Definition
- A progressive wasting and emaciation, primarily in infants and young children, due to lack of adequate caloric intake.

Etiology
- Marasmus or energy (calorie) malnutrition is the more common type of malnutrition in many parts of the world today.
- Marasmus is more prevalent in younger infants and children (vs. kwashiorkor which is more common in slightly older children).

- Most common in nonbreastfed children or in those who were breastfed for just a few months.
- Marasmus is a form of starvation and as some believe an adaptation to the lack of adequate food.

Symptoms and Signs

- A marasmic patient is a hungry, thin, wasted, and stunted child with vacant eyes.
- In the majority of cases, it is the diarrhea which brings the child to the hospital.
- Oral thrush, diaper rash, and at times pressure sores are not uncommon.
- Skin changes such as those found in kwashiorkor as well as purpura can be seen.

Treatment

- Hospitalization, age-appropriate food which should look and taste good, vitamins, treatment of possible infections, and training of parents.

MARASMIC KWASHIORKOR

- These children are very thin, stunted, and edematous. Symptoms, signs, and treatment are same as in other types of malnutrition.

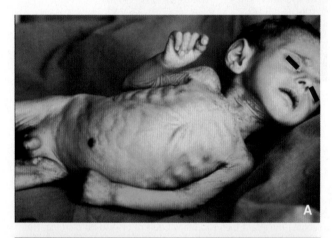

Figure A: An 11-month-old boy with severe calorie malnutrition. Extremely thin, lethargic, and with severe muscle atrophy. The ribs and distended loops of bowl are visible. The skin, paper-thin, with numerous wrinkles on his arms and legs.

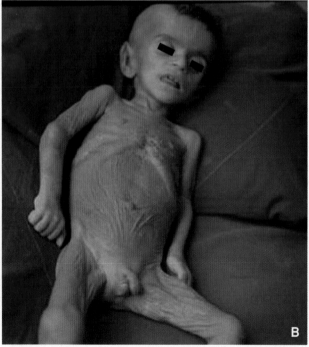

Figure B: A 16-month-old boy with calorie malnutrition (on his way to recovery). Very thin, particularly arms and legs, paper-thin skin with many wrinkles and a new lighter, healthier skin growing on his chest, creating some hyperkeratotic, hyperpigmented scaling, which peels-off like "flakes of paint", called mosaic skin, or "crazy pavement."

figures continues

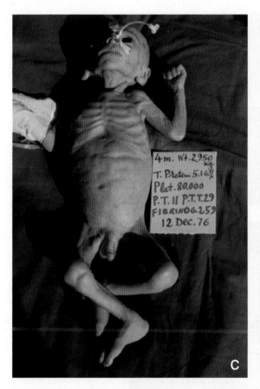
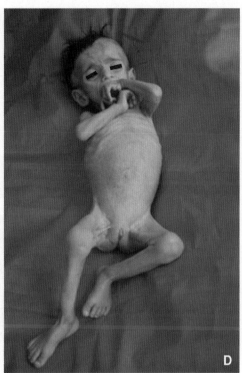

(figures cont.) **Figure C:** A 4-month-old boy, weighing 2.9 kg, with distended abdomen, visible loops of bowl and rib cage, and a few purpuric spots on the abdominal wall. Low total protein of 5.1 g, platelets 80,000, PT 11, PTT 29, and fibrinogen 2.59. The daily sign next to the patient records any change in the amount of purpura as an indication of his condition getting better or worse.

Figure D: Calorie malnutrition in a 14-month-old girl, with distended abdomen, muscular atrophy, and purpura. The presence of purpura on her abdominal wall is an ominous sign.

MARCUS GUNN JAW-WINKING SYNDROME

Definition
- Marcus Gunn jaw-winking syndrome presents as various degrees of blinking in the resting position when there is stimulation of the ipsilateral pterygoid muscle.

Etiology
- Often sporadic, but autosomal dominance inheritance pattern has been reported.

Symptoms and Signs
- This can happen bilaterally or unilaterally.
- Chewing, swallowing, sucking, and opening of the jaw can stimulate this reflex and cause blinking.
- It causes nursing infants to have a rhythmic upward jerking movement of the upper eyelid while feeding (synkinesis).
- An unintentional movement accompanying a volitional movement.
- There appears to be a connection between some branches of the trigeminal nerve innervating the external pterygoid muscle and the oculomotor nerve that innervate the levator superior muscle of the upper eyelid.

Treatment
- Treatment is usually unnecessary.
- Eye surgery may be done in severe cases.
- Figures A–D.

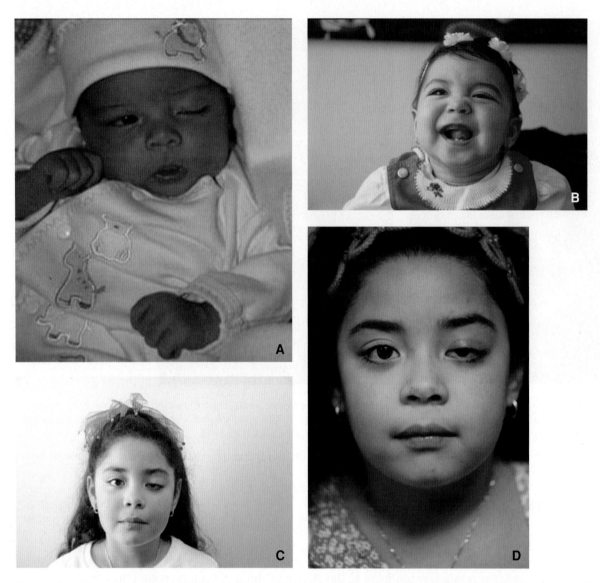

Figures A–D: This newborn, the only child of young parents, had an uncomplicated and normal delivery, no consanguinity or family history of ptosis, and was born with ptosis of the left upper lid. Her left upper lid moved up and down, synchronized with her jaw movements, when nursing and when sucking on the bottle. She was otherwise well. She is 6 days old in **Figure A**, 2 years old in **Figure B**, and 4 years old in **Figure C**. 5 years old and post-blepharoplasty with marked improvement in **Figure D**. A video of the actual jaw-and-eye movements is available online.

MARFAN SYNDROME

Definition
- A congenital disorder of connective tissue characterized by abnormally long extremities, subluxation of the lens, and other abnormalities.

Etiology
- Autosomal dominant inheritance with almost complete penetrance, but variable expressivity.
- Approximately 15% to 30% of cases are sporadic and arise out of a new mutation.

Symptoms and Signs
- The clinical manifestations are divided into major and minor criteria.

M

Major criteria:

- Skeletal system:
    - Pectus carinatum (pigeon chest).
    - Pectus excavatum (funnel chest) severe enough to require surgical correction.
    - Reduced upper-to-lower body segment ratio or arm-span to height ratio greater than 1.05.
    - Wrist sign or thumb sign (Steinberg sign).
    - Scoliosis >20 degrees or spondylolisthesis.
    - Reduced extension at the elbows <170 degrees.
    - Pes planus.
    - Protrusio acetabuli.
- Ocular system:
    - Ectopia lentis (dislocation of lens).
- Cardiovascular system:
    - Dilatation of the ascending aorta with involvement of the sinus of Valsalva or dissection of the aorta.

Minor criteria:

- Moderate degree of pectus excavatum; joint hypermobility, high narrow palate, abnormal facial appearance (dolichocephaly, malar hyperplasia, enophthalmos, retrognathia, and antimongoloid slants).
- Flat cornea, increased axial length of globe, and hypoplastic iris or ciliary muscle resulting in decreased miosis.
- Mitral valve prolapse, dilation of pulmonary artery, calcification of the mitral annulus before the age of 40 years, and dilation or dissection of descending aorta before the age of 50 years.
- Striae atrophicae (stretch marks) not associated with marked weight changes or pregnancy and incisional hernias.

Diagnosis

- In the presence of a positive family history, diagnosis is based on the presence of one major criterion in an organ system plus the involvement in a second organ system (the second organ system can be a major or minor criterion).

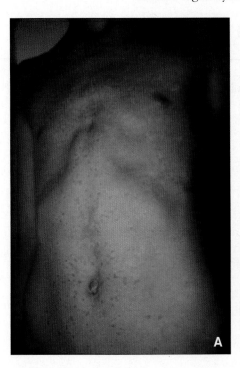

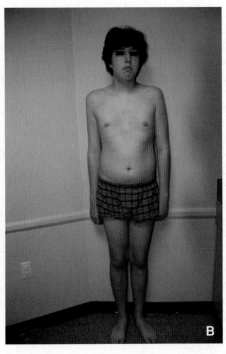

Figure A: A 13-year-old boy who was brought in for skin rash (pityriasis versicolor). He is above the 90th percentile for height for age, has long fingers, high arch palate, lax joints, myopia (but no other eye problems), flat feet, and pectus carinatum. Arm-span/height = 1.06.

Figures B–E: A 14-year-old boy without family history of Marfan syndrome. He has pectus excavatum, pes planus, arachnodactyly, reduced extension of the elbow, flat cornea, and mitral valve prolapse.

figures continues

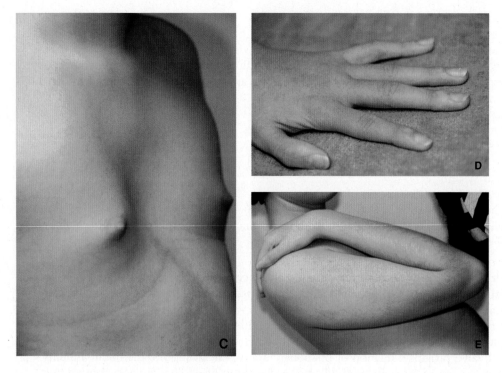

(figures cont.) **Figures C–E**

- In the absence of a clear family history, one major criterion in each of two or more different organ systems plus involvement of a third organ system (the third organ system can be a major or minor criterion).

Treatment
- There is no specific treatment.
- Monitoring of the congenital abnormalities.

MASTITIS

Definition
- An inflammatory condition of the breast, which may or may not be accompanied with infection.
- Breast abscess is a severe complication of mastitis.

Etiology
- *Staphylococcus aureus* is the main pathogen. Gram-negative bacilli and group A streptococcus are the less common pathogens.

Symptoms and Signs
- Mastitis is more common in the first few months of life and during the pubescent and postpubescent periods. It is also more common in girls than boys.
- Rarely, spreads bilaterally or beyond the extra mammary tissue.

Treatment
- Incision and drainage should be avoided, if possible, since it may cause permanent damage and deformity.
- Early aggressive intravenous antibiotic therapy obviates the need for surgery.
- Figures A and B.

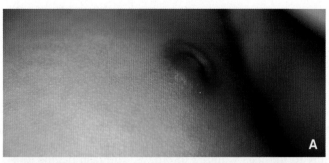

Figure A: A 6-month-old boy with increasing swelling of the left breast for 2 weeks, worse for the last 2 days. He looked well and afebrile. His left breast was red, swollen, warm, tender and the nipple was bulging. He was treated successfully with oral antibiotic.

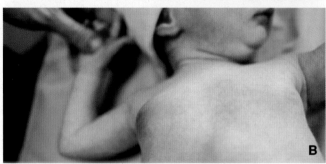

Figure B: A 10-day-old boy with a few hours history of swelling of the right breast. The right breast was swollen, red, warm, but nontender to palpation. His nipple was bulging, he was afebrile, and otherwise looked well. He was treated successfully with oral antibiotic.

MEASLES (RUBEOLA)

Definition
- Measles is an exanthematous disease characterized by fever, coryza, and cough with predictable stages of disease. Measles can have severe and life-threatening complications.

Etiology
- Measles is caused by paramyxovirus, genus morbillivirus.

History
- Measles has been responsible for the death of millions of children throughout the centuries. Successful immunization programs had almost eradicated this disease from the industrialized countries in the last century. But the unfortunate and unsubstantiated claim linking the measles vaccine with the rise in autism caused a decline in the number of children immunized. This drop in immunization in the developed world was soon followed by a rise in the disease itself.
- Overcrowding, under nutrition or malnutrition, vitamin deficiencies (particularly Vitamin A deficiency), and the higher incidence in the younger age group makes this disease more deadly in the developing world.
- The author has been witness to the tragic consequences of measles, a preventable disease, in Tehran/Iran. Blindness following measles's encephalitis. Ear drainages that never seem to end, laryngotracheobronchitis which left a young couple to mourn the loss of their child. Pneumonia complications resistant to all available antibiotics available in Iran. I have witnessed countless tragic deaths as a result of measles epidemics in Iran.

Symptoms and Signs
- Measles is highly contagious with the maximum dissemination of the virus by droplet spray during the prodromal period.
- Measles has three stages:
  - Stage 1. The initial incubation period lasting 10 to 12 days. Patients may transmit the disease from the seventh day.

- Stage 2. The prodromal period (can be severe) lasting 3 to 5 days with low to moderate fever, coryza, dry cough, photophobia, and conjunctivitis. This is followed by Koplik spots. Koplik spots, the pathognomonic sign of measles, are grayish-white spots, mostly the size of grains of sand with reddish areolae which appear opposite the lower molars, but may be elsewhere on the oral mucosa. Koplik spots appear 2 to 3 days before the measles rash and fade within 12 to 18 hours of their appearance.
- Stage 3. The final stage begins with a sudden high fever and rash. The rash begins with faint macules on the upper lateral parts of the neck, along the hair line, and behind the ears, and on the posterior parts of the cheeks and then spreads to the arms, chest, abdomen, and finally to the legs within 2 to 3 days. The rash begins to fade from head and neck and toward the feet, in the same order that it appeared.
- The rash is more confluent and more prominent in the more severe cases of disease.
- Otitis media, pneumonia, and encephalitis are the most common complications of measles. Hemiplegia, cerebral thrombophlebitis, Guillain–Barré syndrome, and retrobulbar neuritis are rare complications.
- Measles manifestations are more severe and complications are more fatal in HIV positive as well as in the malnourished child.
- Measles can aggravate existing tuberculosis.

Treatment

- Supportive treatment.
- Vitamin A supplementation should be considered in the treatment of children 6 months to 2 years of age.
- Prevention is possible with the administration of two doses of the measles vaccine as part of the MMR vaccine at the age of 12 to 15 months and at 4 to 6 years.

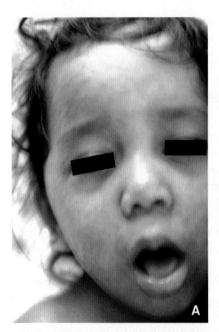 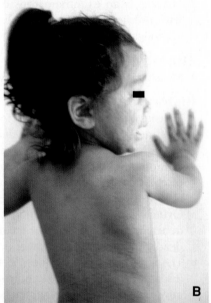

Figures A–B: This 2-year-old girl was brought in for 5 days of increasing fever, cough, runny nose, loss of appetite, and increasing rash. The rash had started the previous day on her face and then spread to the chest and to the extremities over a 3-day period. She had been previously healthy, immunizations were up-to-date except for her MMR (Mumps, Measles, and Rubella) vaccine. The mother refused MMR due to the fear of autism. Patient looked ill. Her temperature was 39.7°C, injected conjunctivae and pharynx and inflamed oral mucosa. Her entire body was covered with a maculopapular rash. There were a few small palpable lymph nodes in the groins. No Koplik spots. Her lungs were clear and her chest x-ray was negative. Her measles's IgM titer was positive and her IgG titers were negative.

figures continues

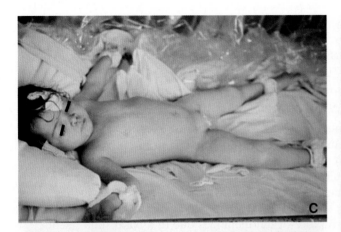

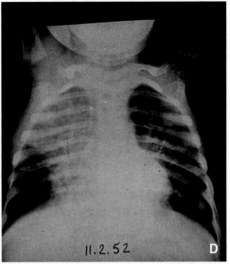

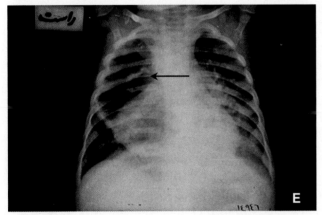

(figures cont.) **Figures C–E:** This 10-month-old girl was admitted with a 3-day history of high fever, a 1-day history of shortness of breath, and a husky voice. Her lungs were clinically clear. No Koplik spots. Both tympanic membranes were inflamed. Initial chest x-ray was negative. She was placed in an oxygen tent, humidifier and given broad spectrum antibiotics. Her condition worsened 2 days later with elevated temperature and a diffuse maculopapular rash. Her breathing became more labored, rapid, and shallow. Subsequent chest x-ray showed a large right upper lobe consolidation compatible with pneumonia **(Figure D)**.

Figure E: A chest x-ray, a few days later, demonstrates a lucent area in the location of the pneumonia. This finding is most compatible with a pneumatocele which is a thin-walled cyst commonly due to infection or trauma.

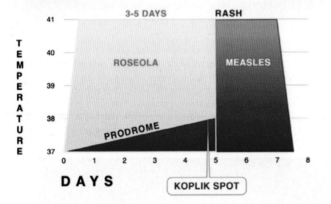

Fever pattern and rash in measles and roseola.

MENINGITIS

Definition
■ Meningitis is the infection and inflammation of the meninges or spinal cord by a microorganism.

Etiology
■ Viruses, bacteria, fungus, and protozoa can cause meningitis.
■ The bacterial etiology in meningitis is age-dependent:

1. <1 month: Group B streptococcus, *Escherichia coli*, *Listeria monocytogenes,* and *Streptococcus pneumoniae.*

2. Four to six weeks: *Haemophilus influenzae* type b, *E. coli, S. pneumoniae,* and group B streptococcus.

3. Six weeks to six years: *S. pneumoniae, Neisseria meningitidis, H. influenzae* type b.

4. >6 years: *S. pneumoniae* and *N. meningitidis.*

- Many viruses such as herpes, mumps, and coxsackie can cause meningitis.
- Tuberculosis and tuberculous meningitis have been on the rise in recent years. Tuberculosis mostly affects children from 6 months to 6 years of age. This is accompanied with miliary tuberculosis in 50% of cases.
- Certain factors such as close contact, lack of immunity to certain pathogens, living in dormitories and overcrowding, specific host defects, splenic dysfunction, asplenia, T-lymphocyte defects, CSF leaks, rupture of the meninges due to a basal skull fracture, lumbosacral dermal sinus, and meningomyelocele and CSF shunt all increase the risk of meningitis.

Symptoms and Signs

- A few days of upper respiratory infection symptoms, fever, vomiting, headache, backache, irritability, myalgia, arthralgia, tachycardia, purpura, bulging fontanelle, neck rigidity, Kernig's sign, Brudzinski's sign, lethargy, potentially seizure, and coma.
- This course may run much faster in some cases and lead to death.
- The triad of fever, headache, and vomiting, which is common in a variety of other diseases, should always bring the possibility of meningitis to mind. If the triad is accompanied by nuchal rigidity or a bulging fontanelle, meningitis needs to rise to the top of the list of possible diseases.
- Lumbar puncture and the examination of the CSF are essential for proper diagnosis, although in potentially serious cases, treatment may have to be initiated before the LP is done.
- The CSF changes are different in each of bacterial, viral, fungal, protozoal, and tuberculous meningitis.

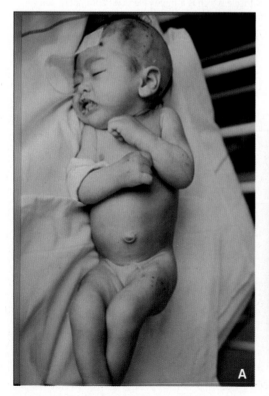

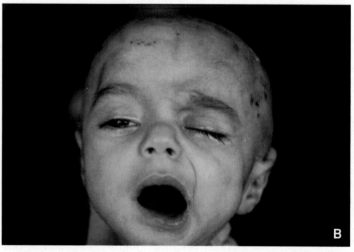

Figures A–B: This 10-month-old girl was brought in for vomiting and diarrhea of 2 days duration, and "for teething," according to the parents. She was lethargic and in the state of shock on admission, had depressed fontanelle and all her veins were collapsed, making it very difficult to start an IV. Her CSF was turbid, with low sugar, high protein, and high WBCs (mainly polymorphs). The gram stain and culture of the CSF showed H. flu. She was treated successfully **(Figure A)**. **Figure B** demonstrates a right sided facial palsy postpneumococcal meningitis.

figures continues

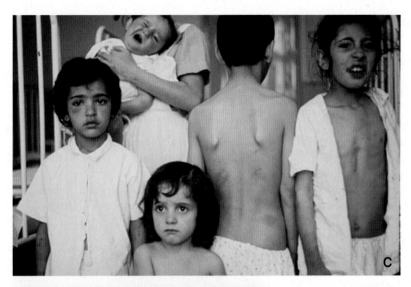

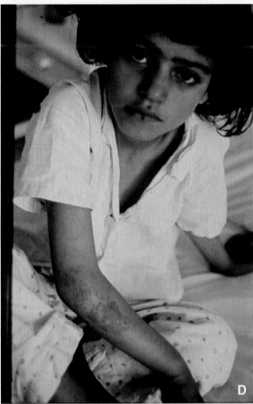

(figures cont.) **Figures C–D:** Reactivation and eruption of herpes simplex on the lips, around the mouth, below the right eye, on the back, below the left jaw, and right arm a few days after the onset of meningococcal meningitis. This was during an epidemic of meningococcal meningitis in Tehran, Iran. We were forced to admit 535 children to a 40-bed Children's Hospital during this epidemic. Many were kept in the ER. Many mothers served as "nurses" to help the under-staffed medical team. Note, left facial palsy in one of the children **(Figure C)**.

Treatment
- Treatment depends on the age of the child and on the offending pathogen.
- Supportive care, adequate IV fluid intake, electrolyte assessments, regular neurologic examinations, adequate ventilation, and cardiac support.
- Regular immunization for *N. meningitidis, S. pneumoniae,* and *H. influenzae* has reduced the incidence of these types of meningitis in the developed world.

MENINGOCELE

(See Neural Tube defect).

MICROPHTHALMIA (MICROPHTHALMOS)

Definition
- Any congenital abnormality, or pathology, causing a smaller size eye or eyes.
- It may present with abnormalities of cornea, lens, or retina.

Etiology
- Ocular disease, inflammation, or developmental defect.
- Persistent hyperplastic primary vitreous can cause microphthalmia with cataract and retinal or optic nerve abnormalities.
- Fetal alcohol syndrome, infections during pregnancy (e.g., rubella, herpes simplex, cytomegalovirus), and genetic syndromes (e.g., trisomy 13, triploid syndrome).

Symptoms and Signs
- A small globe inside the orbit.

Treatment
- Management of the underlying etiology.
- Orbital expanders and prosthesis.

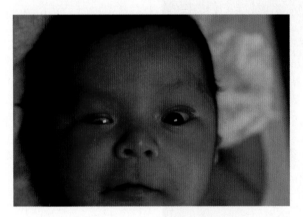

Right microphthalmia. He also has oculoauriculo-vertebral spectrum. There are additional images of him in that section.

MICROTIA

(See Congenital External Auditory Canal Stenosis/Atresia).

MILIA (L. Pleural of milium)

Definition
- Milia are small, white cysts commonly found on the skin and on the oral mucosa at any age, but most commonly in the newborns.

Etiology
- Retention of laminated, keratinized material.

Symptoms and Signs
- Milia are characterized by 1 to 2 mm in diameter, opalescent white, pearly, firm lesions.
- In the neonates, milia are scattered on the face, mostly on the nose and the gingiva.
- Milia present in the midline of the palate are called Epstein pearls.

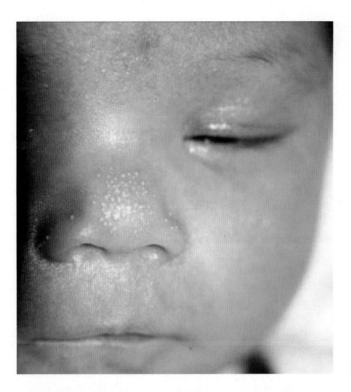

Milia in a 5 day old infant.

Treatment

- Milia are self-limiting.
- Persistent milia in older children are a cosmetic concern and can be drained.

MILIARIA (Milium L., millet)

Definition

- Cutaneous changes associated with sweat retention and leakage at different levels of the dermis.

Etiology

- Prolonged sweating with keratin plugging of sweat glands and the interruption of the normal flow of sweat into the skin.

Symptoms and Signs

- Miliaria is a papulovesicular rash which can present as the three following types:
  1. Miliaria rubra (prickly heat): The most common type found mostly on the occluded areas of the skin and especially the upper trunk. Discrete, but closely aggregated small erythematous papules or papulovesicles. Heat, swaddling, and high fever can lead to miliaria rubra (Figure A).
  2. Miliaria crystallina: These are asymptomatic, 1- to 2-mm, thin-walled, clear, noninflammatory vesicles seen on healthy looking skins, in crops, occurring most frequently on the intertriginous areas.
  3. Miliaria profunda: These are 1- to 3-mm papules, related to a deeper level of obstruction, seen mostly in the tropics, following repeated crops of miliaria rubra. Rare in infants and children.

Treatment

- Miliaria is a self-limited disease.
- Prevention of heat, humidity, and overclothing is all that is needed.

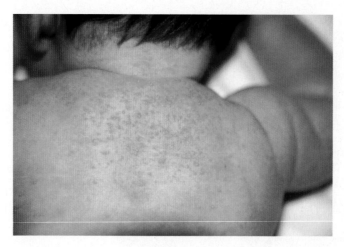

Miliaria in a 7 day old infant.

MILROY'S DISEASE

Definition
- A hereditary abnormality of the lymphatic system; most commonly affecting the lower extremities.

Etiology
- Milroy's disease is inherited in a dominant form with the possibility of skipped generations. Approximately 85% to 90% of individuals who have FLT4 develop lower limb lymphedema. FLT4 is the only known gene associated with this disease.

Symptoms and Signs
- Uncomplicated Milroy's disease is often asymptomatic.
- The most common finding in this disease is lymphedema of the lower limbs, mostly bilateral, and usually present at birth or soon after birth.
- Edema varies in severity and improves with time.
- Hydrocele, prominent veins, and upslanting toenails can be seen in some cases.

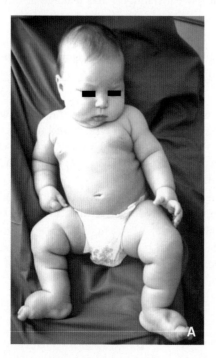

Figure A: This infant was born with pitting edema of both legs and arms which gradually increased over the first 10 months of life and has since diminished. Her mother has lymphedema of the left leg that she claims followed a febrile illness at the age of 20 years. The baby's 7-year-old cousin was born with bilateral edema of the legs. She looked clinically well, had a systolic murmur suggestive of peripheral pulmonary stenosis. Urinalysis, serum protein, and karyotype were normal. 41 days old **(Figure A)**, 3 months old **(Figures B and C)**, 2 years old **(Figure D)**, and 3 years and 10 months old **(Figure E)**.

figures continues

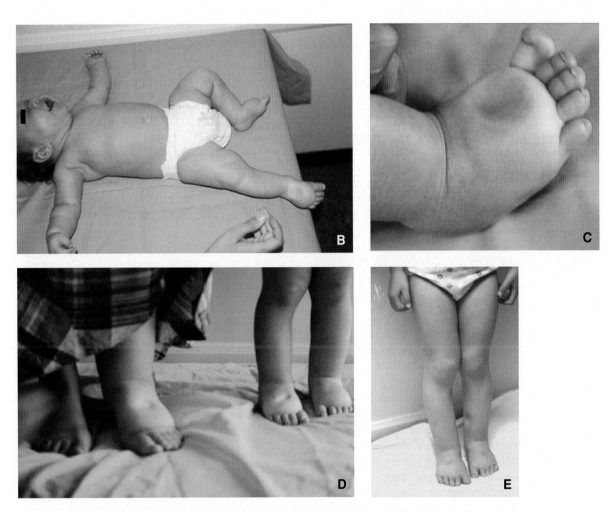

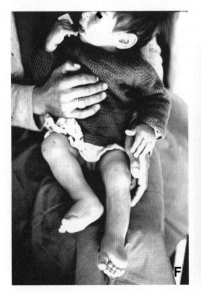

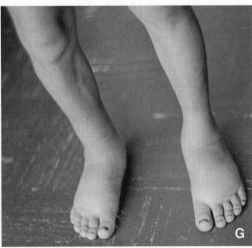

(figures cont.) **Figure D:** Pitting edema of the legs in this 2-year-old girl and edema of the left leg in her mother.

Figures F–G: A 6-month-old girl with pitting edema of the feet since birth. Otherwise well. She had edema of both legs up to below the knee **(Figure F)**. Her serum protein, karyotype, and urine analysis were normal. She is 7 years old, with some edema on the dorsum of her feet and visible veins on her legs **(Figure G)**.

Treatment

■ Treatment is mostly the management of the edema by massage and fitting stockings.

PIGMENTED MOLES AND NEVI

(Mole, a.s. spot).

MELANOCYTIC NEVUS (NEVOCYTIC NEVUS)

Definition

■ A nevus is a type of hamartoma representing a well circumscribed and stable malformation of the skin, or less frequently, oral mucosa, which is believed to be hereditary.
■ Pigmented moles and nevi are the most common neoplasms found in humans.
■ Just over 1% of babies are born with nevi, but they are more common in black babies.

Etiology

■ Genetics and sunlight.

Symptoms and Signs

■ The most common types of moles are skin tags, raised moles, and flat moles.
■ They can be flat, slightly elevated, dome shaped, nodular, verrucous, polypoid, or papillomatous.
■ Benign moles are normally circular or oval, not very large, some may have coarse hair.
■ The incidence increases throughout life until puberty and gradually fades in later life.
■ The pigmentation and size of the nevi increase at puberty, with pregnancy, and with the use of steroids and estrogen.
■ Melanocytes may remain in the dermis after birth and cause mongolian spots, blue nevi, the nevi of Ota and Ito.
■ There are three types of nevi:
  1. Junction nevi with nevus cells located at dermoepidermal junction.
  2. Intradermal nevi with nevus cells within the dermis.
  3. Compound nevi which is a combination of the above.

Treatment

■ Exposure to sunlight should be limited, particularly in children with lighter skin color.
■ A biopsy may be necessary whenever there is a suspected malignancy in a mole.
■ Moles should be regularly checked for any changes in size, shape, color, texture, spontaneous bleeding, or itching. The mole should be removed if signs or symptoms suggestive of malignancy are present.
■ Figures A–H.

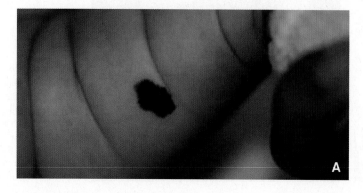

Figure A: A 6 × 12 mm black, flat, congenital melanocytic nevus in a 2-month-old girl.

figures continues

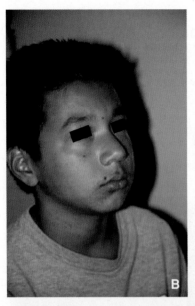

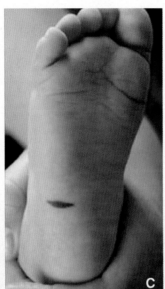

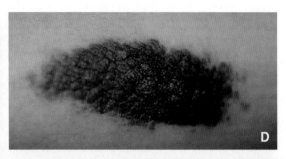

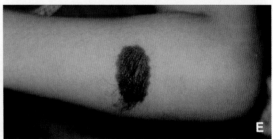

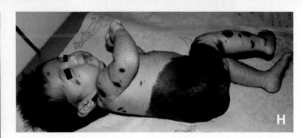

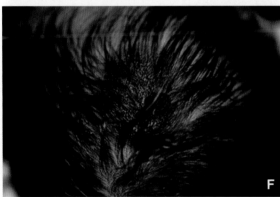

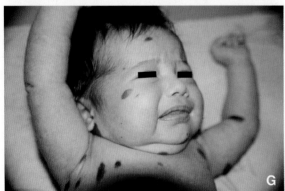

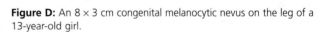

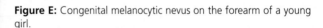

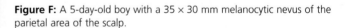

(figures cont.) **Figure B:** A 12-year-old boy with multiple melanocytic nevi on his face and neck.

Figure C: Nevus on sole of foot of a 1 year old girl.

Figure D: An 8 × 3 cm congenital melanocytic nevus on the leg of a 13-year-old girl.

Figure E: Congenital melanocytic nevus on the forearm of a young girl.

Figure F: A 5-day-old boy with a 35 × 30 mm melanocytic nevus of the parietal area of the scalp.

Figures G–H: A 2-month-old infant with many congenital pigmented nevi of different sizes and shapes and a large bathing trunk nevus.

BECKER'S NEVUS (BECKER'S MELANOSIS)

Definition
- A congenital or acquired benign nevus found more commonly during adolescence mostly on the chest and shoulder.

Etiology
- Unknown.

Symptoms and Signs

- Becker's nevus is an irregular, hyperpigmented patch with occasional hypertrichosis occasionally surrounded by hyperpigmented islands without any other abnormality. More common in males.
- It begins as an irregular, brown, pigmentation on the back, chest, or upper arms and then expands to 10 to 15 cm in size.

Treatment

- Laser treatment can occasionally be helpful.

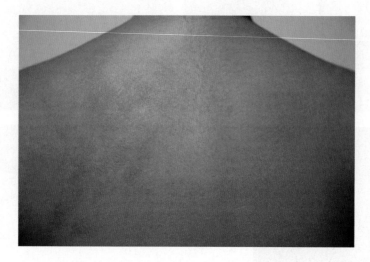

This 14-year-old boy has recently noted this hyperpigmented patch on the left side of his back.

LINEAR SEBACEOUS NEVUS

Definition

- Nevus sebaceous of Jadassohn is a common congenital lesion, predominantly composed of sebaceous glands.
- Linear sebaceous nevus syndrome and epidermal nevus syndrome are often used interchangeably, but are not identical lesions.

Etiology

- A congenital hamartoma.

Symptoms and Signs

- A well-circumscribed plaque, mostly solitary, which appear mainly on the face and scalp.
- The lesions are hairless, yellow to tan-colored plaques, oval or linear, with a surface that can be velvety or rough, and from a few millimeters to several centimeters in size.
- Other abnormalities may be found in other organs including the central nervous system, skeletal, and cardiovascular system with multiple linear sebaceous nevus as part of the epidermal nevus syndrome, called Schimmelpenning syndrome.
- Figures A–C.

Treatment

- Surgery.

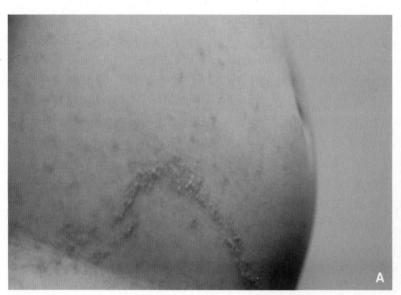
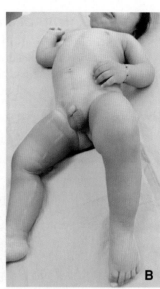

Figures A–B

FRECKLES (EPHELIDES, Gr. Ephelis)

- Freckles are found mostly in fair skin or red-hair children commonly around 2 to 4 years of age, become more conspicuous during the summer, fade during the winter and adult life. These light-brown macules are <3 mm in diameter, present mostly on sun-exposed areas of the face, and have an increased risk of developing into a melanoma. Treatment is by avoidance of sun exposure, full spectrum sun screens, and laser.
- Figures A and B.

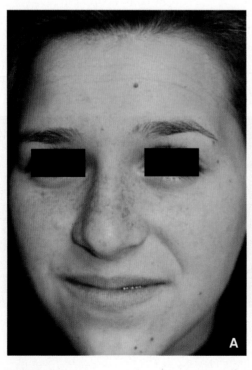
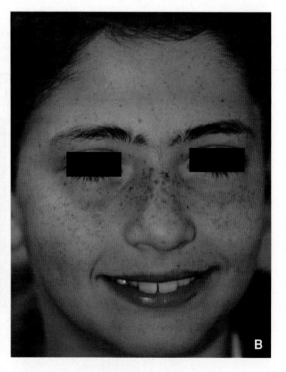

Figures A–B

NEVUS, INTRADERMAL

- Acquired nevi also known as moles are composed of melanocytes. These cells are grouped in collections within the first and second layers of the skin. They have a wide range of presentation and can occur on any surface of the skin or mucous membranes including the nail beds (Figure A).

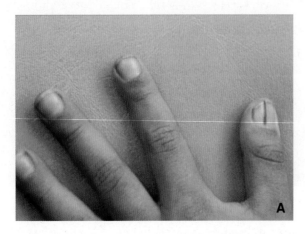

Figure A: A uniform linear band of pigment within the nail plate.

NEVUS OF OTA (NEVUS FUSCOCERULEUS OPHTHALMOMAXILLARIS, OCULODERMAL MELANOSIS)

Definition

- Nevus of Ota is a hamartoma of dermal melanocytes.

Etiology

- Nevus of Ota mostly affects Asians, is congenital in approximately 50% of the cases. In others it often develops in the second decade of life.

Symptoms and Signs

- Nevus of Ota is mostly unilateral, blue, bluish-gray, or brown in color, irregularly patchy, discoloration of the eye and face in the dermatomes supplied by trigeminal nerve's first and second division.
- The periorbital region, the malar area, the forehead, the temple, and the nose are the areas most often involved (Figures A and B).

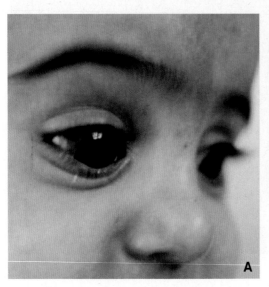

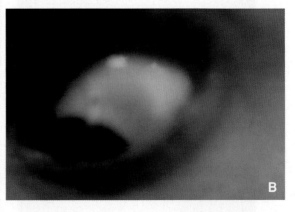

Figures A–B: Nevus of Ota in the right eye of a 1-year-old girl.

- Rare, but possible associated disorders are cutaneous, ocular or intracranial melanosis, intradermal melanocytosis, ipsilateral glaucoma, nevus flammeus, cutis marmorata telangiectasia congenita, Sturge–Weber syndrome, and Klippel–Trenaunay syndrome.
- Lesions are permanent, but the intensity of the color may change.

Treatment
- Laser therapy if required for cosmetic reasons.

MOLLUSCUM CONTAGIOSUM

Definition
- Molluscum contagiosum is a common skin infection.

Etiology
- It is caused by the molluscum contagiosum virus, a member of the Poxviridae. The incubation period is 2 to 6 months.
- Overcrowding and poor hygiene increase the prevalence. Direct contact, fomite, and autoinoculation are the main causes of transmission. Swimming pools and public bath have been implicated in some cases.

Symptoms and Signs
- Molluscum contagiosum is characterized by sharply circumscribed, dome shaped, centrally umbilicated, 1 to 5 mm papules with waxy surfaces. They can be pruritic and may number from one to hundreds (Figures A–E).
- Spontaneous regression may take months or years; often leaving no scar after regression.

Treatment
- If required, includes curetting, freezing with liquid nitrogen, electrocautery, CO_2 laser, and cantharidin.

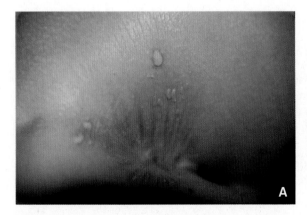

Figure A: A 2-year-old girl with a 2-week history of rash in the diaper area. Biopsy confirmed the clinical diagnosis of molluscum contagiosum. Our investigation of possible sexual abuse was unsuccessful.

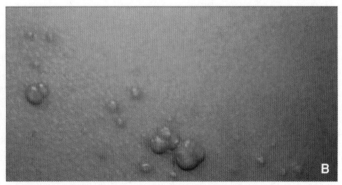

Figure B: Close-up view of a few molluscum lesions.

figures continues

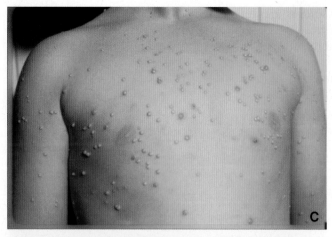

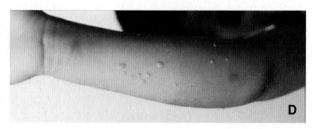

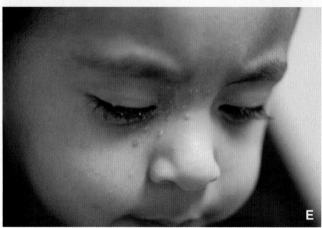

(figures cont.) **Figures C–D:** Dry and eczematous skin and constant itching, helped autoinoculate and spread molluscum throughout the body.

Figure E: Increasing molluscum contagiosum around the eyes of a 21-month-old boy. The eczematous skin and constant rubbing have contributed to the spread of infection.

MONGOLIAN SPOTS (CONGENITAL DERMAL MELANOCYTOSIS)

Definition
- Mongolian spots are benign, congenital, hyperpigmented macules that are present at birth.

Etiology
- Melanocyte produces melanin and transfers it to the keratinocytes and hair cells. Melanocytes migrate from the neural crest, where they originate, with the nerves to the skin. Mongolian spots are melanocytes that have remained in the dermis.

Symptoms and Signs
- Mongolian spots are bluish-grey in color, found in different shapes and sizes, very common in Chinese, Japanese, Africans, and Mongols; and much less common in Caucasians (Figures A–C).

Treatment
- Reassurance.
- Mongolian spots fade before the age of 3 years and rarely last up to 10 years of life.

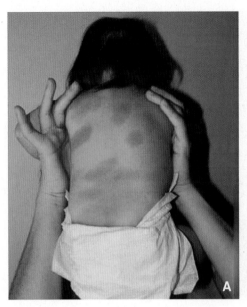 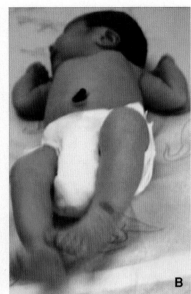 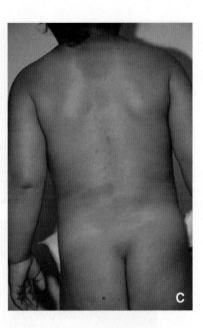

Figure A: Several mongolian spots on the back of a 3-week-old newborn.

Figure B: The parents of this 2-week-old boy believed the band the Nursery personnel put around his ankle had stained his skin.

Figure C: This baby girl was born with several mongolian spots, most of them have faded. But she still has a few at the age of 2 years.

MONILIASIS

(See Candidiasis).

MORPHEA (LOCALIZED SCLERODERMA)

Definition
- Morphea is a localized, circumscribed, nontender, hardening, depigmentation, and atrophy of the skin.

Etiology
- Unknown.

Symptoms and Signs
- An uncommon skin disorder, seen mostly in children and young adults.
- Morphea is ivory colored in the center and surrounded by a violaceous halo.
- The disorder can be divided into five subtypes: Plaque, localized, generalized, linear, and deep.
- Plaque morphea may evolve into generalized morphea.
- Linear morphea is typically unilateral.

Treatment
- There is no satisfactory treatment for morphea; however, the majority of the lesions resolve spontaneously within 3 to 5 years.

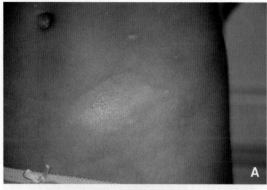

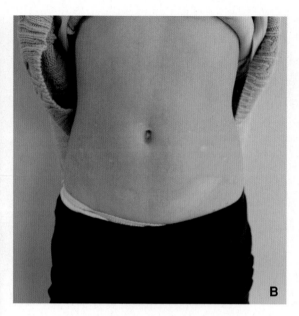

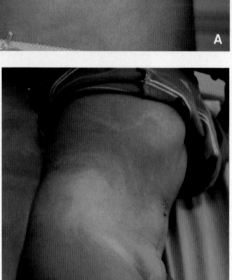

Figures A–B: The lesions were an incidental finding in this 9½-year-old girl who had noticed this asymptomatic, expanding white spot on her abdominal wall for the past 4 years. The smaller satellites are more recent. On examination, a silver–ivory plaque was noted on her abdominal wall with a few satellites around it. She presented with a 2-day history of abdominal pain. No fever, diarrhea, vomiting, or urinary symptoms. She looked well and her abdomen was soft and nontender. Her urinalysis showed four-plus sugar and her blood sugar was in the 400s.

Figure C: Morphea in a 2-year-old.

MUCOCELE

Definition
- Mucoceles are mucous retention cysts.

Etiology
- Trauma may cause rupture of the mucous duct and extravasation of sialomucin into the surrounding tissue.

Symptoms and Signs
- Asymptomatic, soft, translucent, whitish-blue, solitary lesions, often less than 1 cm in size and predominantly on the mucous surface of the lower lip (Figures A and B).
- It can also be seen on the gingivae, buccal mucosa, and the tongue.

Treatment
- Lesions often rupture spontaneously.
- Incision and drainage, surgical excision, and laser ablation.

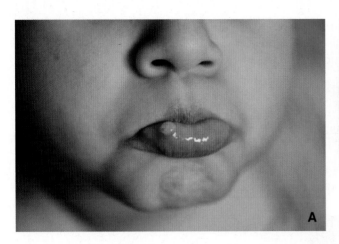

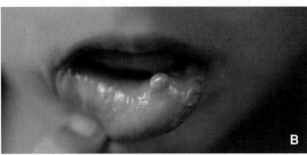

Figures A–B: Asymptomatic mucocele on the lower lip of two toddlers.

MUCOPOLYSACCHARIDOSIS

Definition
- The mucopolysaccharidosis is a heterogeneous group of metabolic disorders caused by the deficiency of lysosomal enzymes needed to degrade glycosaminoglycan. The disorders are characterized by intralysosomal accumulation of glycosaminoglycans causing impairment of cellular function.

Etiology
- Mucopolysaccharidoses involve deficiency of the enzyme needed to break down glycosaminoglycans (long chains of carbohydrates). Hurler syndrome is the best known and most severe form of the mucopolysaccharidoses. It is secondary to alpha-L-iduronidase deficiency and is inherited in an autosomal recessive pattern.
- Sphingolipidoses, or lipid storage disease, include Gaucher's, Niemann–Pick, Tay–Sachs, and leukodystrophies.
- Glycoproteinoses, resulting from defects in glycoprotein breakdown, include sialidosis, mannosidosis, and fucosidosis.
- Defects involving targeting of glycoproteins for lysosomes (mucolipidoses) and lysosomal membrane transport disorders (cystinosis).
- Each disorder has many known mutations and some patients are compound heterozygotes for rare alleles.
- The metabolism of dermatan sulfate, keratan sulfate, or heparan sulfate depends on the enzyme deficiency.

Symptoms and Signs
- Varies depending upon the exact nature of the enzymatic defect.
- Neurologic regression, progressive hepatosplenomegaly, coarsening of facial features, movement restriction of joints, peripheral neuropathy, and ataxia are some of the more common findings.
- Infants with Hurler syndrome typically look normal at birth; often presenting with umbilical or inguinal hernia. However, parents note the slow growth rate and progressive developmental delay by the end of the first year of life.
- Coarse facial features, flat midface, depressed nasal bridge, broad nose, prominent forehead, large tongue, and occasionally large tonsils become more evident by the second year of life.
- Heart disease, hepatosplenomegaly, dwarfism, corneal clouding, degeneration of retinas, and skeletal abnormalities known as the dysostosis-complex are the common findings.

- Death occurs by 10 years of age from a variety of complications.
- Diagnosis of lysosomal storage disease requires specific enzymatic assay on samples of urine, serum, white blood cells, or skin fibroblasts.
- Figures A–D.

Treatment
- Depends on the specific disease.
- There are no cures for these groups of disorders, and therefore, treatment is aimed toward alleviation of symptoms.
- Bone marrow transplantation and enzyme replacement therapy have become successful treatment options in certain disorders.

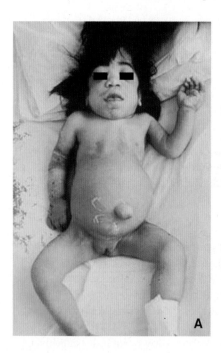
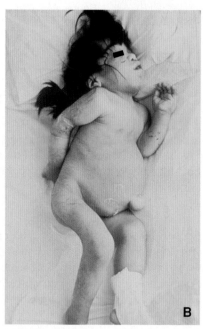

Figures A–B: This 18-month-old girl was brought in for severe developmental delay and an umbilical hernia. She was the product of a healthy-looking and young parents and an uncomplicated delivery. Her parents denied any similar cases in the family. She was delayed developmentally. Had coarse features, large head, hypertelorism, depressed nasal bridge, hepatosplenomegaly, thick lips, a prominent forehead, low-set-ears, gibbus, contracture of the hips and knees, broad hands, umbilical hernia, and hirsutism.

The following are blood smears of the above patient **(Figures C–D).**

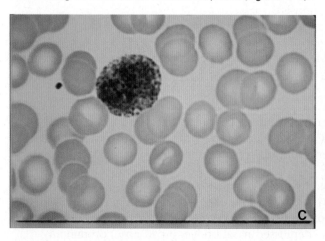
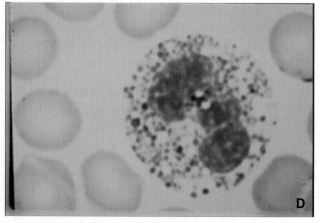

Figure C: Segmented neutrophil containing Alder's anomaly inclusions. Large, coarse, purple granules representing lysosomes filled with undegraded mucopolysaccharides.

Figure D: Alder's anomaly inclusion in a neutrophil that resembles toxic granulations. Alder's anomaly differs from toxic granulation in that all the neutrophils are affected. Alder's anomaly is associated with mucopolysaccharidosis, that is, Hurler syndrome.

MULTIPLE HEREDITARY EXOSTOSES

Definition
- A rare genetic disorder of the bone metaphases.

Etiology
- An autosomal dominant disorder.

Symptoms and Signs
- Multiple osteochondromas, short stature, deformity of upper and lower extremities, inequality of limb length, and premature partial physeal arrest.
- Exostoses can be cartilaginous or osteocartilaginous growth.
- The lesions may be solitary or multiple, usually located on the metaphyseal areas of long bones with the apex of long bone directed toward the diaphysis, which are benign, with rare cases of sarcomatous changes.
- Exostoses can be asymptomatic, or may cause pressure on the tendon, nerve, or interfere with the joint function.
- The main radiographic distribution of the exostoses in order of frequency is distal femur, proximal tibia, proximal humerus, scapula, distal radius, distal ulna, and proximal fibula.

Treatment
- Surgery to remove the exostosis when symptomatic. Recurrence is common.
- Figures A–F.

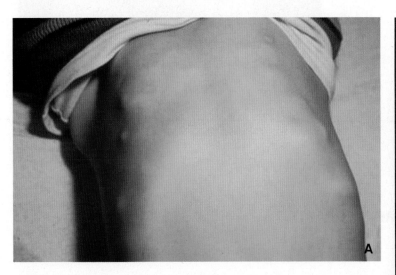

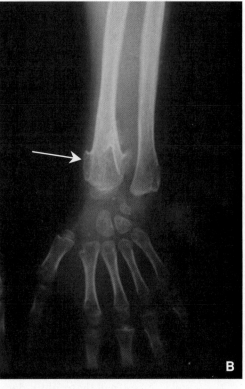

Figure A: Multiple congenital exostoses of the ribs in an 11-year-old boy.

Figures B–C: Wrist x-rays: Multiple bony exostoses which are continuous with the bone cortex and medullary marrow space (*hallmark*). Note how these pedunculated exostoses are directed away from the joint space, which is characteristic of this type. This benign lesion ceases to grow after skeletal maturation. Malignant transformation is rare (3% to 5% in MHE), however should be suspected if growth continues after skeletal maturation or if pain is present in the absence of fracture, bursitis, or nerve compression.

figures continues

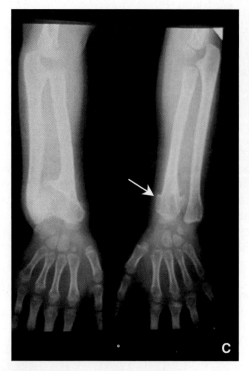

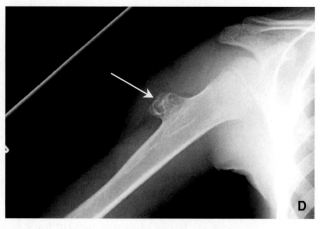

(figures cont.) **Figure D:** Humerus x-ray: Another example of a pedunculated exostosis of the proximal humerus (arrow).

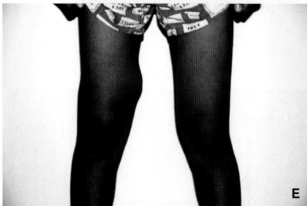

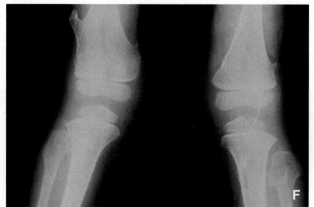

Figures E–F: Exostosis at the distal end of the right femur.

MULTIPLE LENTIGINES SYNDROME (LEOPARD SYNDROME)

Definition
■ A rare disease with multiple organ system involvement.

Etiology
■ An autosomal dominant disease with variable expression.

Symptoms and Signs
■ Skin changes include lentiginosis, café-au-lait spots, axillary freckling, onychodystrophy (nail dystrophy), dermatoglyphics, interdigital webs, hyper elastic skin, pectus abnormalities, and steatoma multiplex.

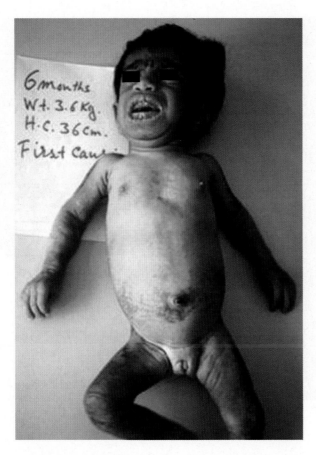

This infant girl was brought in for diarrhea and oral thrush. Note skin changes (lentiginosis), hypertelorism, and pectus carinatum. She also had pulmonary stenosis.

- Abnormalities of cardiovascular system (i.e., hypertrophic cardiomyopathy, conduction defects, and pulmonary stenosis), genitourinary system (i.e., cryptorchidism and hypospadias), growth retardation, sensorineural deafness, and hypertelorism.
- Leopard syndrome and Noonan syndrome are allelic disorders.

Treatment
- These children need several referrals to different specialists related to their abnormalities.

MUMPS

Definition
- Mumps is an acute infectious disease of primarily the parotid glands.
- In the pre-vaccine era, mumps used to be a common cause of pediatric illness and of severe epidemics. Mumps remains a problem in primarily unvaccinated children and in the developing countries.

Etiology
- Mumps virus is an RNA virus from the genus Paramyxovirus.

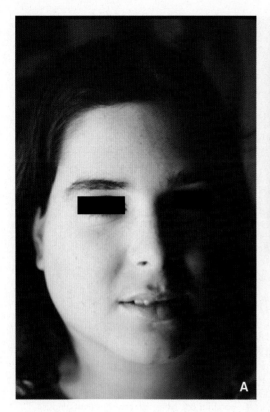

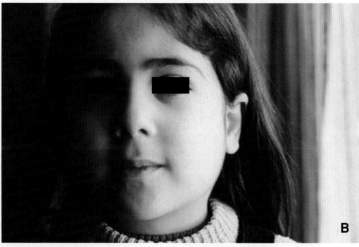

Figures A–B: Swelling of the right parotid gland in **Figure A** and the left parotid gland in **Figure B**. Both girls contracted mumps in the pre-vaccination era.

Symptoms and Signs

- The incubation period is from 14 to 24 days.
- Pain and swelling in one parotid gland, followed in 2 to 3 days with swelling of the other parotid gland.
- The swelling of the parotid gland is tender and unilateral in approximately 25% of cases.
- Swelling subsides within 3 to 7 days in the majority of cases.
- Redness and swelling may be present at the opening of Stensen duct.
- Swelling of the submandibular glands, edema of the homolateral pharynx and palate, and low-grade fever are other manifestations of the disease.
- Mumps spreads through direct contact and by contaminated fomites.
- Diagnosis is primarily clinical.
- A rise in the IgM antibody titers occurs within the first few days of disease and a four-fold rise in the IgG antibody titers is considered diagnostic.
- Mumps virus can be cultured from the saliva, urine, blood, and CSF.
- Complications are meningoencephalomyelitis (the most common complication), orchitis, epididymitis, oophoritis, pancreatitis, arthritis, thyroiditis, myocarditis, deafness, and dacryoadenitis.
- Figures A and B.

Treatment

- Symptomatic treatment with acetaminophen and ibuprofen.
- Prevention is by administration of the mumps vaccine at 12 to 15 months and a booster at 4 to 6 years of life.

MUSCULAR DYSTROPHY (Trophe Gr., nourishment)

DUCHENNE MUSCULAR DYSTROPHY (DMD), BECKER MUSCULAR DYSTROPHY (BMD)

Definition
- Muscular dystrophy refers to a group of progressive, degenerative, and inherited disorders of primary myopathy leading to progressive muscular weakness.

Etiology
- X-linked recessive with mutation in dystrophin gene in about 70% of cases and new mutations in 30% of the cases.

Symptoms and Signs
- Carriers are normally asymptomatic.
- Affected girls (based on the Lion theory of dormant healthy X chromosome) are much less symptomatic than boys.
- The majority of asymptomatic carriers have high serum creatine phosphokinase (CK).
- In infancy: Hypotonia and poor head control.
- In toddlers: Hip girdle weakness, lordotic posture, Gowers' sign, and hip waddle (Trendelenburg gait).
- Scoliosis, which rapidly worsens after the child is wheelchair bound.

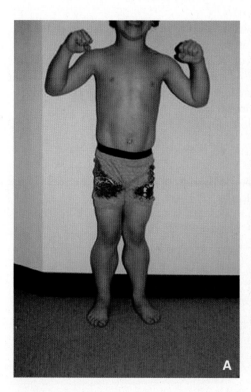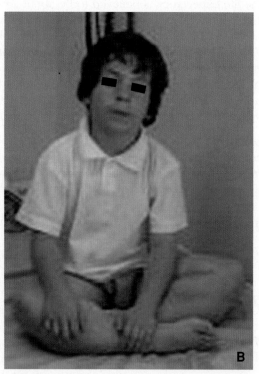

Figures A–C: The mother of this 6-year-old Caucasian boy had noticed her son's progressive weakness and his difficulty standing up from a sitting position. But she was always told "he is fine." No family history of myopathy. He looked healthy and muscular with pseudohypertrophy of the calves and forearm muscles. He had some degree of waddling gait and the Gowers' sign. His serum creatinine kinase was >5,000 (normal 23 to 200), CK index >300 (normal 0 to 10.4), AST (SGOT) 423 (normal 10 to 42), ALT (SGPT) 514 (normal 0 to 42). Duchenne–Becker muscular dystrophy deletion analysis: Mutations detected showed deletion of exons 45 to 52. Interpretation: Affected with DMD/BMD.

figures continues

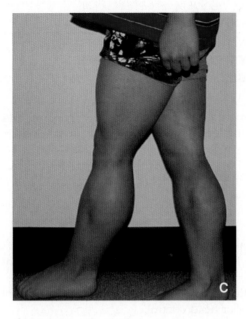

(figures cont.) **Figure C**

- Weak cough and pulmonary infections due to the involvement of the respiratory muscles.
- Aspiration, urethral and anal incontinence, contracture deformities, enlargement of the calves (pseudohypertrophy), and wasting of thigh muscles.
- Hypertrophy and fasciculation of the tongue, cardiomyopathy, and intellectual impairment.
- The life expectancy is believed to be about 25 years.
- High serum CK and other lysozyme enzymes such as aldolase and aspartase, muscle biopsy, and molecular genetics are very helpful in the diagnosis.
- DNA analysis of chorionic villi by southern blot or PCR for prenatal diagnosis is available as early as the 12th week of gestation.
- In Becker muscular dystrophy, life expectancy is slightly longer, there is severe learning problem and the disabilities manifest later than in DMD.
- Figures A–C (also an electronic video is available online).

Treatment
- Supportive treatment only.
- Treatment of pulmonary infections, cardiac decompensation, physiotherapy and delaying of scoliosis, immunizations, and adequate nutrition.

MYOTONIC CHONDRODYSTROPHY

(See Schwartz–Jampel syndrome).

MYOTONIA CONGENITA (THOMSEN DISEASE)

Definition
- Myotonia congenita is a rare genetic disease.

Etiology
- A genetic channelopathy (chloride channels).

Symptoms and Signs
- Characterized by hyper excitability, myotonia (tonic spasm and rigidity of certain muscles when an attempt is made to move them after a period of rest), and muscular hypertrophy.

M

- After a period of inactivity, the muscles stiffen and are difficult to maneuver but improve with increasing use and movement to near normal.
- Two types of myotonia congenita are recognized:
  1. Thomsen disease: Inherited as an autosomal dominant in which symptoms may present much earlier and even as early as during infancy.
  2. Becker disease: Transmitted as an autosomal recessive and may become symptomatic in later childhood.

Treatment
- The majority of patients improve with time.
- Figures A–C.

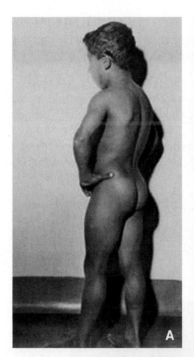
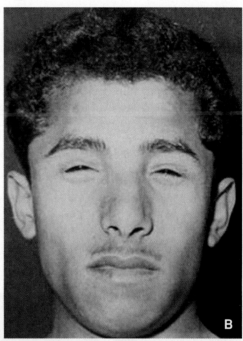
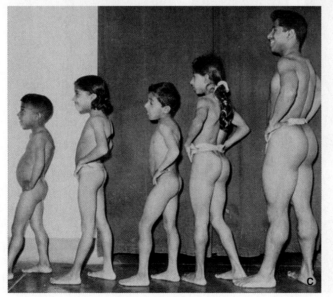

Figures A–C: The older brother had noticed the same problems in his younger siblings. They all had difficulty getting up from the sitting position on the floor. But once up and moving, they had fewer problems. The older sister's eyelids were also affected. They were all very thin and yet seemed to have areas of significant muscular hypertrophy. The oldest sibling had difficulty opening his eyes in the morning and also after closing them for a few minutes during the day **(Figures A and B)**. His sister, next to him in **Figure C**, had the same but less severe problem with her eyes. Parents were first cousins themselves and there were several generations of intermarriages in their families.

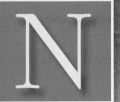

NEONATAL SEBACEOUS GLAND HYPERPLASIA

(See Milia).

NEPHROTIC SYNDROME

Definition
- Nephrotic syndrome is defined as a glomerular disorder with heavy proteinuria, hypoproteinemia, hypercholesterolemia, and edema.

Etiology
- Ninety percent of pediatric nephrotic syndromes are idiopathic, of which 85% are minimal change diseases, 5% are mesangial proliferation, and 10% are focal segmental glomerulosclerosis.
- Ten percent are secondary nephrotic syndromes, related to glomerular diseases (e.g., membranoproliferative glomerulonephritis and membranous nephropathy).

Symptoms and Signs
- The age range in idiopathic nephrotic syndrome is mostly between 2 and 6 years, with a peak incidence at 3 years.
- It is more common in boys (M/F ratio of 2/1).
- A minor infection, an insect bite, bee sting in particular, or poison ivy may precede the disease or future relapses.

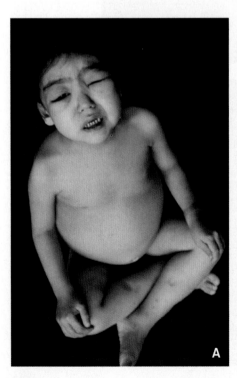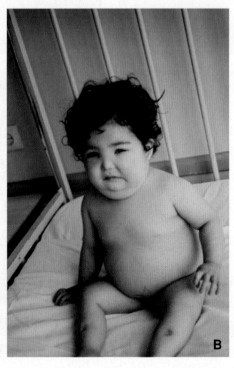

Figures A–B: Two children with nephrotic syndrome. Note the swelling of the face and abdomen, pitting edema, and the cushingoid face in **Figure B.** The child was unresponsive to treatment with steroid.

- Mild edema, as periorbital swelling and edema of the feet and ankles, which may progress to generalized edema, pleural effusion, ascites, and heavy proteinuria.
- Abdominal pain, anorexia, and diarrhea.
- Infrequent hypertension and gross hematuria.
- Serum albumin less than 2.5, high serum cholesterol and triglyceride, and spot urine protein to creatinine ratio exceeding 2.

Treatment:

- Restricted sodium intake, oral diuretics (there is the risk of thromboembolic complications), fluid restriction, intravenous administration of 25% human albumin, steroid for the minimal change disease, and cyclosporine are helpful.
- Angiotensin-converting enzyme (ACE) inhibitors and angiotensin II blockers are useful in children with steroid resistance.
- Relapse is common and an infection can lead to serious complications.

NEURAL TUBE DEFECT, CLOSED (DYSRAPHISM)

Definition
- Neural tube defects are the result of the failure of the neural tube to close properly.
- Anencephaly, myelomeningocele, meningocele, tethered cord, and spina bifida occulta are some of the more common neural tube defects.

Etiology
- Etiology is unknown, but chemicals, drugs, radiation, genetics, folate deficiency, and malnutrition are among the suspected causes.

Symptoms and Signs
- The presence of midline abnormalities in the back, such as a skin tag, a hemangioma, a hairy patch, or a subcutaneous lipoma, may suggest an underlying defect.

Treatment
- Early diagnosis and treatment is essential in preventing possible neurologic complications.

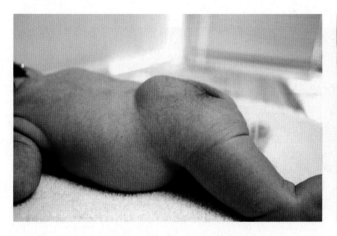
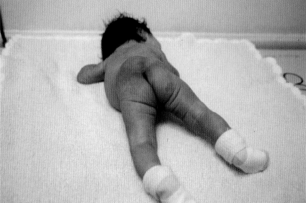

A 2-week-old baby girl with a subcutaneous lipoma on her back and covered by a small hemangioma. No neurologic findings.

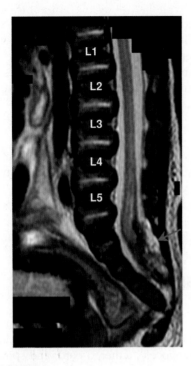

MRI lumbar spine (*white arrow*). Tethering of the cord to the L5–S1 level. The spinal cord should not extend below the inferior endplate of L2. Significant spinal dysraphism with an associated 1.3-cm intraspinal lipoma (*red arrow*) is causing tethering of the cord.

NEUROBLASTOMA

Definition
- Neuroblastoma is the most common and most deadly solid tumor of childhood.
- These tumors may regress spontaneously, especially in infants, may mature to a benign form of ganglioneuroma, or may be metastatic, unresectable, and ultimately fatal.

Etiology
- The majority of cases occur sporadically and some have a predisposition for the disease with malignant transformation possibly arising from the interaction of common DNA.

Symptoms and Signs
- Neuroblastoma can arise from any site within the sympathetic nervous system.
- They usually occur in the abdomen, and occasionally, the primary tumor cannot be found.
- The age at diagnosis is often around 5 years.
- Metastasis is through the lymphatic or the homogenous route.
- Symptoms are related to the location of the tumor.
- Figures A and B.

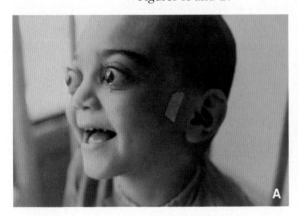
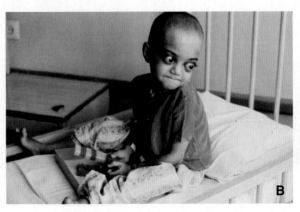

Figures A–B

Treatment

- Staging is very important in planning appropriate therapy (surgery, chemotherapy, or radiotherapy may be selected).

NEUROFIBROMATOSIS

Definition

- Neurofibromatosis is a multisystem disorder involving the nervous system with dermatologic manifestation. It may be present at birth.

Etiology

- Neurofibromatosis is an autosomal dominant disorder.

Symptoms and Signs

- Two distinct types are recognized: Neurofibromatosis 1 (NF1, also known as von Recklinghausen disease or generalized neurofibromatosis) and neurofibromatosis 2 (NF2, also called central or bilateral acoustic neurofibromatosis).
- Two out of the following seven features are necessary for the diagnosis of neurofibromatosis 1:
  1. Six or more café-au-lait spots equal to or greater than 5 mm each in the longest diameter in prepubertal children and 15 mm in the longest diameter in postpubertal patients (Café-au-lait spots may increase in size and number during early childhood).
  2. Two or more neurofibromas of any type or one plexiform neurofibroma.
  3. Freckling in the axillary or inguinal regions.
  4. Optic glioma (optic pathway glioma).
  5. Two or more Lisch nodules (iris hamartomas).
  6. A distinctive osseous lesion, such as sphenoid wing dysplasia or cortical thinning of the cortex of long bones, with or without pseudarthrosis.
  7. A first-degree relative (parent, sibling, or a child) with NF1 (Figures A–G).

Treatment

- Management is based on early detection, symptomatic treatment, and surgical removal of tumors, whenever possible.

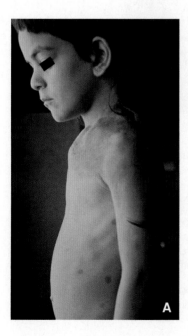

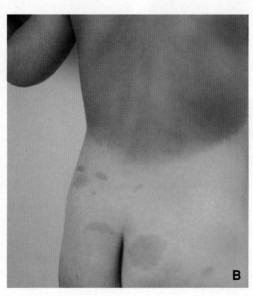

Figures A–B: Café-au-lait spots of different sizes and shades in a teenage boy and girl.

figures continues

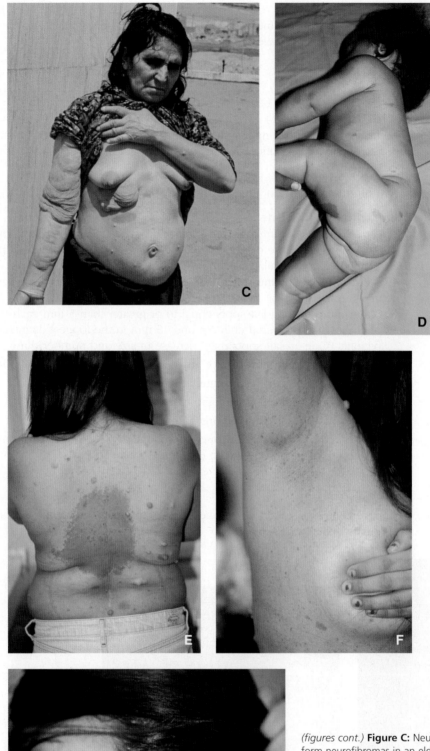

(figures cont.) **Figure C:** Neurofibromas and plexiform neurofibromas in an elderly woman.

Figure D: An asymptomatic 8-month-old girl,
with many café-au-lait spots and no other signs
of neurofibromatosis.

Figures E–G: Café-au-lait spots, axillary freckling,
and neurofibromas on the back and temporal
areas in a 19-year-old girl.

NEUROTIC EXCORIATION (PSYCHOGENIC EXCORIATION, DERMATITIS ARTEFACTA)

Definition
- Neurotic excoriations are self-induced skin lesions due to an irresistible urge, conscious or subconscious.

Etiology
- It is found mostly in patients with mood disorders, obsessive compulsive disorder, anxiety disorder, depressive disorder, borderline personality disorder, and impulse disorder.

Symptoms and Signs
- It may start with an itching rash or acne, but scratching or picking will continue long after the lesion has healed.
- Abrasions, excoriation, crusting, necrosis, purpura, and ulcers.
- Injuries are mostly inflicted with nails, teeth, and fingers. Patients may also use other tools to inflict harm.
- Lesions can be more common on one side of the body than the other, depending on the handedness of the patient.
- The out-of-reach parts of the body are mostly spared (Figures A and B).

Treatment
- They are mostly resistant to therapy, but treatment of the underlying lesion is the first step.
- Successful use of Unna's boot has been described.

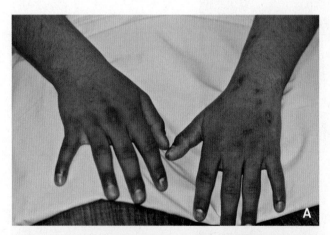

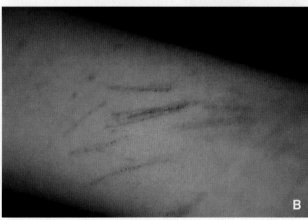

Figures A–B

NEVUS

(See Moles).

NOMA (Gr., eating sores), CANCRUM ORIS, AND GANGRENOUS STOMATITIS

Definition
- Gangrene of mouth and face.

Etiology
- *Fusiform bacilli, Bacteroides melaninogenicus,* and *Treponema vincentii.*

Symptoms and Signs
- It begins as a small vesicle on the gingiva, mostly in malnourished children, ulcerates, and causes necrosis, rapidly destroying large areas of the oral mucosa and face.

Treatment
- Appropriate and speedy antibiotic therapy.

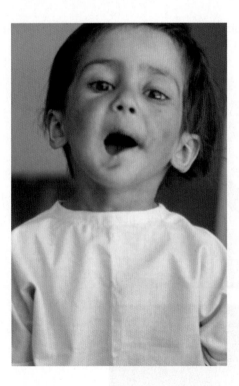

Destruction and deformity of the oral mucosa, lower jaw, and face in a severely malnourished child who developed some swelling of the jaw following a few days of toothache. She had a tactile fever and could not eat. Her face and jaw were badly damaged by the time she got to the hospital.

NOONAN SYNDROME

Definition
- Noonan syndrome, called after Dr. Jacqueline Noonan who first described the syndrome, is a clinically heterogeneous condition characterized by short stature, distinctive facial features, congenital heart disease, chest deformity, and other abnormalities.

Etiology

- It is an autosomal dominant disorder with complete penetrance and variable expressivity (in 61%, a genetic mutation is identifiable).

Symptoms and Signs

- The facial features are diagnostic. The characteristic features are more obvious during infancy, becoming more subtle later in adulthood.
- A large head, small face, tall forehead, narrowing at the temples, hypertelorism, epicanthal folds, ptosis, horizontal or down-slanting palpebral fissures, and a short, broad nose with depressed root and full tip.
- Posteriorly rotated, oval low-set ears, with thickening of the helix.
- Deeply grooved philtrum with high, wide peaks to the vermilion of the upper lip.
- Short neck with excess skin and low posterior hair line.
- Pectus carinatum superiorly and pectus excavatum inferiorly.
- Cardiovascular abnormalities: Pulmonary valve stenosis, atrial septal defect (ASD), and hypertrophic obstructive cardiomyopathy.
- Learning disability, lymphedema, and malignant hyperthermia can be seen.
- There is a remarkable change in the facial expression and features as these children march through infancy, toddlerhood, puberty, and adulthood (Figures A and B).

Treatment

- Genetic counseling; management of individual defects; periodic and regular supervision; and treatment of comorbidities.

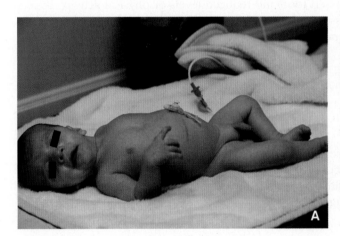 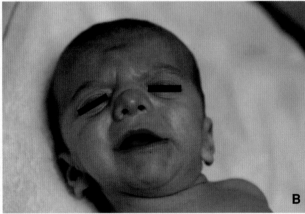

Figures A–B: This 4-month-old boy has young healthy parents and a healthy older sister. His mother had polyhydramnios. He had intestinal malrotation at birth. He has a short, broad nose with depressed root and full tip, low-set ears, cryptorchidism, and posteriorly rotated ears with thick helix. He has subaortic stenosis, hypertrophic cardiomyopathy, is a poor feeder, has GERD, has had Ladd's procedure, and required a gastrostomy tube placement. His diagnosis was confirmed by the Noonan sequential panel test.

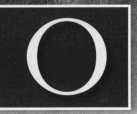

OBESITY (L. Obesus, fat)

Definition
- Obesity is the accumulation of excess fat in the body.
- World Health Organization definition of obesity:

BMI	Classification
<18.5	Underweight
18.5–24.9	Normal weight
25–29.9	Overweight
30–34.9	Class I obesity
35.5–39.9	Class II obesity
≤40	Class III obesity

Etiology
- Large-portion, high-calorie, processed food and reduced levels of physical activity (reducing physical education classes and increasing reliance on cars).
- Premature babies have an accelerated growth around 8 to 14 years of age and at risk of obesity.
- Insufficient sleep.
- Leptin and ghrelin, the two hormones that control appetite do not seem to have a major role in obesity.

Symptoms and Signs
- The obesity epidemic encompasses all age groups.
- Increasing weight for height (as above), acanthosis nigricans, stria, and high blood pressure.
- Elevated inflammatory markers, linked to heart disease later in life, are present in children as young as 3 years of age.
- Figures A–D.

Treatment
- Obesity in the first 6 months of life is associated with the highest prevalence of obesity as well as high blood pressure 5 to 10 years later.
- Treatment of obesity in children is frustrating for both parents and pediatricians. Therefore prevention becomes a priority. Parental awareness of the risks and metabolic consequences of obesity are important. Parents need to know the risk when solids are introduced to an infant early, again at the 1-year checkup, and regularly thereafter when we want to prevent a disease which is increasing in incidence, difficult to treat, and easier to prevent.
- Identification of infants at high risk of obesity is important.
- Most of these children miss breakfast, have a small lunch, and eat from the moment they get home until they go to bed. This is a habit that should be broken.
- Family, psychologist, nutritionist involvement, reward system, and daily regular physical activity are all helpful.

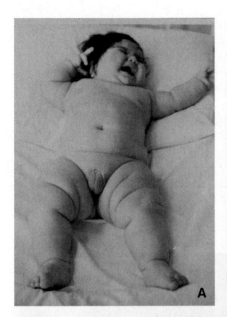

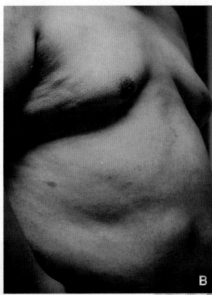

Figures A–B: A 1-year-old boy weighing 19.2 kg **(Figure A)** and an overweight teenage boy **(Figure B)**. Note the large abdomen and gynecomastia.

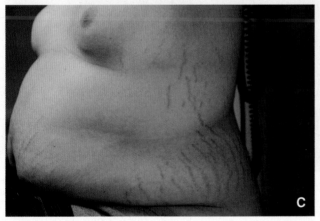

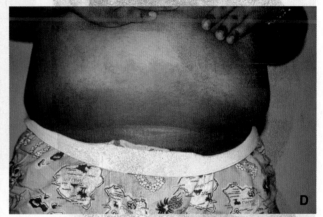

Figures C–D: A large abdomen, gynecomastia and stria in obesity **(Figure C),** and acanthosis nigricans **(Figure D)**.

OCULO-AURICULO-VERTEBRAL SPECTRUM (OAVS) (GOLDENHAR SYNDROME)

Definition
- Oculo-auriculo-vertebral syndrome and hemifacial microsomia are called the oculo-auriculo-vertebral spectrum.
- OAVS is a rare congenital defect characterized by epibulbar dermoids, auricular deformities, and vertebral anomalies. The spectrum includes additional findings.

Etiology
- Unknown.

Symptoms and Signs
- An often one-sided (more frequently right-sided), incomplete development of ear, soft palate, lip, nose, and mandible.
- Approximately 50% have additional abnormalities.

- Maxillary, temporal, and zygomatic hypoplasia; coloboma of the upper eyelid; periauricular appendages; esotropia or exotropia; external ear deformities; external auditory canal stenosis or atresia; and cleft lip with or without cleft palate.
- Hydrocephaly, microcephaly, and seventh cranial palsy.
- Hemivertebrae; cervical vertebral fusion; butterfly, fused, or hypoplastic vertebrae; and scoliosis.
- Tetralogy of Fallot, ventricular septal defect, and dextrocardia.
- Renal and other anomalies have been described in OAVS.

Treatment

- Cooperation of pediatricians, reconstructive surgeons, dietitians, and therapists is required.

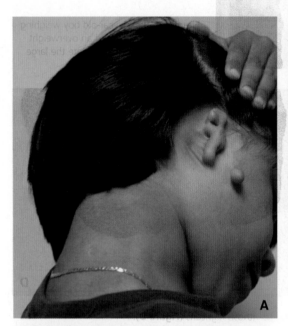

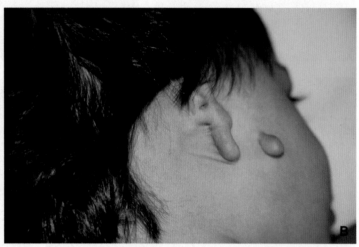

Figures A–B: Ear deformities and appendages in OAVS.

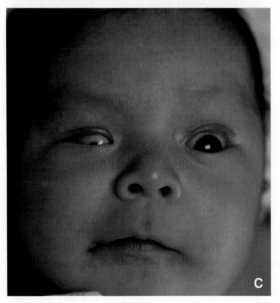

Figures C–F: This Hispanic boy was born by C-section due to maternal high blood pressure. Birth weight was 3 kg, height 46 cm, and head circumference 33 cm. The maternal grandparents were fourth generation cousins. No parental consanguinity. He is now 2 years old and developmentally delayed with several "febrile seizures." He is hypotonic and has microcephaly, right hemifacial microsomia, microphthalmia, cataract, persistent hyperplastic primary vitreous, and ciliary body detachment. Bilateral accessory tragus, one skin-tag intraorally on the right lateral aspect of the lip border. Hypoplastic mandible, right malar flattening, and right lateral cleft mouth. His CBC, metabolic panel, renal ultrasound, and EEG are normal. His ECG shows right axis deviation and no other abnormality and cardiac echocardiogram is normal. His microarray showed a loss of approximately 3.95 Mb at 14q24.2q24.3. This deletion is expected to cause phenotypic and developmental abnormalities. The MRI without contrast showed abnormal dysplasia of the right optic nerve and left optic tract which can associated with congenital pituitary anomalies. Has an associated absent right lens. The pituitary gland was slightly small for his age and asymmetric decreased size of the left gyrus. Same patient after his skin tag was removed **(Figure F).**

figures continues

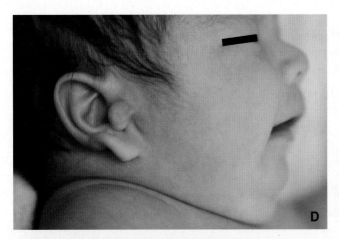

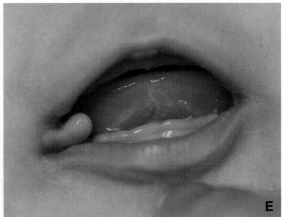

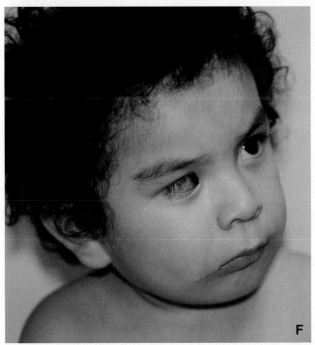

(figures cont.) **Figures D–F**

OMPHALITIS (Omphalos, Gr., navel)

Definition
- Omphalitis is an infection of the umbilical stump. The infection can begin as a superficial infection and then progress to necrosis, myonecrosis, and sepsis.

Etiology
- The majority are polymicrobial with about 85% aerobic organisms (mostly gram-positives) such as *Staphylococcus aureus,* group A Streptococcus, and gram-negative enteric bacilli such as *Escherichia coli.*
- Anaerobic bacteria, *Bacteroides fragilis* and *Clostridium perfringens* are less common.
- *Clostridium tetani,* a gram-positive anaerobic bacilli, may contaminate the umbilicus and is mostly found in the developing countries. These babies are often born at home by uneducated individuals and the umbilical cord is then covered with unsterile material once the baby is brought home.

Symptoms and Signs
- Depend on the severity of the infection. Include abdominal tenderness, periumbilical erythema, edema, malodorous and purulent discharge (Figure).

Treatment
- Debridement of the wound and appropriate broad-spectrum antibiotics should be started pending culture and sensitivity studies.

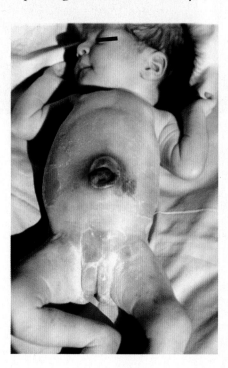

Omphalitis in a newborn, whose malodorous, erythematous umbilical stump was covered with mercurochrome, an antiseptic used in some developing countries (no longer in use in the United States due to its mercury content).

OMPHALOCELE (UMBILICAL EVENTRATION)

Definition
- Omphalocele is a birth defect in which part of the intestine is protruded through a large defect in the abdominal wall at the umbilicus and covered by a thin transparent membrane composed of amnion and peritoneum.

Etiology
- Some are due to genetic disorders such as trisomy 13 and trisomy 18.

Symptoms and Signs
- A central abdominal-wall deformity resulting from central defects in the medial and lateral wall folds and umbilical rings.
- A sac with an outer amniotic and inner peritoneal layer is covering the protruding organs.
- The size of this defect varies from an umbilical hernia to a large defect that may contain the intestine and the liver.
- There is always the possibility of other coexisting congenital abnormalities.

Treatment
- In a small omphalocele, the exposed organs can be returned to the abdominal cavity and the herniation can be surgically closed.
- In a larger omphalocele, the exposed organs are covered with a protective wrap allowing gravity to return the organs into the abdominal cavity with surgical closure.

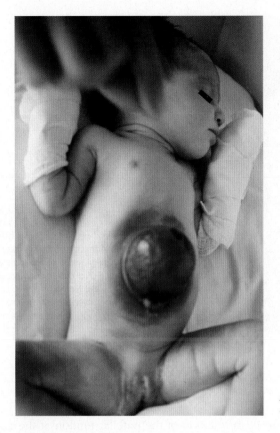

A newborn with an omphalocele covered with mercurochrome in Iran.

ONYCHOMYCOSIS

(See Tinea unguium).

OPIUM ADDICTION

Definition
■ According to the World Health Organization, addiction is "A cluster of physiological behavioral and cognitive phenomena of variable intensity, in which the use of a psychoactive drug (or drugs) takes on a high priority. The necessary descriptive characteristics are preoccupation with the desire to obtain and take the drug and persistent drug-seeking behavior. Determinants and problematic consequences of drug dependence may be biological, psychological, or social and usually interact."
■ Opium is one of the least frequently reported drugs in use over the last decade.

Etiology
■ Parental or caregiver exposure of children to opium.

Symptoms and Signs
■ These children are asymptomatic and fairly content as long as they receive their daily opium.
■ They become symptomatic when they are weaned off opium, developing withdrawal or an abstinence syndrome: Yawning, lacrimation, mydriasis, insomnia, cramping of the voluntary muscles, goose flesh, tachycardia, systolic hypertension, and rarely seizure.

Treatment
■ Methadone, a synthetic opiate, is the drug of choice.
■ A short course of diazepam may be helpful.

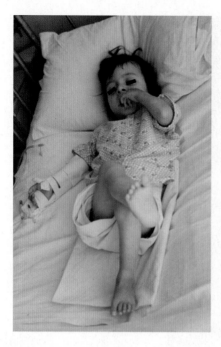

This is a 2-year-old boy whose mother asked a neighbor to baby-sit while she was at work. The neighbor had her own children at home. She sedated this 2-year old daily with PO opium. He was opium-addicted when admitted to the hospital for post-measles pneumonia. His babysitter, aware of his addiction, visited the hospital daily to give him a piece of opium. She was caught feeding the child opium by the hospital staff. He was restless, coughing, sneezing, and developed diarrhea when weaned off opium. He was treated with diazepam. In the photograph, this otherwise active 2-year-old toddler is calm and sedated due to the opium effect (before diagnosis).

OSGOOD–SCHLATTER DISEASE

Definition
- Osgood–Schlatter disease is an irritation of the patellar tendon at the tibial tuberosity.

Etiology
- The tibia tubercle, which is an extension of epiphysis, the area that the patellar tendon inserts into, is vulnerable to microfractures during childhood and adolescence.

Symptoms and Signs
- Intense knee pain, which occurs during sport activities like jumping, running, or even going upstairs or downstairs worsen with acute impact.

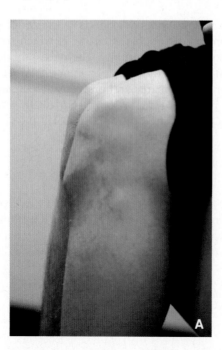

Figure A: This 16-year-old boy had pain in the left knee for nearly 4 months, mostly on running and touching. But pain was continuous for 1 day and he came in for evaluation. There was a tender area of swelling on the left tibial tuberosity.

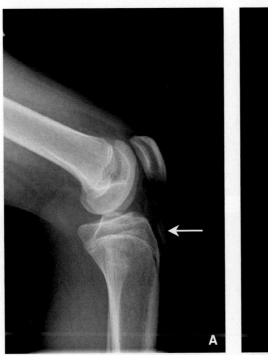
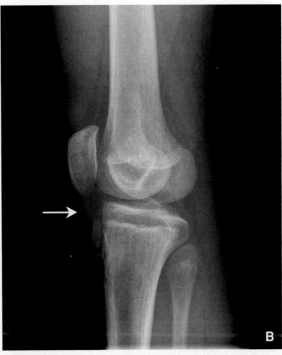

Figures A–B: Lateral **(A)** and oblique **(B)** views of the left knee: There is irregularity of the tibial tuberosity (*arrow,* **A**) with thickening of the patellar tendon and soft tissue swelling around the patellar ligament (*arrow,* **B**).

- Pain is mild and intermittent early in the course, but eventually severe and continuous.
- Increased prominence, swelling, and tenderness of the tibial tubercle.

Treatment
- This is usually a self-limiting disease.
- Rest and knee immobilization can help.
- Complete resolution may take up to 2 years.

OSTEOCHONDROMA (Gr., Osteon, bone; Chondros, cartilage)

Definition
- Osteochondroma is a benign tumor consisting of bone and cartilage attached to a bone with a stalk, and one of the most common benign tumors of children.

Etiology
- Unknown.

Symptoms and Signs
- The majority are asymptomatic, mostly arising from the metaphysis of long bones: Distal femur, proximal humerus, and proximal tibia.
- In most cases, a painless and asymptomatic bony structure is noticed by the child or a parent.

Treatment
- Surgery in cases of rapid growth, or if symptomatic.
- Osteochondromas can rarely degenerate into osteosarcoma in children.

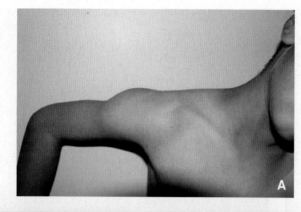

Figure A: A 12-year-old boy had pain and a mass in the right upper arm for 2 months which got worse after a fall last week.

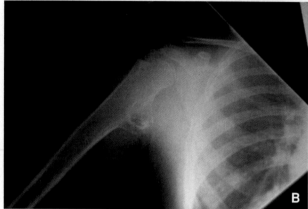

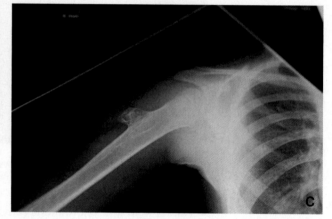

Figures B–C: Internal and external rotation x-rays of the right shoulder demonstrate a bony exostosis which is continuous with the bone cortex and medullary marrow space (hallmark). The lesion is directed away from the joint space which is characteristic of this type.

OSTEOMYELITIS AND SEPTIC ARTHRITIS

Definition
- Osteomyelitis and septic or suppurative arthritis are infections of the bones and joints.

Etiology
- *Staphylococcus aureus* is the most common causative organism and is responsible for 90% of the cases.
- *Streptococcus pyogenes, Haemophilus influenzae,* Group B streptococcus and *Escherichia coli* (in newborns), Salmonella (in children with sickle cell disease), and *Pseudomonas aeruginosa* (puncture wounds to the foot).
- *Mycobacterium tuberculosis,* less common bacteria, as well as fungal and viral infections can be the causative organism in osteomyelitis.

Symptoms and Signs
- Fever, unwillingness to move the affected extremity, swelling, warmth, and tenderness of the skin over the infected bone.
- Neonates can be afebrile and may present with pseudoparalysis.
- Long bones are affected most frequently with over 60% involvement of the tibia, femur, and humerus.

- High ESR and C-reactive protein, leukocytosis, blood culture, bone aspirates, plain x-rays (it may take 1 to 2 weeks to show changes, by which time about 30% to 50% of the bony matrix is destroyed), CT scan (80% accurate), radionuclide, and MRI (best demonstrates the details of bone destruction).
- Positive PPD test in TB osteomyelitis.
- Figures A–D.

Treatment

- Immediate empiric treatment with broad-spectrum IV antibiotics until etiology is confirmed through cultures. Immediate treatment is important to minimize the bone and particularly growth-plate destruction in young infants and children.
- Salmonella coverage for children with sickle cell disease and gram-negative coverage for neonates is important.
- The course of treatment is 4 to 6 weeks and change to oral antibiotic may be possible once the result of culture and sensitivity is available.

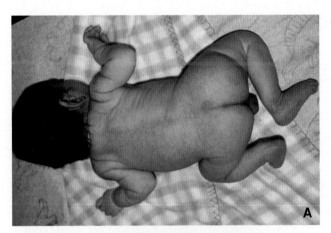

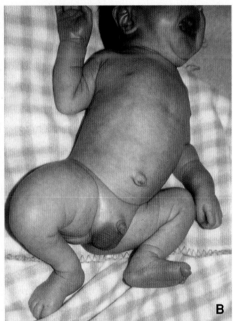

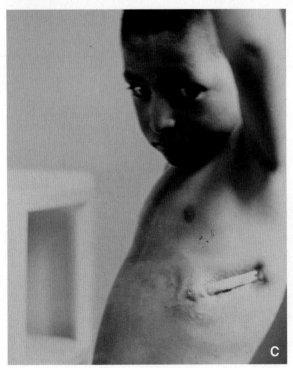

Figures A–B: This 20-day-old boy was brought in for a regular checkup. He was born by normal spontaneous vaginal delivery to a 17-year-old mother and a 21-year-old father. Birth weight 2.72 kg. He had mild meconium aspiration and spent 2 days in the newborn intensive care unit to rule out sepsis. His weight here in the office was 3.45 kg, length 47 cm, head circumference 34 cm, and temperature 38° C. He was obviously in pain and crying. His right thigh and left wrist were tender and swollen. He was hospitalized with the diagnosis of septic arthritis.

Figure C: This boy lived in a remote part of Iran and had difficulty reaching medical attention. The infection started as a boil on his chest and then progressed to cellulitis and osteomyelitis of his rib by the time he was able to reach medical attention. Ribs are one of the least common sites of osteomyelitis.

figures continues

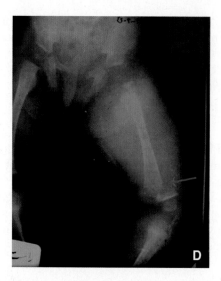

(figures cont.) **Figure D:** There is a displaced fracture of the distal portion of the left femur. Note the irregularity and erosive changes of the fracture margins suggesting that this is a pathologic fracture secondary to patient's known osteomyelitis.

OVERRIDING OF THE TOES (OVERLAPPING TOES)

Definition
- Overriding of the toes is not an uncommon congenital deformity; the fifth toe is the most commonly affected one.

Etiology
- Some cases are familial. The mode of inheritance is not clear.

Symptoms and Signs
- It can be unilateral or bilateral.
- It is an adduction and at times rotation of a toe, covering part of the adjacent toe.
- Most cases are asymptomatic unless the mispositioned toe is under pressure in a shoe. It can also be of cosmetic concern.

Treatment
- Taping in the newborns.
- Various spacers may correct the overriding in the newborn.
- Surgical correction if symptomatic or for cosmetic reasons.
- Figures A–E.

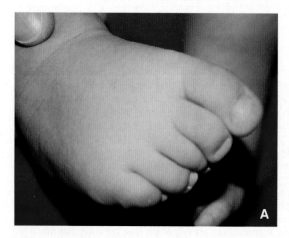

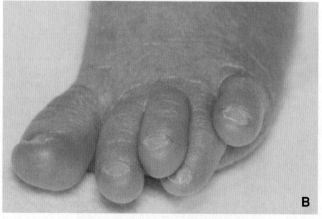

Figure A: Overriding of the second toe.

Figure B: Overriding of the third and fifth toe.

figures continues

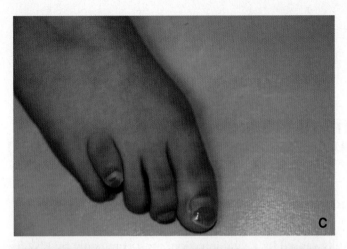

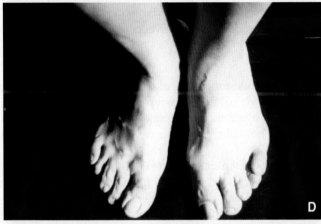

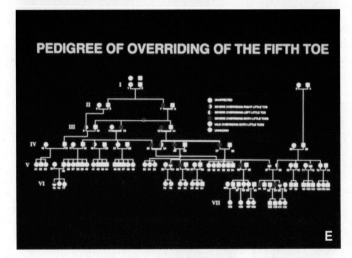

(figures cont.) **Figure C:** Overriding of the fourth toe.

Figures D–E: Overriding of the fifth toe **(Figure D)** and a pedigree of a family with the overriding of the fifth toe **(Figure E)**.

PAPULAR ACRODERMATITIS OF CHILDHOOD (PAC) (GIANOTTI–CROSTI SYNDROME, PAPULOVESICULAR ACROLOCATED SYNDROME)

Definition
■ A self-limited exanthematous disease of childhood.

Etiology
■ PAC is typically caused by a viral infection, most commonly by EBV and hepatitis B. CMV, enteroviruses, RSV, adenovirus, parvovirus B19, and rotavirus are less frequently involved.
■ PAC has been temporally associated with vaccine administration. However, direct causality remains unproven.

Symptom and Signs
■ More commonly seen in children aged 1 to 6 years but can rarely be seen in adults. The rash is typically preceded by either URI symptoms or a GI illness during the previous week.
■ Symmetrical eruption of small, multiple, pink-brown, papulovesicular lesions that are distributed on the face, buttocks, and the extensor surfaces of the upper and lower extremities.
■ The rash may appear on the trunk, but spares the mucosal surfaces and nails.
■ The rash is often asymptomatic other than the majority of patients experience mild pruritus. Hemorrhagic changes, including development of petechia, and purpura occur occasionally.
■ Other findings may include lymphadenitis, anicteric hepatitis, and splenomegaly.

Treatment
■ None, as spontaneous remission is the rule.
■ Symptoms may last from 5 days to 12 months.
■ Complications are related to the underlying etiology, including hepatitis B infection, or infectious mononucleosis.

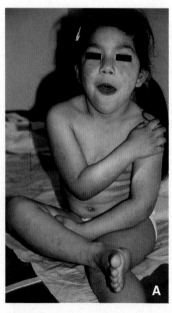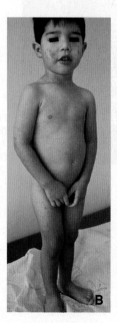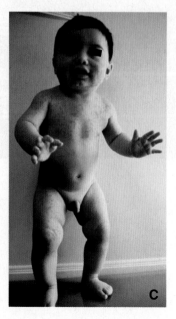

Figures A–C: Papular acrodermatitis of childhood (PAC) in a 6-year-old girl. Note the symmetrical, edematous, erythematous rash on her face and extensor surface of the upper and lower extremities. The lesions appear coalesced on her legs **(Figure A)**. Two toddlers with PAC in **Figures B** and **C**. The child in **Figure C** has the uncommon finding of a truncal rash.

PAPULAR URTICARIA

Definition
- Papular urticaria is a common skin reaction to insect bites in children.

Etiology
- Hypersensitivity to insect bites such as fleas, bedbugs, mosquitoes, and mites.

Symptoms and Signs
- Symmetrical distribution of multiple, small papules or papulovesicles with or without an erythematous, urticarial flare. Lesions commonly appear during spring and summer.
- Lesions typically appear on the exposed, extensor surfaces of the extremities.
- They are usually localized to the site of the insect bite but may also be found over the entire body.
- Lesions are intensely pruritic and scratching may lead to secondary impetigo.
- Papules usually resolve within days to weeks. Scratching may lead to postinflammatory hyperpigmentation or scarring.

Treatment
- Symptomatic treatment includes oral antihistamines and steroid creams.
- Environmental control and eradication of the offending insects for prevention of recurrences.

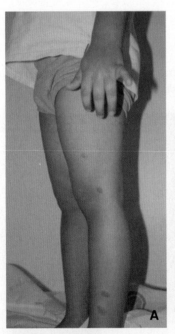
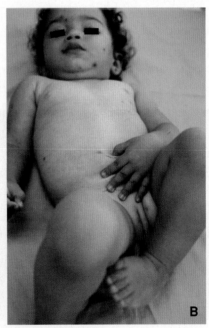
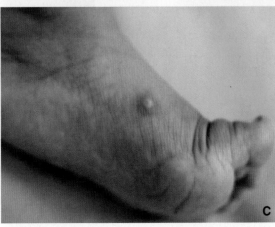

Figures A, B, and **C** demonstrate papular urticaria in three children. Note the papules with a surrounding urticarial flare in **Figure C**.

PARONYCHIA (Gr. Onychos, nail)

Definition
- Paronychia is an infection of the skin or soft tissue surrounding the nail.

Etiology
- Damage to the cuticles, the protective seal which surrounds the nail, allows microorganisms to enter the skin and cause an infection.
- Aggressive manicuring, thumb-sucking, nail-biting, occupations in which the hands are frequently immersed in water, diabetes mellitus, and other causes of immunodeficiency are predisposing factors.
- *Staphylococcus aureus* and other skin and oral flora are the predominant organisms responsible for acute paronychia.
- Tuberculosis and HSV are less frequently involved.
- Candida and fungal infections may play a role in the development of chronic paronychia. However, recent studies suggest that chronic paronychia may be due to an eczematous process.

Symptom and Signs
- Acute paronychia presents with the acute onset of redness, swelling, and pain in the periungual area.
- In chronic paronychia, there is erythema of the periungual area with nail plate ridging, dystrophy and cuticle loss.

Treatment
- In acute paronychia, application of warm compresses and administration of oral antibiotics with anti-*Staphylococcus aureus* activity.

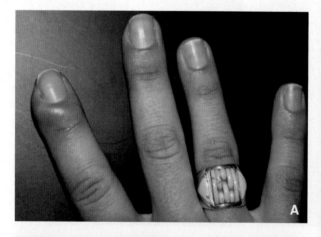

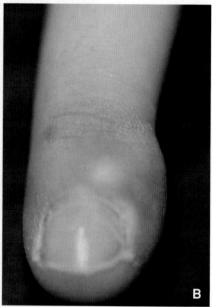

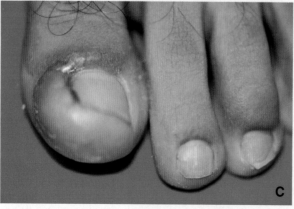

Figures A–B: Paronychia of the fingers.

Figure C: Paronychia of the toe.

- If there is evidence of abscess formation, incision and drainage is indicated along with oral antibiotic therapy.
- Chronic paronychia may be treated with topical corticosteroids and avoidance of allergens and irritants. If all measures fail, antifungal therapy may be warranted.

PAROTITIS, RECURRENT

Definition
- Recurrent unilateral or bilateral inflammation of the parotid glands.

Etiology
- Definite causative factors have not been identified.
- Congenital ductal malformations, hereditary–genetic factors, viral and bacterial infections, allergies, autoimmune disorders, and immunodeficiencies have been proposed as unproven etiologic factors.
- It is difficult to distinguish recurrent parotitis from mumps at the initial presentation.

Symptoms and Signs
- Recurrent and painful swelling of one or both parotid glands.
- More frequent in males. Symptoms may appear by 16 months of age and typically disappear during puberty.
- Episodes may last from 3 days to 3 weeks.

Treatment
- Conservative therapy with massage, warm compresses, chewing gum, or sour candies.
- Antibiotics may be given prophylactically early in the course of an attack or in case of a superimposed infection.

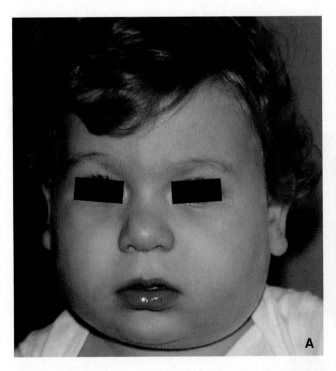 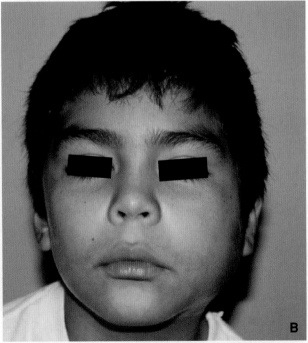

Figures A–B: Recurrent parotitis in a previously healthy 2-year-old male. His MMR was up-to-date. He presented with a low-grade fever, bilateral swelling, discomfort, and tenderness of the parotid glands. The swelling subsided within a week **(Figure A)**. The second episode of unilateral parotitis in a male teenager who was up-to-date with the MMR vaccines. He was afebrile and had painful swelling of the left parotid gland. The serum amylase level was elevated. The swelling lasted approximately 10 days **(Figure B)**.

- Endoscopic evaluation of the parotid gland with irrigation, dilatation of strictures, and injection of steroids.
- Recalcitrant cases may be referred for parotidectomy or ductal ligation.

PECTUS CARINATUM (L. Pectus, front of the chest; Carina, keel)

Definition
- Pectus carinatum, also known as pigeon chest, is a chest wall deformity which is characterized by a prominent sternum and lateral depression of the ribs.

Etiology
- It may be present at birth as an isolated finding. Affected infants have an increased incidence of a positive family history.
- Excessive growth of cartilage, sternum, and ribs.
- Also found in association with other genetic disorders including trisomy 21, trisomy 18, Marfan syndrome, osteogenesis imperfecta, multiple lentigines syndrome, and homocystinuria.
- Other causes include open heart surgery and vitamin D deficiency rickets.

Symptoms and Signs
- Forward protrusion of the sternum that may become apparent during the adolescent growth spurt.
- Pectus carinatum is more common in males and has two subtypes depending on the site of the greatest protrusion:
  1. Chondrogladiolar prominence, the most common type: Protrusion of the middle and lower portions of the sternum.
  2. Chondromanubrial prominence: Anterior protrusion of the upper portion of the sternum.
- Asymptomatic in mild cases, but may cause the following symptoms in severe cases: Dyspnea on exertion, decreased lung compliance, emphysema, hypoxemia, mitral valve prolapse, cardiac rhythm disturbances, decreased myocardial contractility, and scoliosis.
- Cosmetic appearance may have a negative psychosocial impact on children.
- Figures A–D.

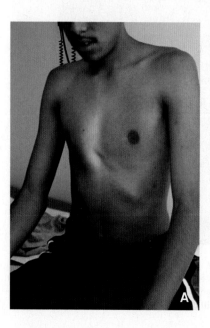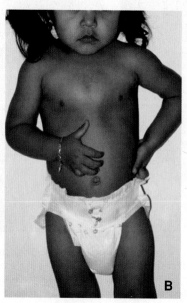

Figures A–D: Four asymptomatic children with chest deformities of pectus carinatum.

figures continues

P

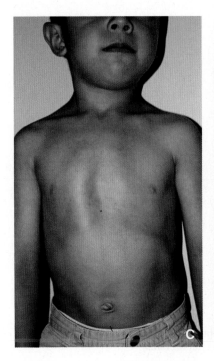
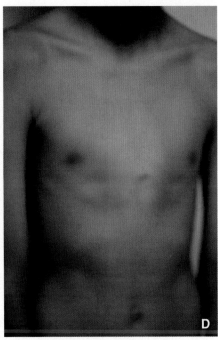

(figures cont.) **Figures C–D**

Treatment
- Bracing and surgery are considered safe and effective treatment modalities.
- Bracing appears to be effective in children who have flexible chest walls.
- Skeletally mature children with a rigid chest wall are more likely to improve with surgery versus bracing.

PECTUS EXCAVATUM (FUNNEL CHEST)

Definition
- Pectus excavatum is the most common congenital deformity of the anterior chest wall. It is seven times more prevalent than pectus carinatum.

Etiology
- Unknown. Genetic factors may play a role. Approximately one out of three patients has a first-degree family member who has pectus excavatum.
- Connective tissue disorders: Marfan syndrome, Ehlers–Danlos syndrome, and osteogenesis imperfecta.
- Neuromuscular disorders: Spinal muscular atrophy.
- Other genetic syndromes: Noonan syndrome and Turner syndrome.
- Pulmonary disease: Repaired congenital diaphragmatic hernia, subglottic stenosis, and chronic lung disease.
- Other causes include rickets and celiac disease.

Symptoms and Signs
- A sunken appearance of the chest wall and sternum. It may be apparent at birth but worsens during the adolescent growth spurt.
- Patients typically present with symptoms of exercise-intolerance or cosmetic concerns.
- Cardiovascular findings may include right axis deviation, conduction abnormalities, mitral valve prolapse, and right ventricular outflow obstruction. These findings are thought to be secondary to the displacement of the heart.
- Pulmonary function tests typically reveal normal lung volumes. However, impairment may be noted during exercise testing, which correlates to the severity of pectus excavatum.

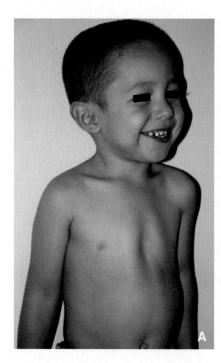
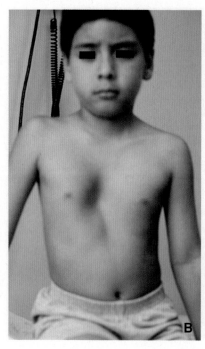

Figures A–B: Two asymptomatic males with pectus excavatum.

Treatment

- Most patients will not need surgical correction. However, patients should be monitored closely for progression of deformity during periods of rapid growth.
- Corrective surgery is indicated in cases of cardiopulmonary symptoms or for cosmetic reasons.

PEDICULOSIS (LICE)

Definition

- Infestation of the human head, body, or pubic area with lice.

Etiology

- Lice are most commonly found among people who live in overcrowded conditions (schools and various institutions) and among the homeless.
- These parasites require human blood meals for existence. They press their mouths against the human skin, pierce the surface, and ingest human blood. An anticoagulant is injected into the skin in order to assure continued blood flow.
- Three species of lice infest humans:
  1. Pediculus humanus corporis (the body louse). It is the only louse that can carry human diseases including epidemic typhus, louse-borne relapsing fever, and trench fever. It lives on clothes and bedding. Poor hygiene and communal bedding are the major risk factors for transmission.
  2. Pediculus humanus capitis (the head louse) is transmitted by close contact or fomites (comb, brush, hats, and headgear).
  3. Pthirus pubis (the pubic or crab louse) is considered a sexually transmitted disease since the majority of cases are transmitted by close body contact. Rarely, transmission can be through an object such as a toilet seat, bathing suit, bedding, or towels.

Symptoms and Signs

- Itching, excoriation, secondary infection, and lymphadenopathy are the most common symptoms and signs.

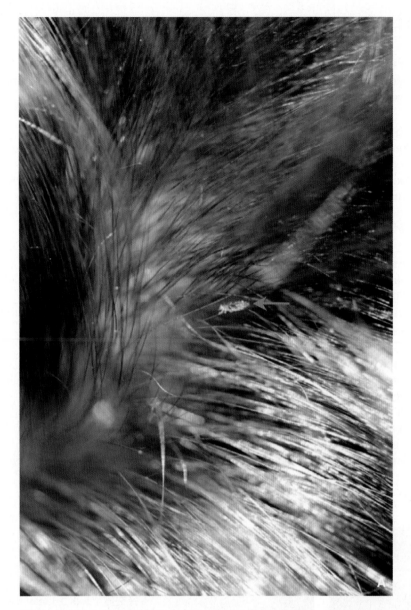

Figure A: A louse (*arrow*) with numerous ova glued to the hair of a teenage girl.

- Head lice are seen infrequently. However, the nits which are the egg cases are abundant. They are whitish-gray spots which are tightly attached to the hair shaft and close to the scalp.
- Head lice can easily be mistaken with dandruff (seborrheic dermatitis).
- Figure A.

Treatment

- Permethrin 1% cream rinse (Nix), Permethrin cream 5%, Benzyl alcohol 5% lotion, and occlusive agents including petroleum jelly. A second course of treatment, 1 week after the initial treatment, is recommended by some experts.
- In pediculus capitis, fine combing of the hair to remove all nits is very important.
- All clothing, bedding, and headgears should be washed in hot water and dried in high heat (e.g., a drier).
- Close family members should be examined and treated if necessary.

PERIORBITAL CELLULITIS (PRESEPTAL CELLULITIS)

Definition
- Periorbital cellulitis is an acute infection and inflammation of the anterior portion of the eyelid and the surrounding skin.

Etiology
- Intrinsic causes of periorbital cellulitis may arise from pre-existing sinusitis or hematogenous spread of bacteria.
- Extrinsic causes include foreign body trauma and insect or animal bites to the surrounding tissue of the eyelids.
- Etiologic organisms include *Staphylococcus aureus, Staphylococcus epidermidis, Haemophilus influenzae,* and *Streptococcus pneumoniae.*

Symptoms and Signs
- Tender, erythema, edema, induration, and warmth in the area which surrounds the orbit (Figures A and B).
- Unlike in orbital cellulitis, there is no evidence of proptosis, ophthalmoplegia, loss of vision, or painful eye movements in periorbital cellulitis.

Treatment
- Periorbital cellulitis must be immediately distinguished from orbital cellulitis which may require surgical treatment.
- CT scan may help distinguish findings between the two conditions.
- Intravenous antibiotics for younger and ill-appearing children. Empiric treatment should provide coverage against *S. aureus* and other causative organisms.
- Oral antibiotic coverage may be adequate for older and well-appearing children.

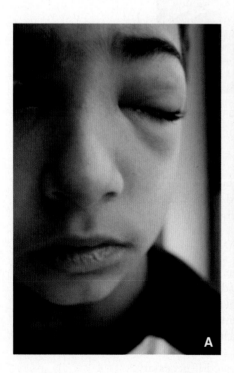
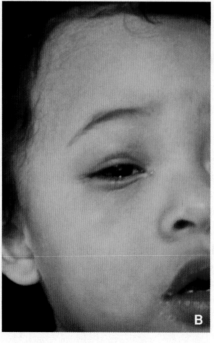

Figure A: This 8-year-old male presented with 3 days of fever and increased swelling of the eyelids. Physical examination revealed a warm and violaceous discoloration and swelling of the left eyelid which extended to the nose and limited movement of the left eyeball. CT scan indicated extensive inflammatory disease involving the frontal sinuses and the left ethmoid sinus with mild chronic inflammatory changes involving the left maxillary sinus. He was diagnosed with periorbital cellulitis.

Figure B: A 16-month-old male, woke up with a temperature of 37.7° C. Physical examination revealed erythema and swelling of the right eyelid. There was no evidence of ophthalmoplegia. CT scan revealed minimal swelling of the right periorbital area.

PERIORIFICIAL DERMATITIS (PERIORAL DERMATITIS)

Definition

- Periorificial dermatitis is a common, distinctive skin eruption noted around the mouth, nose, and eyes.

Etiology

- Unknown. There is an unclear association of potent corticosteroid use and the development of periorificial dermatitis.

Symptoms and Signs

- Clusters of small, erythematous, or flesh-colored papules, papulopustules, or papulovesicles in the perioral, perinasal, or periorbital areas.
- Lesions may resemble acne, may have mild scaling, and commonly occur in the prepubertal children and young adults.
- Children may complain of a burning sensation or pruritus.
- Figures A–C.

Treatment

- This is a self-limited disease, although resolution may take a few years.
- Discontinuation of topical steroids.
- Topical metronidazole, erythromycin, or oral tetracycline (for children >8 years of age) may be effective in treating this eruption.

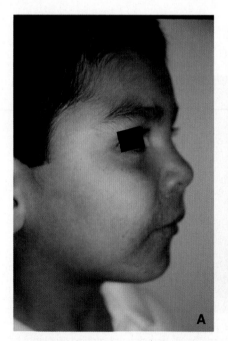 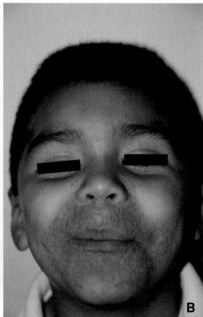 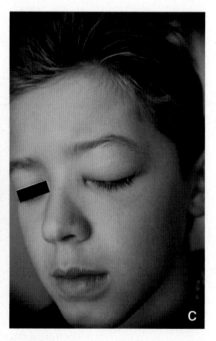

Figures A–B: A healthy 13-year-old male presented with a 9-month history of the rash. Clusters of numerous erythematous papules with mild pruritus were noted around the mouth, nose, and eyes. He responded well to two courses of systemic erythromycin and topical moisturizers.

Figure C: A 13-year-old male with a 2-month history of left periorbital erythema and pruritus.

PERITONSILLAR ABSCESS

Definition
- Peritonsillar abscess or quinsy is a collection of pus in the tonsillar fossa.

Etiology
- It may occur as a complication of partially treated or untreated pharyngitis.
  It is commonly a polymicrobial infection. Group A Streptococcus, *Staphylococcus aureus,* Haemophilus species, and oral anaerobic bacteria are typically the causative bacteria.

Symptoms and Signs
- Sudden onset of fever, dysphagia, a unilateral sore throat with radiation of the pain to the ipsilateral ear.
- Muffled "hot-potato" voice, inability to open the mouth (trismus), drooling, and lymphadenopathy.
- A bulging and fluctuant tonsil with deviation of the uvula to the opposite side.
- Bilateral symptoms are rare.
- Complications may be fatal and include septicemia, airway compromise, and extension of abscess into the adjacent deep neck structures.
- Figure A.

Treatment
- Drainage of abscess accompanied by intravenous antibiotic therapy.
- Immediate surgical intervention if there is evidence of airway compromise.
- Tonsillectomy may be indicated if there is a history of recurrent peritonsillar abscesses.

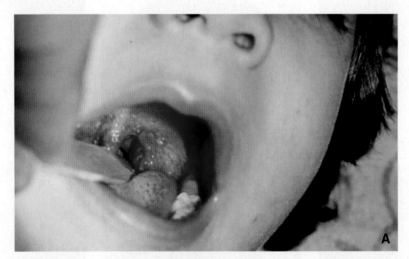

Figure A: This 7-year-old female presented to the ER with a 2-week history of periodic fever and sore throat. Upon presentation, she had a temperature of 38.3° C and a severe sore throat. Her voice was muffled. Her left tonsil appeared large, bulging, and inflamed. The uvula was deviated to the right and bilateral anterior cervical lymphadenopathy was present. Her WBC was 17.9 with 83% neutrophils and 5% bands. A CT scan of the neck showed "a collection of abscess, 16 mm × 11 mm at left pharynx at the level of the left palatine tonsil." Incision and drainage of the abscess was performed. There was a moderate growth of group A β-hemolytic Streptococcus without anaerobic bacteria.

P

PES CAVUS AND HAMMER TOE

(See Talipes).

PEUTZ–JEGHER SYNDROME (PJS)

Definition
- A genetic disease which is characterized by the development of hamartomatous polyps in the gastrointestinal tract and hyperpigmented macules on the oral mucosa.

Etiology
- Autosomal dominant disorder with high degree of penetrance.
- In most families, a mutation of a chromosome 19 gene, which encodes a serine threonine kinase, has been found to be responsible for PJS.

Symptoms and Signs
- The cutaneous markers of PJS are pigmented mucocutaneous macules that are bluish-brown to black, irregularly oval, and 2 to 5 mm in diameter.
- These pigmentations are found on the perioral region, buccal mucosa, nasal and periorbital regions, hands and feet, and perianal and genital regions.
- Skin findings may appear at birth and can increase in both size and number over time. They subsequently fade after puberty with the exception of those found on the buccal mucosa.
- The characteristic hamartomatous gastrointestinal polyps are found in the stomach, small intestine, colon, and rectum.
- Polyps grow in size during the first decade of life.
- PJS may present with recurrent abdominal pain, obstruction due to intussusception, anemia, melena, or hematemesis.
- PJS is associated with an increased risk of intestinal, pancreatic, breast, and reproductive tract cancers.
- Figures A and B.

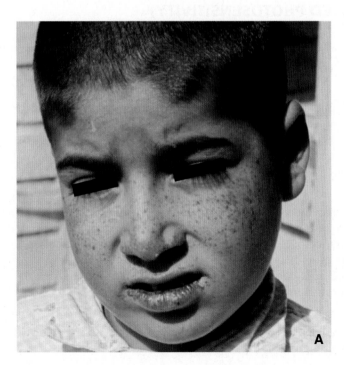

A

Figures A–B: Peutz–Jeghers syndrome (PJS). This child's father had melena and was diagnosed with polyps in his colon. The child was asymptomatic at the time. There were multiple, hyperpigmented macules on his face, lips, oral mucosa, hands, and feet.

figures continues

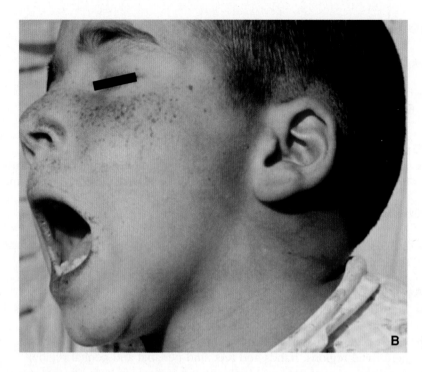

(figures cont.) **Figure B**

Treatment

- Upper endoscopy and colonoscopy surveillance for polyp detection. Recommended to begin at 8 years of age with repeated examinations depending on the specific findings and symptoms.
- Endoscopic polypectomy for polyps greater than 1 cm in size.
- Close evaluation for development of thyroid, breast, testicular, and ovarian cancer.
- Close evaluation of first-degree relatives for PJS.
- Laser and intense pulsed light for treatment of the hyperpigmented cutaneous lesions.

PHYTOPHOTODERMATITIS (PLANT-INDUCED PHOTOSENSITIVITY)

Definition

- Phytophotodermatitis is the most common phototoxic reaction in children.

Etiology

- The majority of cases are due to phototoxic reactions to furocoumarin compounds which are present in certain vegetables and fruits including lime, fig, parsnips, carrots, dill, and parsley.
- Direct contact with furocoumarins, in combination with exposure to UVA radiation, may induce a photosensitivity reaction.

Symptoms and Signs

- Ranges from mild erythema, edema, and bullae in the sun-exposed areas of the skin.
- Lesions commonly appear within 24 hours of sun exposure.
- The lesions may have the appearance of a bizarre linear streak or blotchy configuration in the pattern of contact with the offending object.
- Hyperpigmentation of the affected area commonly occurs after resolution of the original skin findings. Resolution of hyperpigmentation may take months or years.

Treatment

- Symptomatic treatment with oral analgesics or cool compresses.
- Discontinue contact with the offending object if possible.

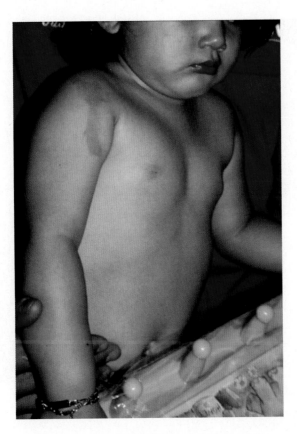

This toddler was running shirtless during a family barbecue. There was spillage of lemon juice on her right shoulder with subsequent development of a hyperpigmented patch the following day.

PICA

(See Hyperphosphatemic tumoral calcinosis).

PILONIDAL SINUS (L. Pilus, hair; Nidus, nest) (SACROCOCCYGEAL FISTULA)

Definition
- A dimple in the intergluteal cleft that often contains hair and skin debris.

Etiology
- Unknown. Originally thought to be a congenital defect. Recent evidence, however, suggests that pilonidal sinus may be an acquired condition.

Symptoms and Signs
- Clinical findings vary widely:
  1. The most benign presentation is an asymptomatic, benign dimple visualized in the intergluteal cleft.
  2. Acute abscesses with sudden onset of pain and swelling. This presentation is more common in adolescence and males.
  3. A chronic, inflammatory, draining cyst.
- Figures A and B.

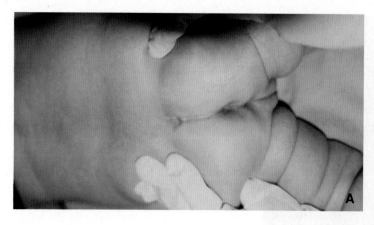

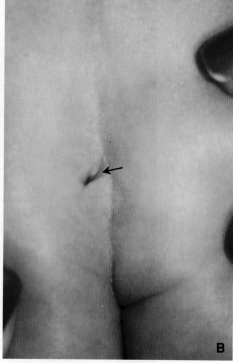

Figure A: Pilonidal sinus in a healthy 1-month-old girl.

Figure B: A symptomatic pilonidal sinus.

Treatment
- Benign dimples do not require treatment.
- Antibiotics and incision and drainage of pilonidal abscesses.
- Surgical excision for the removal of the cysts.

PITYRIASIS ALBA (Gr. Pityrion, bran)

Definition
- Pityriasis alba is a skin condition which is characterized by hypopigmented scaly patches.

Etiology
- A nonspecific dermatitis with postinflammatory hypopigmentation.
- It is associated with atopy, sun exposure, use of public swimming pools, and excessive bathing.

Symptoms and Signs
- Round or oval, scaly, hypopigmented patches, which appear on the face, neck, shoulders, and upper arms.
- The lesions are usually asymptomatic and range from 0.5 to 5 cm in diameter.
- The lesions become more visible after exposure to sunlight, especially in darker-skinned people, since the surrounding healthy skin darkens with the ultraviolet exposure.
- Figures A and B.

Treatment
- No specific treatment is needed, since most patches will resolve over a period of a few months.
- A mild corticosteroid cream, calcineurin inhibitors, and moisturizers may decrease the scaliness of the patches.
- Protection from sun exposure helps minimize the discrepancy between the patches and the surrounding normal skin.

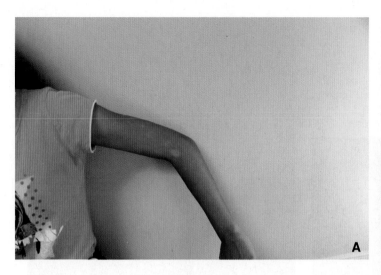
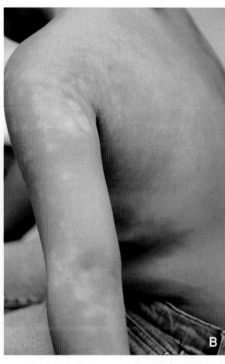

Figures A–B

PITYRIASIS LICHENOIDES

Definition
- Pityriasis lichenoides is an uncommon rash that ranges from a spectrum of acute to chronic forms.

Etiology
- Unknown.
- Current theories include abnormal immune response to a viral infection, an immune-complex–mediated hypersensitivity vasculitis, or a benign T-cell lymphoproliferative disorder.

Symptoms and Signs
- Pityriasis lichenoides et varioliformis acuta (PLEVA, also known as Mucha–Habermann disease) is the acute form.
  - Reddish-brown patches that evolve into papules are 5 to 15 mm in diameter. Pruritus and burning are common.
  - The rash is typically seen on the trunk and the extremities. The mucous membranes, palms, soles, face, and scalp are typically spared. Occasionally, the rash may be widespread and cover the entire body.
  - Papules can become filled with blood and pus or progress to vesicles and hemorrhagic crusts.
  - Constitutional symptoms and fever are rare with the exception of patients who present with the subtype of PLEVA known as febrile ulceronecrotic PLEVA.
- Pityriasis lichenoid chronic (PLC) is the chronic form. It can follow the acute form or begin de novo. It involves over one-third of the cases.
  - Lesions begin as small, scaly, pink papules that turn reddish-brown in color.
  - They appear over several days or weeks. Various stages of the lesion can be seen at one time.
  - Lesions resolve over several weeks, leaving a hyperpigmented brown mark.
  - Some children may have clinical and histologic presentation of acute and chronic forms.
- Figures A and B.

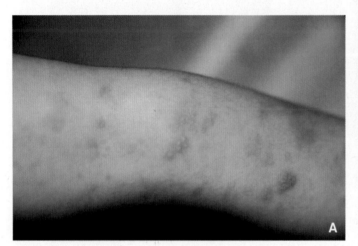

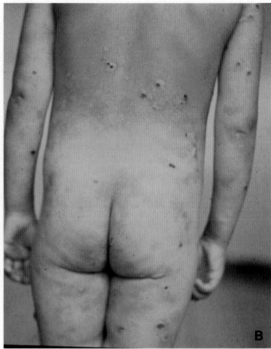

Figure A: Reddish-brown macules and papules on the arm of a 12-year-old boy with PLEVA.

Figure B: This child had a 2-year history of intermittent, pruritic, erythematous rash with depigmented patches. His body was covered with numerous 2 to 5 mm reddish-brown, oval, round, macules, papules, vesicles, and crusted lesions. Areas of hypo- and hyperpigmentation were noted throughout his skin. He was diagnosed with PLC and treated with oral erythromycin. He responded slowly with resolution of the skin eruptions.

Treatment
- Sun exposure may help with resolution of lesions.
- Topical steroids or tacrolimus for reduction of symptoms.
- Systemic antibiotics including erythromycin, azithromycin, and tetracyclines (not indicated in children younger than 8 years of age or in pregnant women) for 1 to 2 months.
- Methotrexate and cyclosporine can be used in resistant cases.

PITYRIASIS ROSEA

Definition
- Pityriasis rosea is an acute, benign, self-limited skin disorder.

Etiology
- Unknown. Suspected viral etiology with human herpesvirus 6 or 7.

Symptoms and Signs
- Can be preceded by fever, headache, lymphadenopathy, and other prodromal symptoms of a viral upper respiratory tract infection.
- The majority of cases begin with a "herald patch," a 2- to 5-cm sized, sharply defined, scaly, oval–round patch that is pink or salmon-colored.
- The herald patch is found mostly on the trunk, upper arm, neck, or thighs.
- The second wave of eruptions begins a few days or up to a few weeks later. Crops of smaller papules appear on the trunk and the proximal extremities. The characteristic ovoid lesions create a pattern similar to a Christmas tree and are best noted on the back.

- In children, lesions may also cover the scalp, face, distal extremities, pubic area, and inguinal and axillary regions.
- Lesions in children may appear vesicular, purpuric, pustular, or urticarial.
- Pruritus occurs in approximately one out of three cases.
- Most lesions clear within 5 weeks to 5 months. Postinflammatory hyper- or hypopigmentation may occur.
- Figures A–H.

Treatment

- Reassurance and patient education.
- Symptomatic treatment of pruritus with topical lubricants, topical steroids, antihistamines, and calamine lotion.
- Ultraviolet light and sunshine may decrease disease severity.

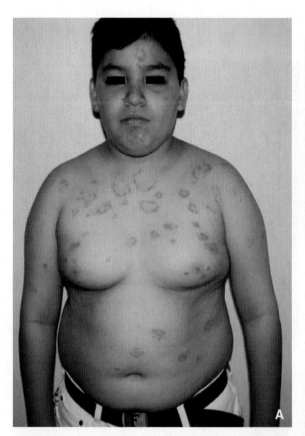

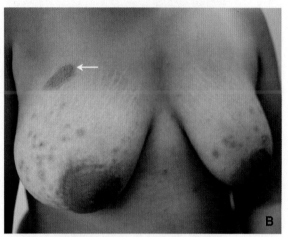

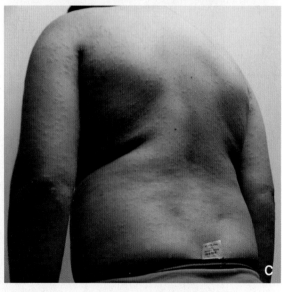

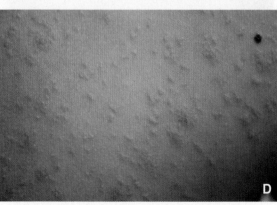

Figures A–H: The characteristic skin eruptions in pityriasis rosea. The arrows point to the herald patch. **Figure A** demonstrates the presence of the rash on an adolescent patient's face. The "necklace of scales" is seen in **Figure F**.

figures continues

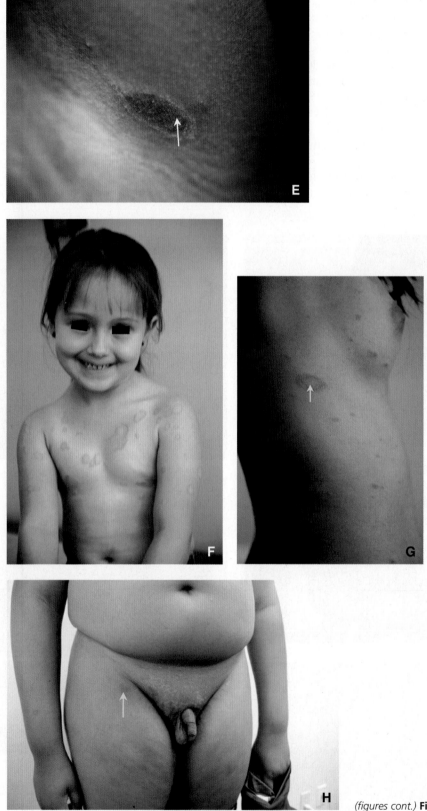

(figures cont.) **Figures E–H**

PLAGIOCEPHALY

- Plagiocephaly is an asymmetrical appearance of the skull and face. This may be the result of in utero positioning, torticollis, as well as the recent and appropriate "back to sleep" recommendations for the prevention of SIDS (Figures A and B).

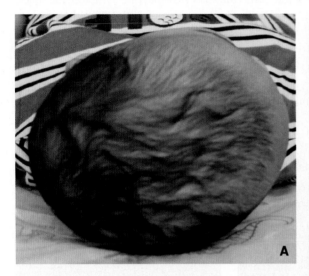

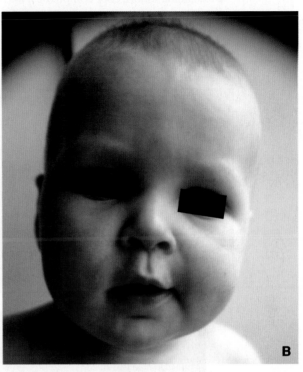

Figure A: Plagiocephaly in a 3-month-old male. Note the forward advancement of the right frontal bone and the reciprocal advancement of the left occipital bone.

Figure B: Plagiocephaly in a 9-month-old female. There is prominence of the right frontal bone and cheek. Note that the head is slightly tilted to the left.

POISON IVY DERMATITIS (RHUS DERMATITIS)

Definition
- Rhus dermatitis refers to a genus of trees and shrubs that belong to the Anacardiaceae family and can cause allergic contact dermatitis. Poison ivy, poison oak, and poison sumac are the most notable members of this plant family.

Etiology
- Sensitization to urushiol, which is the allergenic component of the plants listed.
- Contact with any part of the plant, including the sap, may cause a classic type IV hypersensitivity dermatitis.
- Plants related to the Anacardiaceae may contain allergenic compounds that cross-react with components of urushiol. Japanese lacquer tree, mango rind, oil from the shell of Brazil nut or cashew, and the marking nut tree of India belong in this category.

Symptoms and Signs
- Rhus dermatitis is more frequent during the summer months; this correlates with the increase in outdoor activities.
- Intense itching and redness are the most common presenting signs. Papules, vesicles, and bullae can appear within 8 hours to 3 days in sensitized individuals.
- The eruptions are frequently linear and occur in the area where the plant has come into contact with the skin.
- Untreated lesions may last up to 3 weeks.
- Complications include secondary bacterial infection, nephrosis due to renal immune complex depositions, and postinflammatory hyperpigmentation.

Treatment

- The best mode of management, if possible, is avoidance of the toxic plants.
- Immediate change of clothing and skin washing with soap and water is recommended after a known exposure.
- Barrier creams for prevention of contact dermatitis including bentoquatam.
- Calamine lotion, cool compresses, and topical corticosteroids may provide symptomatic relief.
- In severe cases, especially those which involve the face, systemic corticosteroid treatment may be beneficial.
- Figures A–D.

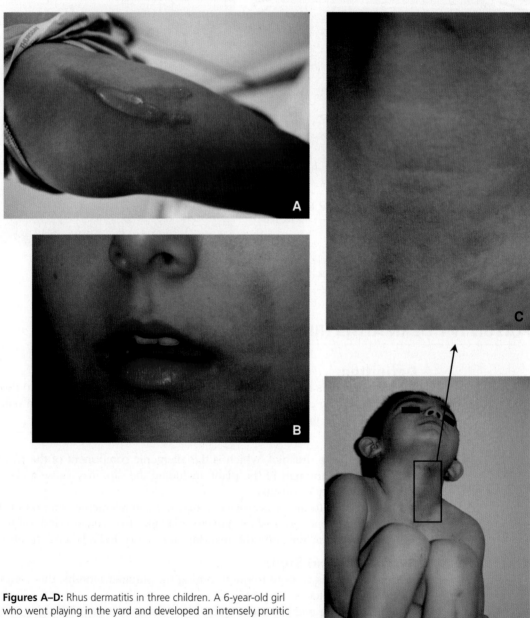

Figures A–D: Rhus dermatitis in three children. A 6-year-old girl who went playing in the yard and developed an intensely pruritic rash the following day. Note, the streak of erythematous papules on her face and right thigh. A large bulla is also noted on the right thigh **(Figures A** and **B)**. An intensely pruritic rash in a 6-year-old male who went hiking the prior day. There is a streak of erythematous papules on his left leg, neck, and face **(Figures C** and **D)**. An enlarged picture of the skin lesion on his neck **(Figure C)**.

POLAND SYNDROME

Definition
- A rare congenital abnormality consisting of abnormal development of the pectoralis muscle.

Etiology
- Unknown. It may be secondary to the interruption of blood flow to the pectoralis muscle during embryonic development.
- Poland syndrome is associated with maternal diabetes. It is three times more common in males, and twice more frequent on the right side.

Symptoms and Signs
- The most frequent and obvious finding is unilateral absence of the pectoralis muscle.
- Associated findings include aplasia of ipsilateral ribs, costal cartilages, and nipples. Abnormalities of the ipsilateral proximal and distal upper extremity and fingers, dextrocardia, diaphragmatic hernia, and renal and biliary tract abnormalities.
- Figures A–E.

Treatment
- Severe chest wall abnormalities may require surgical repair.
- Other accompanying congenital anomalies may require pediatric subspecialty expertise.

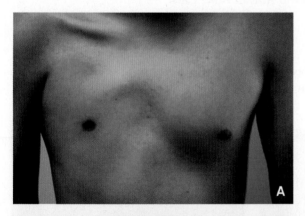

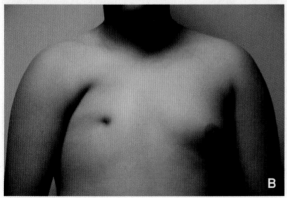

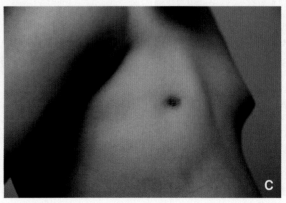

Figure A: An asymptomatic male teenager with the absence of the pectoralis muscles. He had no other associated abnormalities.

Figures B–C: Isolated absence of the pectoralis major muscle in a 13-year-old male.

figures continues

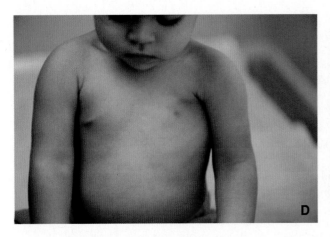

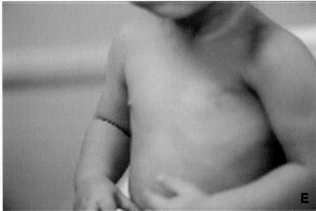

(figures cont.) **Figures D–E:** Absent left pectoralis major and minor muscles in a 14-month-old girl.

POLYDACTYLY AND BIFID DIGITS

Definition
- Polydactyly is defined as the presence of more than the normal number of fingers or toes. A bifid digit is one in which a cleft divides a finger into two digits.

Etiology
- Mode of inheritance can be sporadic, autosomal dominant, or X-linked recessive.
- It may be an isolated finding or part of a genetic syndrome.
- Polydactyly is nine times more frequent in African Americans.

Symptoms and Signs
- Polydactyly and bifid digits may occur in many forms. The severity of the individual case can vary.
- A supernumerary digit is a known subtype of polydactyly. It is a rudimentary, pedunculated digit that is a duplication of the little (ulnar) finger. It is more commonly located on the left hand.

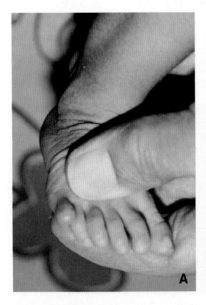

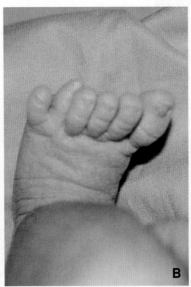

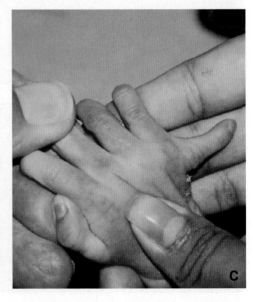

Figures A–D: Figures A and **B** demonstrate polydactyly of the sixth toe. Ulnar polydactyly of the right and left hand **(Figures C** and **D)**. A thin, pedunculated tissue is connecting the supernumerary digit to the fifth (small) finger in **Figure D**.

figures continues

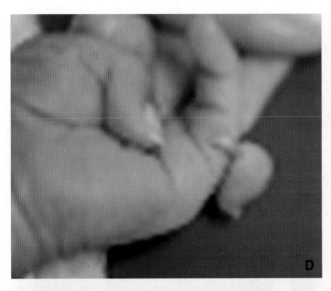

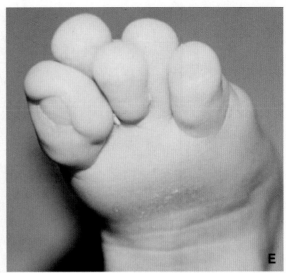

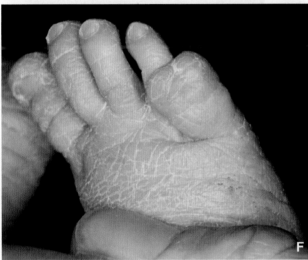

(figures cont.) **Figure D**

Figure E: Bifid right big toe and overriding of the third toe are the only abnormalities found in this newborn female.

Figure F: Bifid fifth toe is a solitary finding in this male newborn.

Treatment
- Radiographic evaluation of the affected digit.
- Removal of the extra digit is usually performed after the first birthday.
- Supernumerary digits may be ligated by a suture at its base. This leads to necrosis and autoamputation.
- In the case of an equally divided bifid thumb, the radial one is usually surgically removed.

PRUNE BELLY SYNDROME

Definition
- Prune belly syndrome is a rare congenital defect which occurs almost exclusively in males. It is characterized by urinary tract abnormalities, deficiency of abdominal muscles, and bilateral cryptorchidism (in males).

Etiology
- Unknown. Proposed mechanisms include genetic inheritance, early urethral obstruction, and abnormal embryonic mesoderm development.

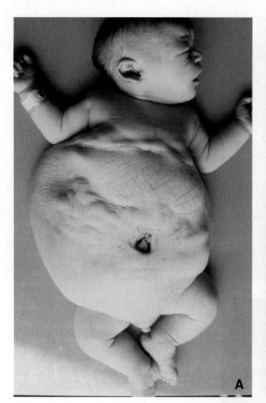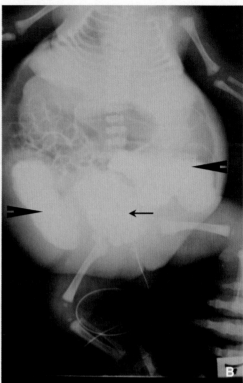

Figures A–B: A stillborn male with prune belly syndrome. Note the floppy, wrinkled abdomen and the bell-shaped thorax. Bilateral cryptorchidism and complete loss of abdominal muscles are also evident **(Figure A)**. AP radiograph of the abdomen taken during a voiding cystourethrogram (VCUG). A grossly dilated bladder (*arrow*) with reflux into the severely dilated ureters (*arrowheads*) **(Figure B)**.

Symptoms and Signs

- Significant renal dysplasia which can lead to pulmonary hypoplasia and end-stage renal disease.
- Aplasia or hypoplasia of abdominal muscles leading to the classic prune belly appearance.
- Unilateral or bilateral abnormalities of the genitourinary tract including megaureter, distended bladder due to abnormal bladder urodynamics, and vesicoureteral reflux.
- Cryptorchidism.
- Skeletal abnormalities secondary to pulmonary hypoplasia.
- Recurrent urinary tract infections.
- Gastrointestinal abnormalities including malrotation, imperforate anus, and constipation.

Treatment

- Management depends on the severity of the renal dysplasia.
- Establishment of urinary drainage by prenatal and postnatal interventions.
- Dialysis and renal transplantation for progressive renal disease.
- Corrective surgery for GI and orthopedic malformations.

PSEUDOHYPOALDOSTERONISM TYPE I

Definition

- It is a rare genetic disorder that is characterized by hyponatremia, hypovolemia, and hyperkalemia.

Etiology
- Mutation in the gene coding for aldosterone receptors. Pattern of inheritance is autosomal dominant and the defective aldosterone receptors are limited to the kidney.
- Mutations in epithelial sodium channels which lead to aldosterone resistance. Pattern of inheritance is autosomal recessive and the defective sodium channels are located in the lungs, kidneys, intestines, and sweat glands.

Symptoms and Signs
- Volume depletion, hyponatremia, hyperkalemia, and metabolic acidosis.
- Patients are usually normotensive.
- Elevated plasma and urinary aldosterone levels.
- Autosomal recessive defect may present with recurrent pneumonia; coughing; wheezing; abnormalities of sweat sodium and chloride concentrations; and pustular erythematous eruptions of the face, trunk, and extremities.

Treatment
- Autosomal dominant disease is a self-limited disorder as symptoms usually resolve by 2 years.
- High sodium diet in both autosomal dominant and recessive conditions.
- High-dose fludrocortisone in autosomal recessive cases which do not improve with high sodium diet alone.

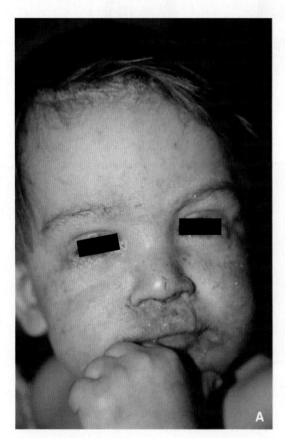

Figure A: This 3-kg male infant was born by repeat cesarean section to a mother with a history of hypertension. He was brought in at 1 week of life with maternal concerns of an "eye infection since birth." The mother's prior pregnancies had resulted in two miscarriages, a stillborn, one healthy male, and a death secondary to pseudohypoaldosteronism. The newborn has lost 336 g since birth. His eyes appeared injected with yellowish discharge. The skin appeared eczematous. Further studies confirmed the clinical diagnosis.

figures continues

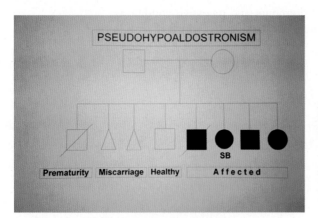

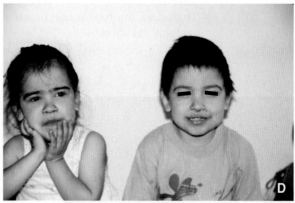

(figures cont.) **Figures B–C:** The sister to the index case was born a year later by cesarean section with a birth weight of 1.5 kg. She was seen in our office with dehydration, dry skin, crusted eyes, hyponatremia, hyperkalemia, and metabolic acidosis. Her skin, eyes, and nasal discharge appeared strikingly similar to that of her brother **(Figures A–F)**. Both are currently receiving sodium chloride, sodium bicarbonate, sodium acetate, florinef, albuterol, and budesonide inhalers.

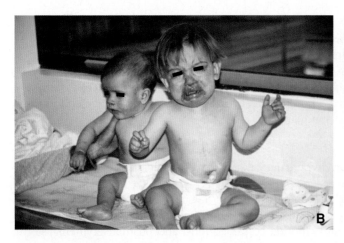

Pedigree of the family with pseudohypoaldosteronism.

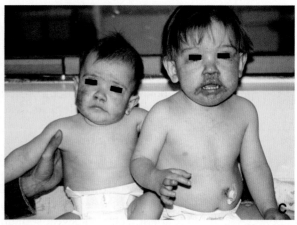

Figure D

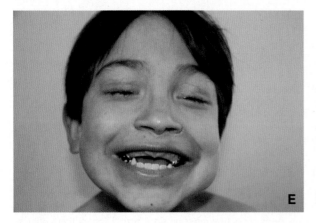

Figure E: He is reportedly doing well in school and is a "straight A student".

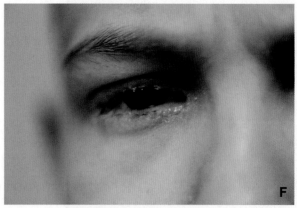

Figure F: Both siblings have dry skin, recurrent conjunctivitis, and erythema of the eyelids.

PSORIASIS (Gr. Psoros, scabby + iasis)

Definition
- Psoriasis is a common, immune-mediated, chronic inflammatory skin disorder that occurs in all ages.

Etiology
- Strong genetic and familial correlation. However, pattern of inheritance remains unknown.
- Environmental factors include skin trauma, various infections, Kawasaki disease, growth hormone and interferon injections, as well as psychological stress.

Symptoms and Signs
- It is more common in Caucasians. Approximately one-third of cases present during the first two decades of life. Overall, it affects 2% to 3% of the general population.
- Psoriasis is very rarely noted during the newborn period, but two forms may be seen during infancy:
  1. Pruritic, erythematous plaques with a silvery scale may affect the diaper area, scalp, and the face.
  2. Pustular psoriasis. Erythematous scales that are peripherally surrounded by pustules.
- In older children and adults, plaque psoriasis lesions are the most common form. They are erythematous, well-marginated, raised plaques that are symmetrically distributed on the body and covered by a grayish-silvery scale.
- Woronoff's ring refers to a peripheral white ring around the lesion and may be the first sign and indication of a lesion due to psoriasis.
- Plaque psoriasis may be seen anywhere on the body including the torso, face, extensor surfaces of elbows and knees, and lumbosacral areas.
- Scalp lesions are common and frequently extend beyond the hairline into the forehead and are rare in the occipital area.
- Other findings may include pitting, hyperkeratosis, and color changes of nail plates; umbilical and anogenital involvement; and geographic tongue.
- Lesions may occur at sites of skin injury as described by the Koebner phenomenon.
- The Auspitz's sign is the fine punctate bleeding points that are created after the removal of the characteristic grayish-silvery scale.
- Inverse psoriasis occurs when lesions are seen on the flexor aspect of the joints, axillae, groin, perineum, and inframammary areas.
- Guttate (drop-like) psoriasis refers to an acute eruption of multiple small plaques. It is more common in children and young adults without a previous history of psoriasis. There is a strong association with a preceding bacterial infection (i.e., Streptococcus).
- Pustular psoriasis presents with widespread erythema, scaling, pustules, and erosions. It may have systemic and life-threatening complications including fever, anorexia, malaise, hepatitis, and acute respiratory distress syndrome.
- Erythrodermic psoriasis is a severe, rare form of psoriasis. It is characterized by extensive erythema and scaling. Infection and electrolyte abnormalities are frequent complications.
- Arthritis, uveitis, and other ophthalmologic abnormalities are among the extracutaneous manifestations of psoriasis.

Treatment
- Topical steroids and emollients are often the first line of treatment in children.
- Liquid carbonis detergens may be added to topical steroids for better disease control.
- Systemic medications (methotrexate, retinoids, and cyclosporine) may be used in refractory cases.
- There are no efficacy or safety data on adult psoriasis medications that are being used for children.

- Patient and parental education regarding the chronicity, spontaneous remissions, and exacerbations of psoriasis.
- Removal of potential triggers including medications (β-blockers, lithium, antimalarial drugs) and sun exposure.
- Avoid irritating soaps, tight clothing, and shoes.
- Antibiotics do not seem to change the course of the disease. However, tonsillectomy may have a beneficial effect in children with chronic psoriasis.

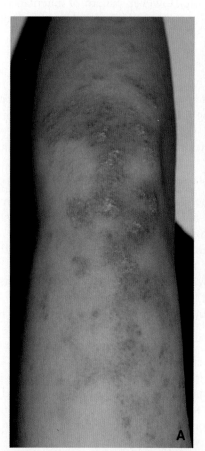

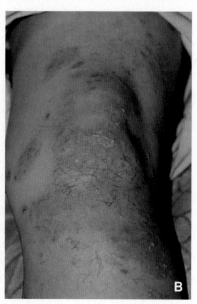

Figures A–B: Erythematous plaques of psoriasis in a 16-year-old male with Down's syndrome, diabetes mellitus, and hypothyroidism.

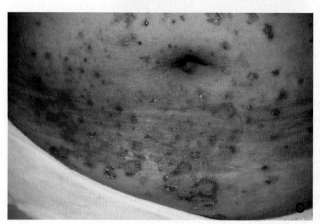

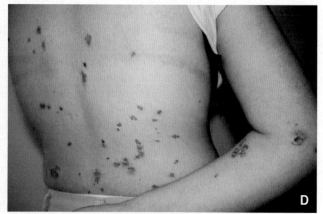

Figures C–E: This 12-year-old female presented with a new body rash. The rash erupted 4 days prior to her visit. She could not recall a recent episode of pharyngitis or URI illness. Her body was covered with 1 to 2 cm salmon-pink macules and papules. Her hands and feet were spared. Her throat culture was negative for β-hemolytic Streptococcus group A. She was diagnosed with psoriasis.

figures continues

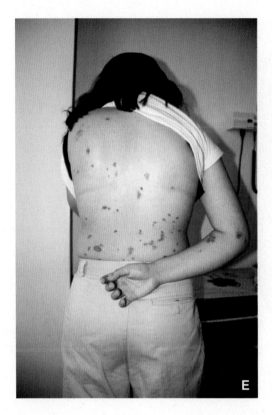

E   *(figures cont.)* **Figure E**

PTOSIS (Gr. Fall) (BLEPHAROPTOSIS)

Definition
- Ptosis is an abnormal lowering of one or both upper eyelids.

Etiology
- Inability of the levator palpebrae superioris muscle to raise the eyelid. Ptosis may be present at birth (congenital) or develop with age (acquired).
- Causes of ptosis include the following:
  - Aponeurotic ptosis: Refers to dehiscence of levator muscle aponeurosis. It may be congenital, secondary to birth trauma, or acquired.
  - Myogenic ptosis: Most common cause of congenital ptosis. It is caused by dystrophy of the levator muscle tissue. Examples are myotonic dystrophy and oculopharyngeal muscular dystrophy.
  - Neurogenic ptosis: Caused by damage to the third cranial nerve which controls the ability of the levator muscle to raise the eyelid. Third cranial nerve palsy, Horner's syndrome, and Marcus Gunn syndrome are included in this category.
  - Neuromyogenic ptosis: Deficit at the neuromuscular junction leads to ptosis. Myasthenia gravis is the most prominent example.
  - Mechanical ptosis: Heavy lesions such as capillary hemangioma may place heavy burden on the eyelid causing it to droop.
  - Pseudoptosis: Apparent drooping of the eyelid is secondary to abnormalities of the globe or ocular adnexa. Microphthalmus, contralateral eye retraction, and exophthalmus lead to pseudoptosis.

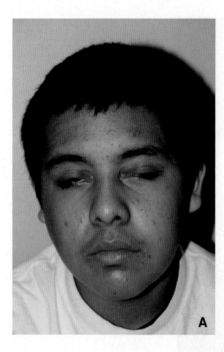

Figure A: Bilateral congenital ptosis in an otherwise healthy 18-year-old male. There was no prior family history of ptosis.

Symptoms and Signs
- Drooping of one or both eyelids. Children may hold their heads up in order to compensate for ptosis.
- Myasthenia gravis should be suspected with ptosis that worsens as the day goes on.
- Ptosis, miosis, anhidrosis, and heterochromia of the iris are classic findings in Horner's syndrome.
- Ptosis may interfere with the visual development of a child and lead to amblyopia.
- Figure A.

Treatment
- Treatment of the underlying disease.
- Surgical indications include amblyopia, abnormal head position, and cosmetic concerns.
- Specific surgical approach depends on the cause of ptosis.

PURPURA (L., purpura, purple)

Definition
- Purpura is characterized by small hemorrhages underneath the skin, mucous membranes, or serosal surfaces.

Etiology
- Platelet disorders: Thrombocytopenic purpura (nonpalpable).
- Vascular disorders: Henoch–Schonlein purpura (palpable).
- Coagulation disorders: Disseminated intravascular coagulation (DIC) and scurvy (palpable).
- Infectious: Meningococcemia.

Symptoms and Signs
- Red or purple discoloration of the skin which measure 0.3 to 1 cm.
- Application of pressure on the skin does not lead to blanching.

- Purpura can be nonpalpable or palpable. See above.
- The anatomic position of purpura may depend on the etiology.
- Figures A–O.

Treatment
- The underlying etiology must be addressed.

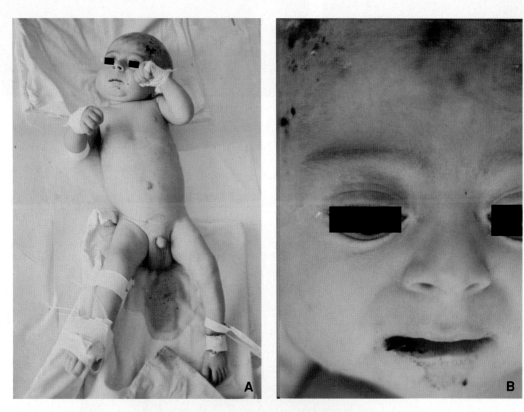

Figures A–B: Purpura in DIC. Note purpura on the abdominal wall, face, right sclera, and hematochezia.

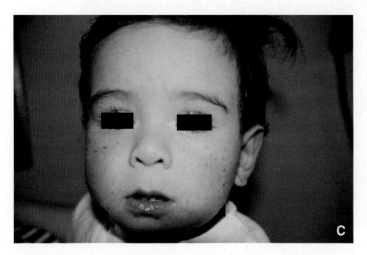

Figure C: Purpura due to breath-holding spells in a 20-month-old male.

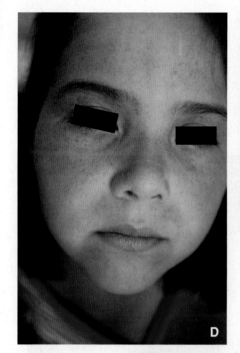

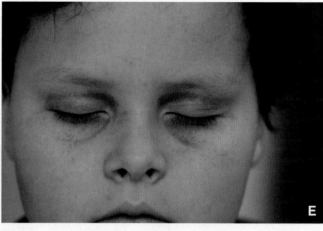

(figures cont.) **Figures D–E:** Purpura following heavy coughing in two school-aged children.

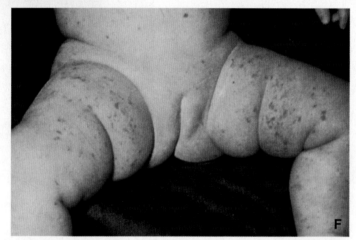

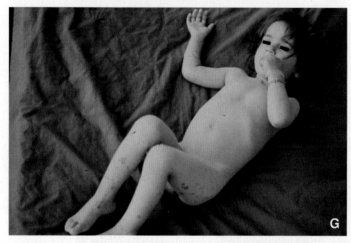

Figures F–G: Purpura in streptococcal infection.

figures continues

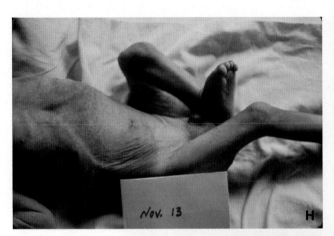

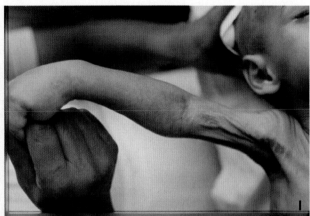

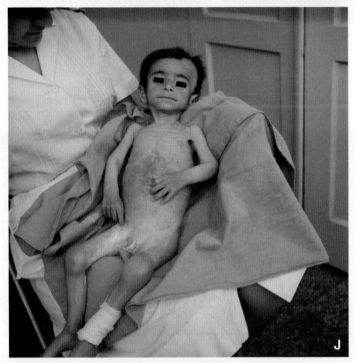

(figures cont.) **Figures H–J:** Purpura in malnutrition is an ominous finding.

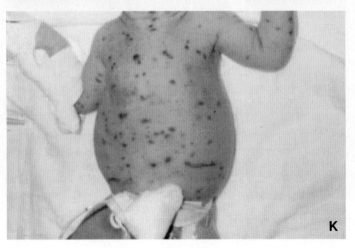

Figure K: Purpura in meningococcal meningitis.

figures continues

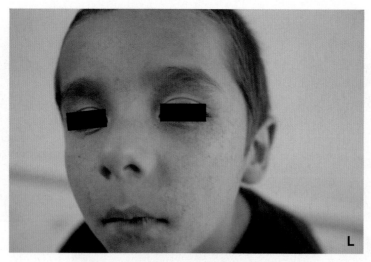

(figures cont.) **Figure L:** This 11-year-old male presented with acute onset of vomiting and rash. He appeared well and was afebrile. His face and neck were covered with purpura. However, none were noted on his extremities. He was diagnosed with vomiting-induced purpura.

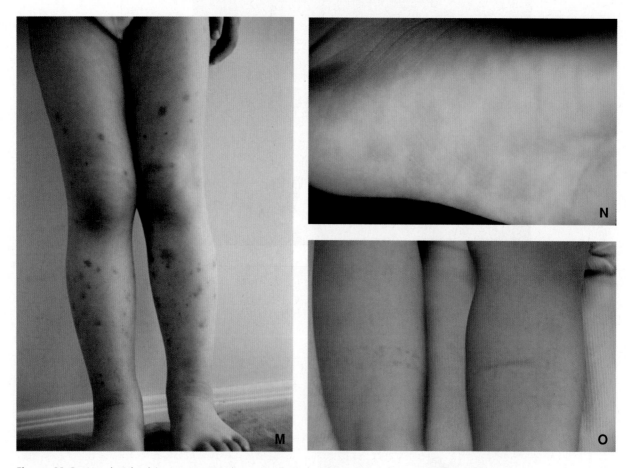

Figures M–O: Henoch–Schonlein purpura. Note linear purpura induced by pressure from socks **(Figure O)**.

figures continues

IDIOPATHIC THROMBOCYTOPENIC PURPURA (ITP)

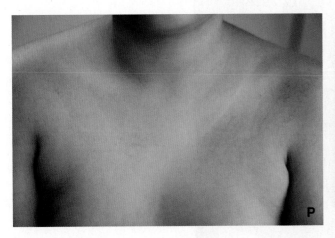
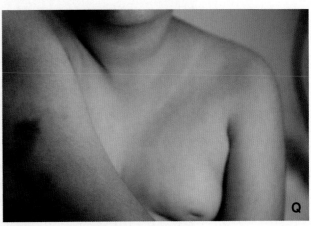

(figures cont.) **Figures P–Q:** This 11-year-old male has had a history of epistaxis which had worsened over the last month. He was well appearing, and purpura and ecchymosis were noted on his chest and right arm, respectively. There was no evidence of lymphadenopathy or hepatosplenomegaly. His platelet count was 14,000. His previous CBCs during his annual checkups were normal.

PYKNODYSOSTOSIS (Gr. Pyknos, thick, dense)

Definition
- Pyknodysostosis is a rare genetic disease consisting of dwarfism, osteosclerosis, and several other bone deformities.
- The disorder is also known by Toulouse-Lautrec syndrome after the French artist Henri de Toulouse-Lautrec who suffered from this disease.

Etiology
- Pyknodysostosis is an autosomal recessive bone dysplasia.
- It is caused by a mutation of the gene encoding the lysosomal cysteine protease known as cathepsin K.
- Cathepsin K is highly expressed in osteoclasts and is thought to play a role in bone remodeling and resorption.

Symptoms and Signs
- Short stature, generalized and diffuse osteosclerosis, hypoplastic clavicles, long bone fractures, rickets, and short, stubby fingers.
- Large skull with fronto-occipital bossing. Large anterior fontanelle with open sutures.
- Characteristic facies of proptosis, maxillary and mandibular hypoplasia, depressed nasal bridge, beaked nose, and a multitude of dental abnormalities.
- Systemic signs may include cardiomegaly and hepatosplenomegaly.
- X-ray of the bone shows a generalized increase in bone density and normal metaphyses.

Treatment
- Treatment is symptomatic.
- Management of fractures and dental problems.
- Overall prognosis is good.

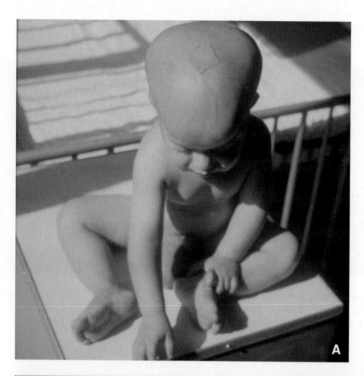

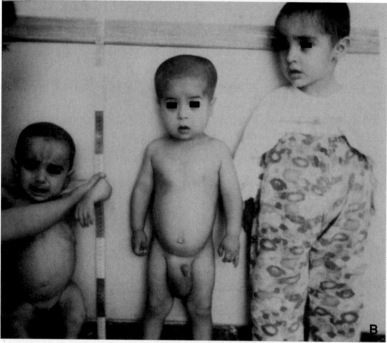

Figures A–B: This 3-year-old child was brought in for his large inguinal hernia. He had short stature, a large skull, a wide anterior fontanelle, occipital bossing, and pectus carinatum. Radiographic studies of his bones and skull revealed increased bone density and widened sutures, respectively. He was diagnosed with pyknodysostosis **(Figure A)**. He is standing next to two children of similar age **(Figure B)**. The child on his right has vitamin D deficiency rickets and the one on his left has primary tuberculosis.

RAYNAUD'S DISEASE

Definition

- Raynaud's phenomenon is a condition resulting from blood vessel spasm, limiting blood flow to the fingers, toes, nose, and the ears as a result of exposure to cold and stress. The vasospasm leads to the discoloration of the affected body part.
- Raynaud's disease (also called idiopathic Raynaud's or primary Raynaud's phenomenon) is a vascular disorder characterized by bilateral attacks of Raynaud's phenomenon.
- Raynaud's syndrome is associated with Raynaud's phenomenon and as part of a connective tissue disease or syndrome. Vascular insufficiency of the extremities, in the syndrome, is secondary to a condition such as scleroderma, rheumatoid arthritis, dermatomyositis, and systemic lupus erythematosus (SLE).

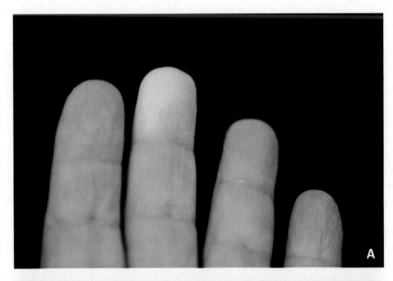

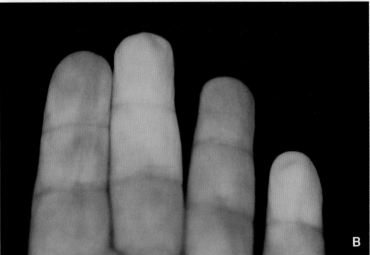

Figures A–C: Different stages of the Raynaud's phenomenon in the fingers of an 80-year-old man with the condition since the age of 15 years.

figures continues

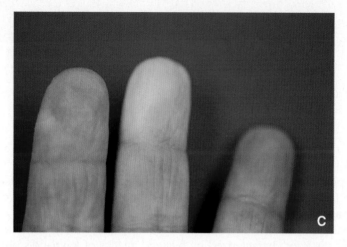

(figures cont.) **Figure C**

Etiology
- Unknown.

Symptoms and Signs
- Raynaud's phenomenon is a vasomotor hyperresponsiveness or hyperactivation of the sympathetic system to cold, emotional stress, and other unknown factors leading to vasoconstriction of the peripheral blood vessels causing hypoxemia.
- An asymptomatic pallor of a finger, often the left third or fifth, begins from the distal phalange and then spreads proximally. Other fingers are soon affected. If the precipitating stimulus continues (stress or cold), the involved fingers gradually feel numb, stiff, and uncomfortable to use. The first fingers and the first toes are the last digits to be affected in the process.
- More common in women than in men.
- Fingers are more often affected than toes.
- Recovery begins in the reverse order of presentation, once the hands and feet are warmed (or other triggers are removed).
- Over 50% of patients with Raynaud's phenomenon have Raynaud's disease.

Treatment
- Avoidance of the triggers and warming up of the affected body part.
- Treatment of the underlying condition.

RETINOBLASTOMA

Definition
- Retinoblastoma is a malignant tumor of the embryonic neural retina and the most common intraocular malignancy in children.

Etiology
- Retinoblastoma often presents at birth and close to 80% are diagnosed before the age of 4 years.
- The majority of cases are sporadic; 40% are hereditary and are transmitted as autosomal dominant.
- Estimated frequency of bilateral retinoblastomas is about 25% to 35%.

Symptoms and Signs
- The most common presenting sign is leukocoria or cat's eye reflex.

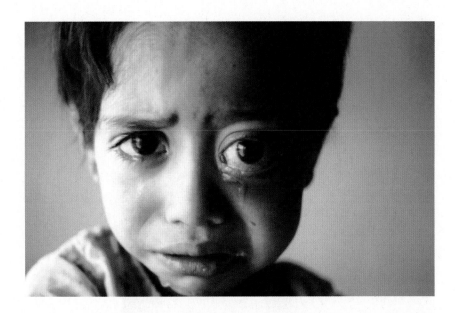

- With hemorrhage, the pupil might have a dark red reflex; heterochromia, and in advance cases glaucoma might occur.

Treatment
- In the early stage of a small tumor, laser photocoagulation.
- Cryotherapy may be helpful for a small peripheral lesion.
- Chemotherapy is the mainstay of therapy.
- Intraocular arterial chemotherapy is used for selective cases.

RHABDOMYOSARCOMA (Gr. Rhabdo, rod; Myos, muscle; Sarkos, flesh)

Definition
- Malignant tumors of the mesenchymal cell origin are called sarcomas. These cells normally mature into skeletal muscles.
- Rhabdomyosarcoma is the third most common extracranial tumor in children (after neuroblastoma and the Wilms' tumor).
- Soft tissue sarcomas consist of different types according to their pathology: Rhabdomyosarcoma, fibrosarcoma, liposarcoma, synovial sarcoma, spindle cell sarcoma, and others.

Etiology
- Alveolar rhabdomyosarcoma has a characteristic translocation of FKHR gene at 13q14 with PAX3 at 2q35 and some rare abnormality.

Symptoms and Signs
- Symptoms and signs primarily depend on the site of the tumor.
- The three main types of rhabdomyosarcoma are embryonal rhabdomyosarcoma (the most common type), alveolar rhabdomyosarcoma, and anaplastic rhabdomyosarcoma.
- Peak age is 2 to 6 years and also again from 15 to 19 years.
- Rhabdomyosarcoma may occur at any anatomic location in the body with skeletal muscle and even in areas without skeletal muscle.

Treatment
- Surgery, chemotherapy, or radiotherapy depending on the stage of the disease.

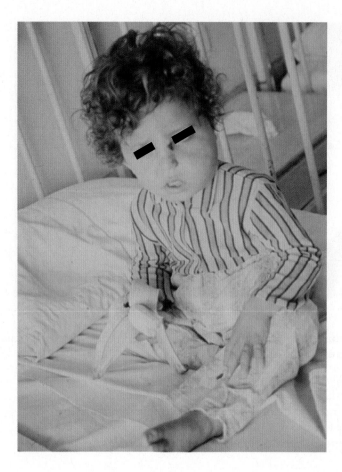

This 3-year-old girl was brought in for a swelling on her face for 2 months. She had a large and visible mass on her left cheek, anterior to the parotid gland, nontender, and without any sign of inflammation or erythema. She otherwise looked well. Biopsy indicated rhabdomyosarcoma, embryonal type.

RHIZOMELIC CHONDRODYSPLASIA PUNCTATA (Gr. Rhiza, root; Melos, limb)

Definition
- Part of a heterogeneous group of disorders with facial features, developmental delay, respiratory problems, skeletal abnormalities, and with impairment in developments of many parts of the body. The specific bone abnormality is chondrodysplasia punctata.

Etiology
- A genetic disease with an autosomal recessive mode of inheritance.

Symptoms and Signs
- Developmental delay, failure to thrive, shortening of bones in the upper arms and thighs, joint deformities, prominent forehead, hypertelorism, midface hypoplasia, small nose, full cheeks, and cataract.

Treatment
- Supportive.

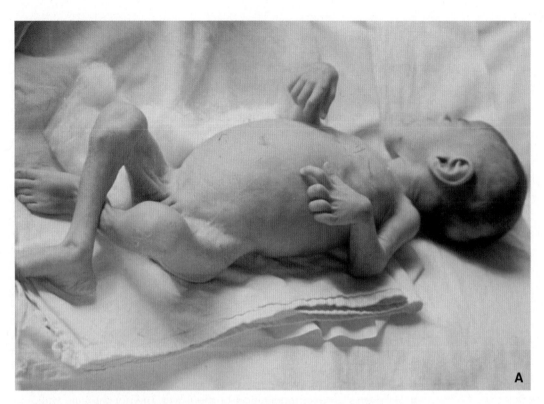

Figure A: This infant girl is the first-born child to young parents who are also first cousins. In Iran, first-cousin marriage is considered "a match made in heavens." This child was brought in for oral thrush and stiff joints. She had calorie malnutrition, contracture deformity of the knees, wrists, and of the elbow joints.

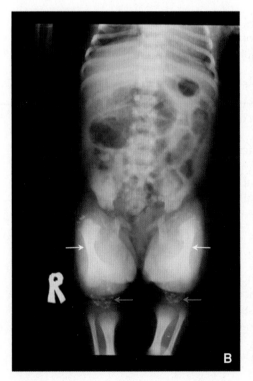

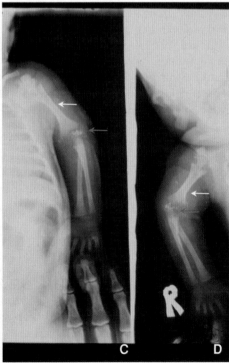

Figures B–D: Frontal x-ray of the torso and proximal lower extremities demonstrate shortening of the proximal portions of the lower extremities (*white arrows*) with a stippled appearance of the epiphyses (*red arrows*) **(Figure B)**. X-rays of the upper extremities demonstrate identical features as described above **(Figures C and D)**.

RICKETS (Gr. Rachitis)

VITAMIN D DEFICIENCY RICKETS

Definition
- Undermineralization and interruption in the development and growth of the bones due to Vitamin D deficiency.

Etiology
- Lack of exposure to adequate sunlight or inadequate intake of Vitamin D.
- Breast-feeding (inadequate amount), having darker skin (interferes with absorption of sunlight and with the synthesis of Vitamin D), drugs such as phenytoin and phenobarbital (activate catabolism of Vitamin D), prematurity, chronic renal insufficiency, biliary atresia and chronic liver disease, and malabsorption (celiac) are all risk factors.

Symptoms and Signs
- Rickets is the failure of mineralization of the growing bone and cartilage.
- The only symptom or sign of rickets which may bring a child to a pediatrician or emergency room is seizure due to hypocalcemia. Most of the other signs are incidental findings.
- Rachitic rosaries: Prominent costochondral junctions.
- Harrison's groove: Indentation of the lower anterior thoracic wall.
- Other features: Bowing of the forearm (if the child is crawling), bowing of the legs, genu varum, and genu valgum (if the child is walking), frontal bossing, craniotabes, and generalized hypotonia.
- Pneumonia is common in advanced rickets, possibly due to the diminished immunity.
- Normal or low plasma calcium and phosphorus, high alkaline phosphatase, low serum 25-hydroxyvitamin D3, and high parathyroid hormone levels.
- Serum calcium, phosphorus, and alkaline phosphatase can be normal if the child has calorie malnutrition.
- Recent studies have shown a high incidence of Vitamin D deficiency and insufficiency in American children; especially in girls, Blacks, Native Americans, Hispanics, and those who spend more than 4 hours a day on a computer, television, or playing video games.
- There is an association between Vitamin D deficiency and cardiovascular risk factors later in life.
- Radiologic changes are evident best in the distal end of radius and include widening of the growth plate, irregular metaphyseal margins that can progress to metaphyseal concavity with fraying of the margins.
- Figures A–R.

Treatment
- 1,000 to 10,000 IU a day until radiologic evidence of improvement is achieved in approximately 1 month. After radiologic evidence of improvement is established, child needs to be placed on a maintenance daily dose of 400 IU.
- We found an IM dose of 600,000 IU to be more effective in the developing world, possibly due to prevalent diarrheal diseases.

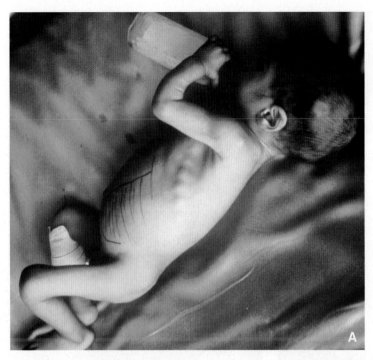

Figure A: Rachitic rosaries, bowing of the forearms, swollen wrists due to flaring of the epiphysis of radius and ulna and hepatosplenomegaly in an infant with rickets.

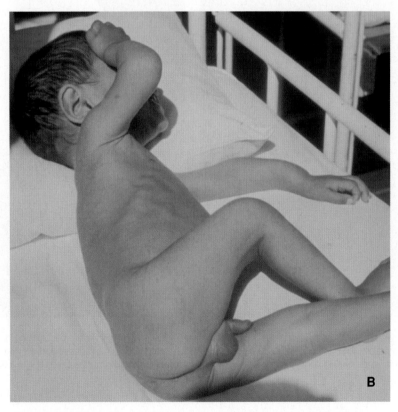

Figure B: Rachitic rosaries, bowed forearms, and swelling of the wrist in rickets.

figures continues

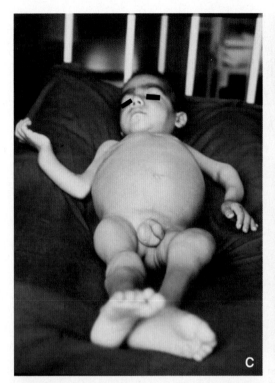

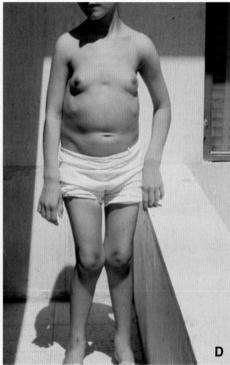

(figures cont.) **Figures C–D:** Potbelly and deformed wrist due to rickets and a greenstick fracture **(Figure C)**. Genu valgum in rickets in a 13-year-old boy who also had gynecomastia **(Figure D)**.

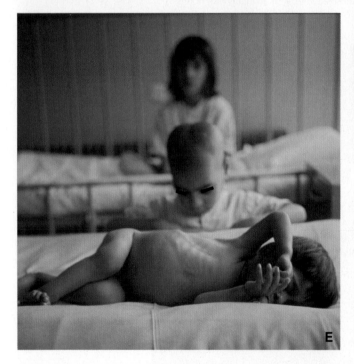

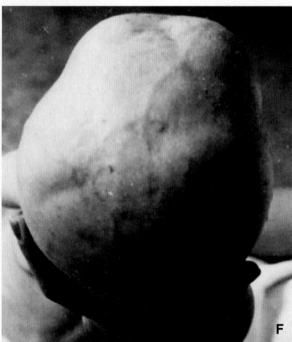

Figures E–F: Chest deformity with bilateral chest depressions and swollen wrists in rickets. The boy in the background had vitamin D deficiency and anemia which led to abnormal skull growth **(Figure E)**. Skull deformity in a 1-year-old who had anemia and vitamin D deficiency rickets, was admitted for diarrhea and vomiting, developed iatrogenic measles while in the hospital and could not be saved **(Figure F)**.

figures continues

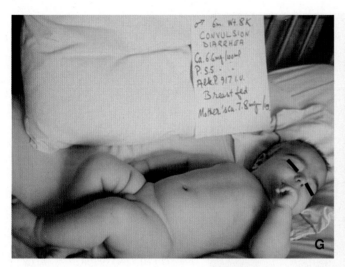

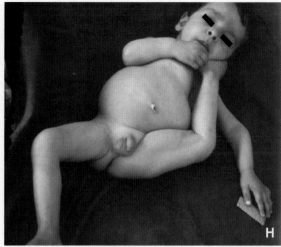

(figures cont.) **Figures G–H:** A well-nourished 6-month-old, breastfed infant who had diarrhea and developed a seizure which brought him into the hospital. He was not given supplemental vitamin D. He weighed 8 kg, had a large anterior fontanelle, and no rachitic rosaries. His plasma calcium was 6.6 mg/dL, phosphorous 5.5 mg/dL, and alkaline phosphatase 917 IU. His mother's plasma calcium was 7.8 mg/dL **(Figure G)**. Deformed chest, hypotonia, and potbelly in rickets. Note, how relaxed and comfortable he is while enjoying a cookie with his hyperextended leg due to severe hypotonia **(Figure H)**.

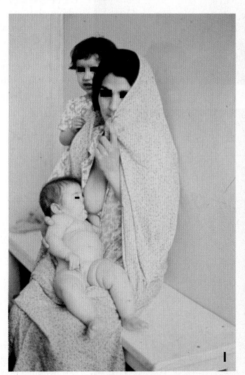

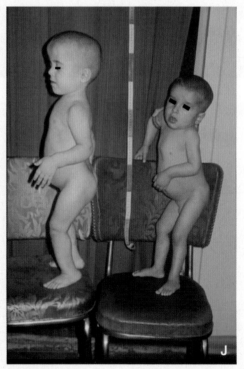

Figures I–J: This 6-month-old exclusively breastfed infant girl and without vitamin D supplementation, was brought to our house one early morning and on a weekend, due to a seizure earlier that day **(Figure I)**. Her older sister, standing behind her mother, was brought to us for the same problem a year earlier. The infant was well-nourished, had a large anterior fontanelle, but no rachitic rosaries or any other features of rickets. Her plasma calcium and phosphorus were low, alkaline phosphatase high, and an x-ray of the wrist showed widened growth plate, irregular metaphyseal margins, but no cupping. Her mother's plasma calcium was 8.1 mg/dL. Two 3-year-old boys are presented in **Figure J**. Their heights are 86 cm and 78 cm respectively (both are below the third percentile for age). Y (front child) has vitamin D resistant rickets and Z (child behind the first) has vitamin D deficiency rickets. Note, both have pectus carinatum (pigeon chest), bowed forearm, swollen wrists, and large abdomen. Y, who has been walking for some time, has bowed legs as well as frontal bossing. Z has severe hypotonia and is unable to walk and therefore there has been no pressure on his legs to bend them.

figures continues

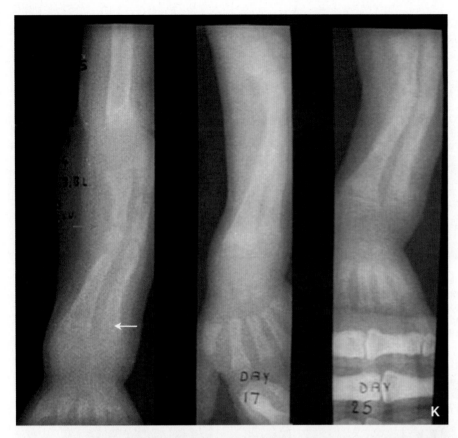

(figures cont.) **Figures K–L:** Two serial x-rays of a 2-year-old boy with advanced vitamin D deficiency rickets and calorie malnutrition, under treatment. In **Figure K**, the progress in 25 days is appreciable, but not complete. In **Figure L**, we have followed up x-rays for up to 87 days following one IM injection of 600,000 IU. On day one, and another one on day 33, of vitamin D. We also have plasma calcium of 9.4, phosphorus of 2.95 mg/dL, and alkaline phosphatase of 1,200 U/L on the same day. Ca of 8 mg/dL, serum phosphorus of 4.63 mg/dL, and alkaline phosphatase had dropped to 200 U/L on day 87. This odd pattern of calcium, phosphorus, and alkaline phosphatase is common in rachitic children with calorie malnutrition.

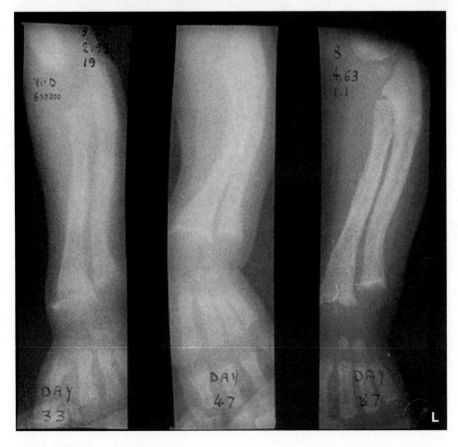

Figure L: Forearm x-rays demonstrate typical findings of rickets with indistinct and widened ends of the long bones (*white arrows*). Also seen is bending deformities and fractures (*red arrows*). The second and third panels demonstrate response to therapy and healing with increased density of the ends and resolving fracture lines **(Figure K)**. Bending deformity persists; however has improved. Continued increased density of the ends of the forearm bones is again observed **(Figure L)**.

figures continues

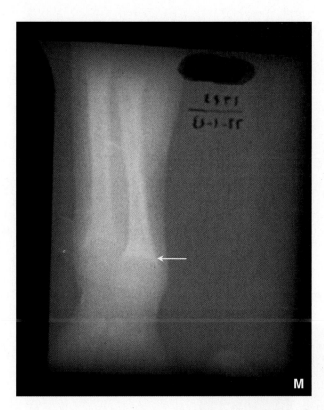

(figures cont.) **Figure M:** Initial wrist x-ray prior to the treatment demonstrates the typical findings of rickets of a cupped, splayed, and frayed metaphysis.

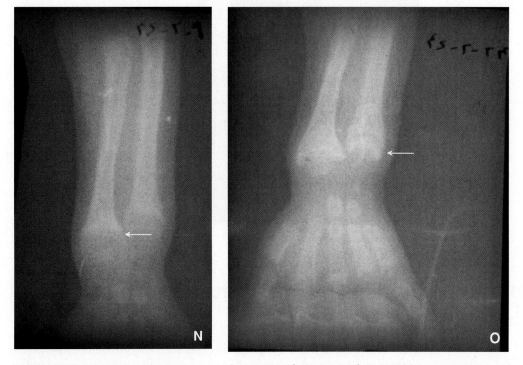

Figure N: Wrist x-ray 6 days after an intramuscular injection of 600,000 IU of vitamin D demonstrates increased density of the abnormal metaphysis.

Figure O: Wrist x-ray at 32 days posttherapy demonstrates continued increased density of the metaphysis.

figures continues

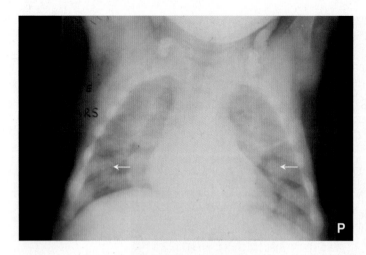

(figures cont.) **Figure P:** Chest x-ray demonstrates the cupping of the rib ends with widening of the rib epiphyseal cartilage giving the "rachitic rosary" of rickets (*arrows*).

ATROPHIC RICKETS

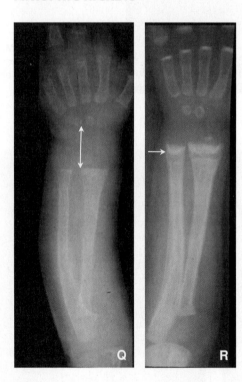

Figure Q: Forearm x-ray shows increased distance from the end of the shaft to the carpal bones suggesting that the metaphysis is uncalcified.

Figure R: Forearm x-ray after therapy now demonstrates increased density in the zone of provisional calcium. Atrophic rickets is seen in severe calorie malnutrition.

ROSEOLA INFANTUM (EXANTHEM SUBITUM, SIXTH DISEASE)

Definition
■ Roseola infantum is a common disease, seen in younger children, characterized by high fever and followed by rapid defervescence and simultaneous exanthema.

Etiology
■ Human herpesvirus 6 and 7, Coxsackievirus A and B, echoviruses, adenoviruses, and parainfluenza virus.

Symptoms and Signs

- Either mild or no prodromal symptoms, high fever for 3 to 5 days which resolves rather rapidly (crisis) or gradually (lysis), eruption of a nonpruritic, slightly raised, rose-colored and discrete rash, which rarely becomes confluent and fades within 1 to 3 days after eruption.
- Seizure may develop in 5% to 10% of the children.
- Encephalitis, meningoencephalitis, hepatitis, and pneumonia may rarely complicate roseola.

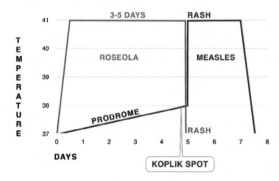

Fever pattern and rash in measles and roseola.

A pink rash appears following 3 to 5 days of fever in roseola infantum; whereas fever peaks after a few days of low-grade fever and coryza, and that is when the measles rash erupts, as the fever continues for a few more days.

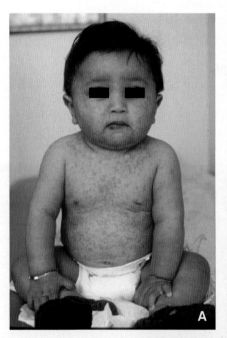

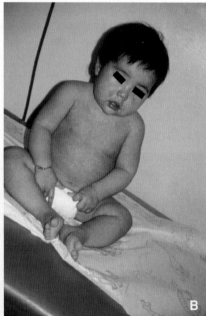

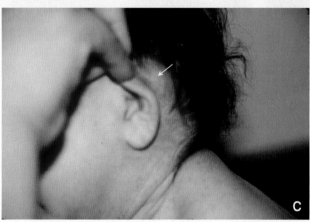

Figures A–C: Two children aged 11 and 10 months old, with the typical rash of roseola infantum **(Figures A and B)**. Retroauricular lymphadenopathy in roseola infantum **(Figure C)**.

Treatment
- Symptomatic.
- Ganciclovir, cidofovir, and foscarnet may be used in the immunocompromised or for complications.

RUBELLA (L. rubellus, reddish) GERMAN MEASLES

Definition
- Rubella, previously a common disease of children and young adults, is now mostly a benign and mild viral infection. In the fetus; however, rubella can develop into a severe multisystem fetal infection, causing a severe and debilitating rubella syndrome.

Etiology
- Rubella is caused by a togavirus, an RNA virus from the genus Rubivirus, which can cause disease only in humans.

Symptoms and Signs
- Rubella is rare in the industrialized countries and may be seen occasionally in the unvaccinated children and young adults.
- Rubella virus spreads either by droplets or passed transplacentally.
- Rubella is contagious from 7 days prior to the eruption of the rash and until 7 to 8 days after the rash has faded.
- The majority of cases are subclinical.
- Retroauricular, posterior cervical, and postoccipital lymphadenopathy are common findings.
- Very mild catarrhal symptoms.

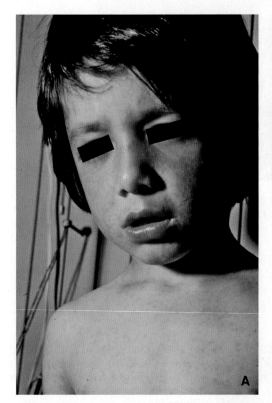

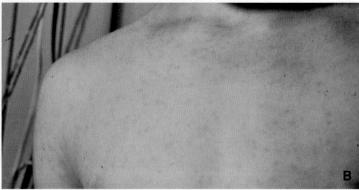

Figures A–B: Rubella in an 8-year-old boy. Note the maculopapular rash on his face and spreading to his chest.

figures continues

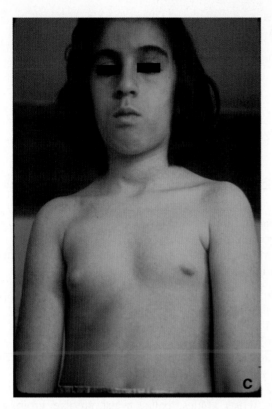

(figures cont.) **Figure C:** Rubella in a 12-year-old girl. Note the maculopapular rash, mostly on the face, spreading to the chest. She had visible lymphadenopathy in her neck which was covered with her hair.

- Forchheimer spot is the enanthem found in about 20% of patients just before the onset of the rash and consists of discrete rose-colored spots on the soft palate.
- A discrete maculopapular rash begins on the face, quickly spreads throughout the body and fades within 3 days.
- A polyarthritis which involves mostly the smaller joints and resolves without any permanent damage may follow rubella.

Treatment
- Symptomatic.

SCABIES (L. Scabere, scratch)

Definition
- A common contagious skin infestation caused by a small species of mite.

Etiology
- *Sarcoptes scabiei,* an obligate human parasite.
- It is more common in women and children.
- Scabies is transmitted through direct skin-to-skin contact with an infected person. Scabies can also spread by sharing clothing and bedding.

Symptoms and Signs
- "The itching in scabies is so intense and majestic that it is only worthy of kings and princesses." King James I.
- The incubation period is 3 weeks.
- Mites burrow into the skin. The mite, their feces, eggs, and larvae irritate the skin and cause an intense itching which is worse at night.
- Papules, nodules, burrows, vesicles, and pustules may be seen.
- Interdigital spaces, palms, wrists, ankles, axillae, waist, areolae, groin, genital, and soles are the most common areas of lesions.
- Head, palms, and soles are often the sites of scabies lesions in infants.
- Norwegian or crusted scabies, seen mostly in the immunocompromised, is scaly and highly contagious.
- Continuous itching and scratching may cause a secondary skin infection with *Staphylococcus aureus* and with group A β-hemolytic streptococci.
- Animal transmitted scabies are short-lived and self-limited.
- Figures A–F.

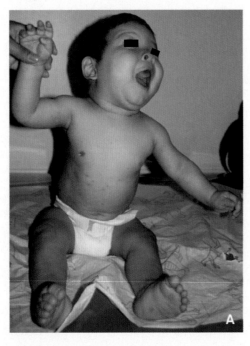

Figure A: Papules and nodules on the chest, palms, and soles.

figures continues

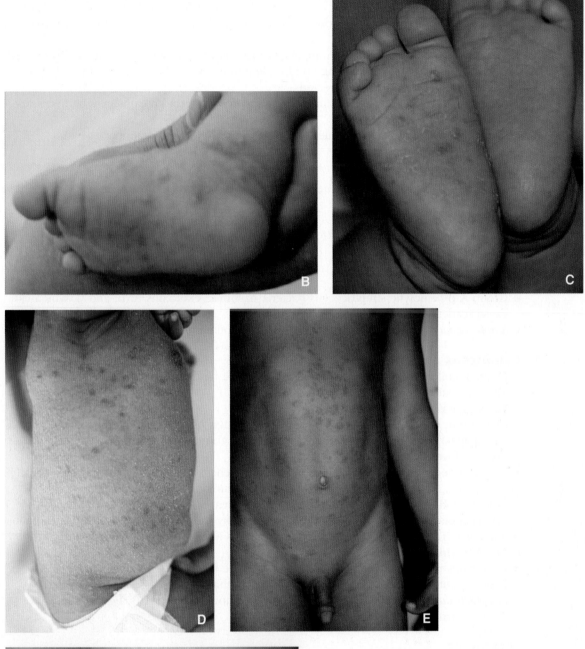

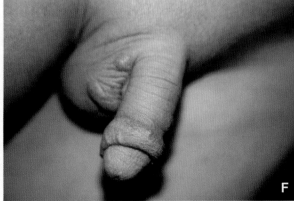

(figures cont.) **Figures B–C:** Papules, vesicles, and scaling of the soles.

Figure D: Papules, macules, and scales in the axillae and trunk in a 4-month-old infant.

Figure E: Papules and nodules on the trunk and the penis.

Figure F: Papules and nodules on the penis and the scrotum.

Treatment

- Permethrin cream, 5% is the drug of choice. Permethrin is not indicated for children younger than 2 months of age. A thin layer is applied from neck to toes, and left on for 8 to 14 hours, washed thoroughly, and followed by a second treatment a week later.
- The scalp should be included in infants, but the mouth and eyes must be well protected from this neurotoxin. All clothing and bedding must be washed and dried in a hot dryer.
- Close contacts should also be treated.
- Symptomatic treatment with antihistamines and corticosteroid creams may be necessary in some cases.
- Symptom of itching may continue for 2 to 6 weeks following treatment.

SCARLET FEVER (L. Scarlet, bright red)

Definition

- Scarlet fever is characterized by fever, pharyngitis, a "sandpaper rash," and cervical lymphadenopathy.

Etiology

- Group A β-hemolytic streptococcus bacteria has three exotoxins A, B, and C, which can cause scarlet fever.
- *Staphylococcus aureus* can cause a rash that can mimic the scarlatina rash.

Symptoms and Signs

- Often in children over the age of 3 years. It is rare before the age of 3 years.
- The incubation period is 1 to 2 days.
- Fever may rise up to 40 °C or higher.
- The rash in scarlet fever is rough and maculopapular on an erythematous base (sandpaper), blanches with pressure and appears about 24 to 48 hours after the onset of fever.
- The rash begins around the neck, spreads to the chest, the extremities, and occasionally to the face. Patients can have flushed cheeks, circumoral pallor (pallor around the mouth), and the rash is more intense along the creases.
- The rash gradually fades in days 3 to 4 followed by the desquamation of the face, palms, and soles. The desquamation begins 1 to 3 weeks after the onset of symptoms.
- Cervical lymphadenopathy.
- Pharyngitis with petechiae on the pharynx and the uvula and a strawberry tongue.
- Pediatric autoimmune neuropsychiatric disorders that are also associated with *Streptococcus pyogenes* (PANDAS): Obsessive–compulsive disorders, tic disorders, and Tourette syndrome.

Treatment

- Timely and appropriate treatment is absolutely important in order to prevent the complications of rheumatic fever, acute postinfectious glomerulonephritis, arthritis, osteomyelitis, otitis media, peritonsillar abscess and cellulitis, sinusitis, meningitis, and brain abscess.
- Treatment can be withheld for a day until the result of the throat culture becomes available.
- A 10-day course of penicillin V is the drug of choice at 250,000 IU three or four times a day. Alternatively, 250,000 IU twice a day for 10 days or amoxicillin in younger children who may not like the taste of penicillin.
- Erythromycin can be used in cases of penicillin allergy.
- Figures A–E.

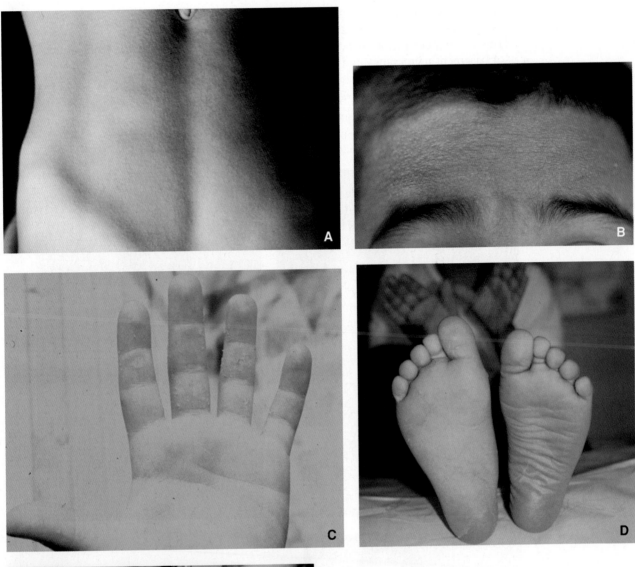

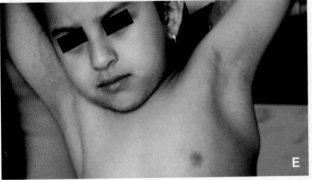

Figures A–E: Sandpaper rash in scarlet fever **(Figures A and B)**. Desquamation of the hands and feet **(Figures C and D)**. The 5-year-old girl **(Figure E)** was brought in for fever and rash. She had a temperature of 39.8 °C and erythema of the axillae and covered with a maculopapular rash. Her throat culture was positive for group A β-hemolytic streptococcus. She was treated with penicillin, the fever and the rash resolved. We had treated her older brother for streptococcus pharyngitis a few days earlier.

SCHWARTZ–JAMPEL DISEASE (MYOTONIC CHONDRODYSTROPHY)

Definition

■ Schwartz–Jampel disease is characterized by generalized muscle hypertrophy and weakness.

Etiology

■ It is a congenital disease possibly inherited as an autosomal recessive.

- The gene defect for type 1A Schwartz–Jampel disease is in 1p34–p36 region of chromosome 1 called HSPG2.
- This is a perlecan gene, which is a heparin sulfate proteoglycan, the major proteoglycan of basement membranes and of cartilage.

Symptoms and Signs
- Some are apparent at birth, but some cannot be diagnosed until later in life.
- Normal intelligence, dwarfism, blepharophimosis, puckered face, pectus carinatum, hypertrichosis of the eyelids, and joint abnormalities are common.
- EMG shows continuous electrical activity in the muscle fibers.

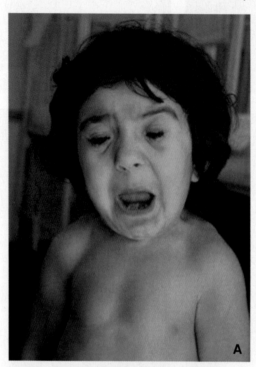

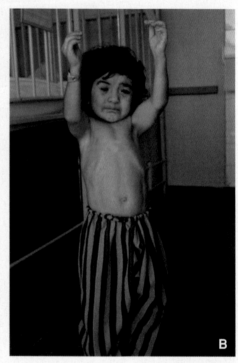

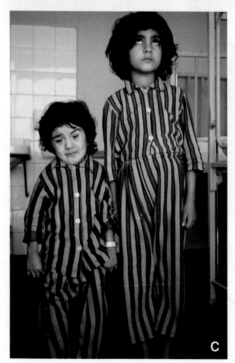

Figures A–C: This girl has most features of Schwartz–Jampel disease: Dwarfism, blepharophimosis, puckered face, hypertrichosis of the eyelids, myotonia (difficulty opening her mouth, her eyes, or raising her arms), and pectus carinatum (pigeon breast) **(Figures A and B)**. She is accompanied by a girl of her age who is much taller than her **(Figure C)**.

Treatment
- These children may require psychosocial support due to their physical appearance.
- Special dental care.
- Figures A–C.

SEBORRHEIC DERMATITIS (L. Sebum, suet)

Definition
- Seborrheic dermatitis is a self-limited, erythematous, scaly, or crusting eruption that is often found in areas of the body with a high concentration of sebaceous glands (i.e., the scalp, face, and retroauricular areas).

Etiology
- Unknown.
- A yeast called Pityrosporum ovale (Malassezia ovalis) found in abundance on the human scalp has been suspected as the cause of adult seborrheic dermatitis.

Symptoms and Signs
- Seborrheic dermatitis presents as a red, scaling rash which involves the scalp (cradle cap), eyebrows, eyelashes, postauricular, and intertriginous areas.
- It can present as early as 1 month of age and disappear before the second birthday.

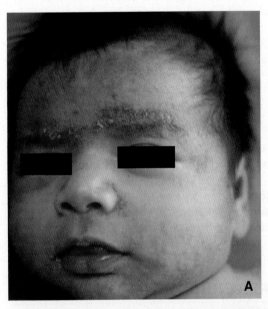

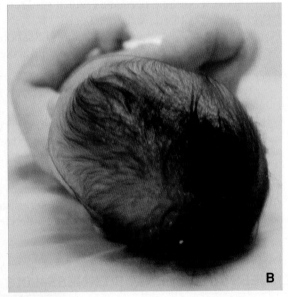

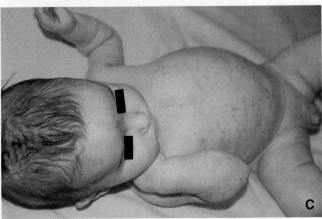

Figures A–C: Seborrhea of the eyebrows and face in a newborn **(Figure A)**. Note the hair loss due to aggressive brushing and shampooing in a 3-month-old infant who has had seborrhea of the scalp (cradle cap) since 1 month of age. The scalp remains salmon color and scaly **(Figure B)**. Seborrhea of the scalp and abdomen **(Figure C)**.

figures continues

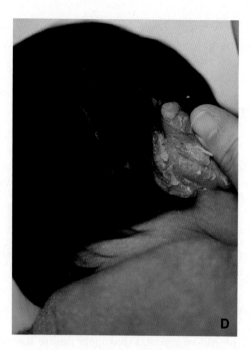

(figures cont.) **Figure D:** Retroauricular seborrheic dermatitis in a newborn.

- Anogenital, groins, umbilicus, trunk, retroauricular, intertriginous, and flexural areas can have seborrheic dermatitis which presents as erythematous, greasy, sharply marginated salmon-colored, scaly patches.
- Dandruff is another manifestation of seborrheic dermatitis during puberty and the middle age. It can present as a dry, fine, and flakey desquamation on the scalp.
- Figures A–D.

Treatment

- Reassurance.
- This self-limiting skin disorder in the newborn responds to frequent shampooing, mild steroid creams, and 1% salicylic acid in aqueous cream BP, and to the ketoconazole shampoo.
- Very dry cradle cups can be softened by warm mineral oil before additional treatment is applied.
- Dandruff can be managed with ketoconazole shampoo and several over-the-counter products such as the Head and Shoulder shampoo, DHS Zinc, Sebulex, Excel, and Selsun.
- Blepharitis can be managed with gentle cleansing of the eyelids with a diluted, nonirritating baby shampoo.

SERUM SICKNESS AND SERUM SICKNESS–LIKE REACTION (SSLR)

Definition

- Serum sickness is an immune system reaction to proteins in antiserums derived from a nonhuman animal source (such as injected proteins or antiserum).
- Serum sickness–like reaction (SSLR) is a reaction to a drug such as cefaclor, penicillin, amoxicillin, sulfa, NSAID, and others, which can cause a serum sickness–like reaction often 1 to 3 weeks after receiving the medication.

Etiology

- A type III hypersensitivity reaction to a foreign protein (or serum).
- Nonprotein drugs can cause a similar reaction (SSLR).

Symptoms and Signs

- Morbilliform, urticarial or purpuric rash, fever, malaise, splenomegaly, lymphadenopathy, arthralgia, and proteinuria.

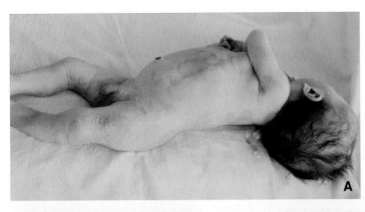

Figure A: Serum sickness in a 3-week-old newborn who received horse antitetanus serum at 1 week of age for the treatment of tetanus. He survived tetanus, but then developed a raised, pinkish-lilac rash throughout his body, with central clearing in a few of the lesions. Also note the site of numerous intramuscular injections on his left thigh.

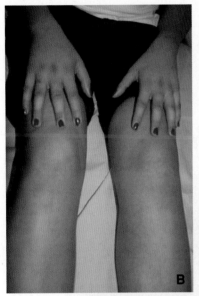

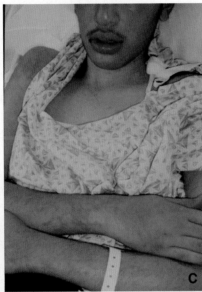

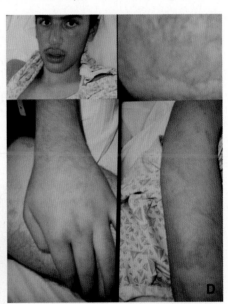

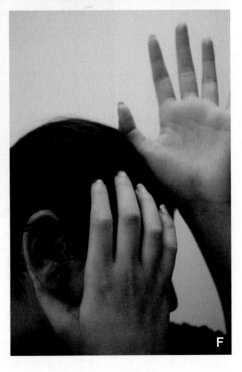

Figure B: This 17-year-old girl developed a rash, pain, and swelling of the knees and of the metacarpophalangeal joints while on minocycline.

Figures C–E: This 17-year-old boy developed symptoms after treatment with oral Prozac (fluoxetine) for 10 days. He developed facial edema, swelling of the lips, rash with central clearing, malaise, and a low-grade fever. He fully recovered a few days later after the discontinuation of Prozac **(Figures C and D)**. Close-up view of the same patient **(Figure E)**.

Figure F: This 18-year-old girl developed rash, swelling of the fingers and toes, erythema of the right auricle, and a few patches of urticaria, a few hours after she took a single dose of NyQuil (acetaminophen, dextromethorphan, and doxylamine succinate). Note erythema of the ear, swelling of the fingers, urticarial rash on the right hand and the left wrist.

- In SSLR, one may see large areas of lilac discoloration (mainly centrally), fever, malaise, symmetrical arthralgia with periarticular swelling involving mostly the knees and the metacarpophalangeal joints, lymphadenopathy, facial edema, headache, myalgia, and eosinophilia.
- Figures A–F.

Treatment

- Improvement can be seen within a few days of discontinuation of the offending drug or agent.
- Antihistamines, nonsteroidal anti-inflammatory drugs, and corticosteroids for severe cases.
- Serum sickness can be a life-threatening condition.
- Epinephrine and IV fluid may be necessary for the treatment of shock.

SKULL CALCIFICATION

(See Calcification in C).

SMITH–MAGENIS SYNDROME

Definition

- The Smith–Magenis syndrome is a developmental disorder that involves many parts of the body.

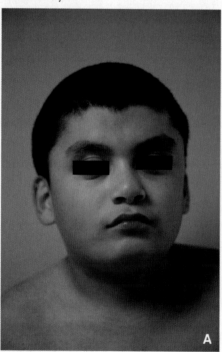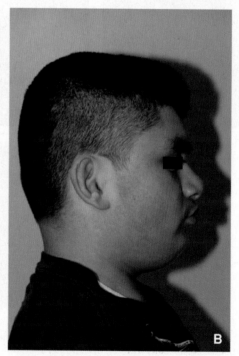

Figures A–C: This currently 8-year-old boy was born by cesarean section to a gravida 1, para 1, 29-year-old mother and a 33-year-old father. Birth weight was 2.7 kg, Apgar scores were 8 and 9. He developed hypoglycemia and respiratory distress in the nursery. Work-up for sepsis was negative. He developed metabolic acidosis at the age of 14 days, which was easily corrected. At the age of 7 months, he developed myoclonic seizures, global developmental delay, and spastic diplegia with a normal EEG. At the age of 18 months, he had a large patent anterior fontanelle, negative brain MRI, and screening for mucopolysaccharidoses was negative. At the age of 3 years, he no longer had seizures, had moderate hearing loss, and mild asthma. Now at age 8 years, he has hypertelorism, large head, brachycephaly, frontal bossing, large mouth, small hands and feet, and clinodactyly of the fifth finger. No hepatosplenomegaly. He has organic aciduria. Chromosome study was negative for Fragile X syndrome, but showed interstitial deletion in the short arm of chromosome 17. Diagnostic of Smith–Magenis syndrome was confirmed.

figures continues

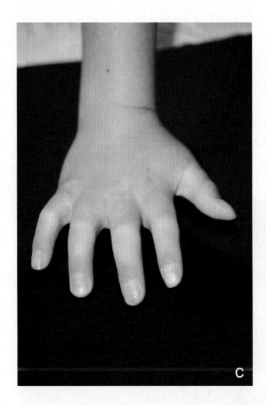

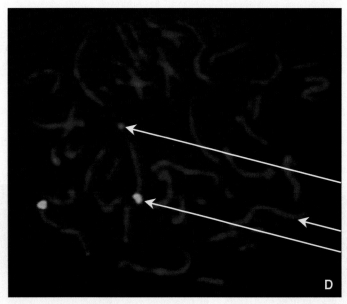

(figures cont.) **Figure D:** Metaphase cell stained with DAPI. FISH study was normal. An abnormal male karyotype with apparent interstitial deletion in the short arm of chromosome 17. Probe of the long arm of chromosome 5 homologues hybridized to the subtelomeric region. Probes hybridized to the subtelomeric region of the short arm of the chromosome 5 homologue.

Etiology
- This disorder is nonhereditary and is caused by the 17p11.2 deletion. A small percentage have a mutation in the RAI1 gene rather than a deletion.

Symptoms and Signs
- Mild to moderate intellectual disability, delayed speech, sleep disturbances (i.e., sleeping during the day and having difficulty falling asleep at night), and behavioral problems (i.e., temper tantrum, outbursts, aggression, anxiety, and impulsiveness).
- Repetitive self-hugging: "lick-and-flip," they lick their fingers and flip pages of books and magazines.
- Brachycephaly, scoliosis, broad square-shaped face, midfacial hypoplasia, deep-set eyes, prominent lower jaw, and full cheeks. The mouth tends to turn downward with a full outward curving upper lip, and ear abnormalities.
- Hoarse voice and reduced sensitivity to pain and temperature.
- Figures A–D.

Treatment
- Management of symptoms, speech therapy, physical therapy, and occupational therapy.

STAPHYLOCOCCAL SCALDED SKIN SYNDROME (SSSS)

Definition
- Staphylococcal scalded skin syndrome is a toxin-mediated epidermolytic disease with extensive erythema, scalding, and exfoliation.

Etiology

■ Certain strains of *Staphylococcus aureus* can cause SSSS through two serologically distinct staphylococcal exfoliative toxins (ETA and ETB). The toxins damage the superficial epidermis, causing separation beneath the granular layer.

Symptoms and Signs

■ Anorexia, fever, malaise, and irritability for a day or two, followed by a painful eruption which begins on the face and neck and then spreads to the entire body.

■ Periorificial and flexural tender erythema with fissuring and crusting around the orifices, eyes, and mouth.

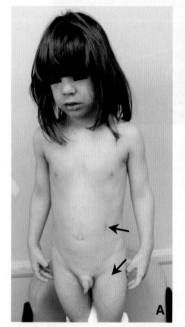
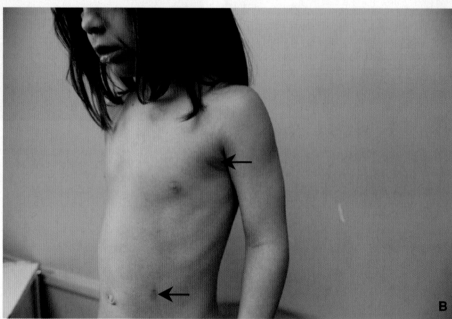
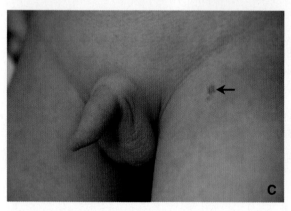
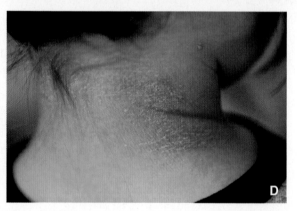

Figures A–L: The visual march of symptoms and signs in two children with SSSS. The photographs in the first patient **(Figures A–G)** are from day 1 to day 6. The patient presented with a 1-day history of low-grade fever, loss of appetite, a slight cough, and a mild rash. The rash was not pruritic, but was *painful*. He did not look well, had a temperature of 37.9°C. He was clearly in pain, but could not point to a specific tender location. He had erythema of the face, mostly around the eyes and more around the right eye than the left, philtrum, neck, axilla, genitalia, and the groins. He had chopped and dry lips and a mild rhinorrhea. He had a few small areas of skin abrasion (*arrows*). No lymphadenopathy. The urine analysis was normal. He was admitted to the hospital immediately. Cultures of the philtrum and nares were positive for methicillin-resistant Staphylococcal aureus. But, his blood culture and throat culture were negative. He was treated with intravenous antibiotic and recovered fully. His peeling of the skin can be seen during the following 6 to 8 days **(Figures A–E)**. The second child is a 6-year-old boy who presented with exactly the same symptoms and signs **(Figures F–J)**. He presented with a small, patchy erythema and skin abrasion which soon spread throughout the body. The erythema worsened, he developed a puffy face, and peeling of the skin. He too fully recovered with IV antibiotics and was discharged home in 2 weeks **(Figures H–L)**.

figures continues

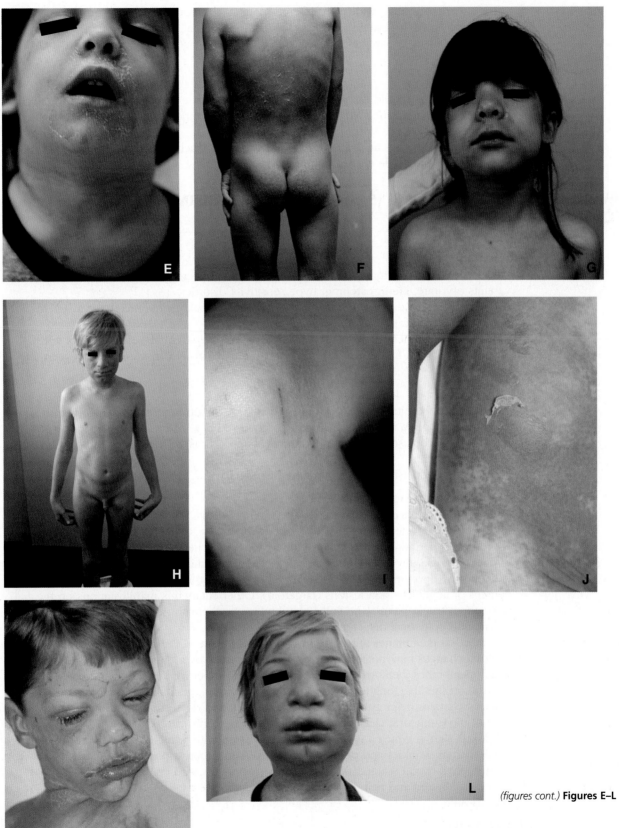

(figures cont.) **Figures E–L**

- Large superficial bullae appear in different parts of the body which may rupture easily and spread laterally, resulting in large sheets of epidermal sloughing (Nikolsky's sign).
- Deeper soft tissue or visceral infections, fluid loss, and poor body temperature control may follow.

Treatment
- Bacterial cultures should be taken from any suspected site of infection including the conjunctivae, nares, nasopharynx, axillae, umbilicus, perineum, urine, and blood (the liquid in the bullae are sterile).
- Appropriate antibiotics against *Staphylococcus aureus* (including resistance strains) and streptococci, and gentle cleansing and bland moisturizers.

STEVENS–JOHNSON SYNDROME (SJS) AND TOXIC EPIDERMAL NECROLYSIS (TEN)

Definition
- Stevens–Johnson syndrome (SJS) and toxic epidermal necrolysis (TEN) are the two variants of a rare, life-threatening, hypersensitivity disorder.
- A rare and serious disease in which the skin and mucous membranes have a severe reaction to a medication or infection.
- Epidermal detachment of <10% is considered SJS and epidermal detachment of >30% is considered TEN. Epidermal detachment of 10% to 30% is considered in between and transitional SJS–TEN.

Etiology
- Sulfonamides, barbiturates, allopurinol, phenytoin, lamotrigine, carbamazepine, NSAID, and acetaminophen are some of the drugs involved.
- Infections; mycoplasma pneumonia, herpes simplex virus, influenza, mumps, and Epstein–Barr virus.
- Vaccination, neoplasia, and autoimmune disorders.

Symptoms and Signs
- The annual incidence is 1 to 3 per 1,000,000 individuals. The incidence is 1,000 times higher in HIV-infected patients (1 to 3 per 1,000).
- A prodromal period of 1 to 14 days with fever, cough, headache, malaise, coryza, sore throat, arthralgia, myalgia, chest pain, diarrhea, and vomiting is not uncommon.
- Patients may develop high fever, epidermal detachment, mucosal erosions, and varying degrees of target-like skin lesions (targetoid). Other cutaneous manifestations on the face, upper trunk, palms, and soles may involve erythematous and purpuric macules, bullae, and epidermal detachment.
- The mucosal membranes are more involved in SJS than in TEN.
- Mucosal changes may precede dermatologic eruptions by a day or two. Bullae, grayish-white membranes, hemorrhagic crusts, and painful superficial erosions and ulcers may be seen on the lips, tongue, buccal mucosa, eyes, nose, genitalia, and rectum.
- Mucosal changes make eating, drinking, urination, and defecation painful and difficult.
- Two or more mucosal changes are required for the confirmatory diagnosis.
- Nikolsky's sign in which a light mechanical pressure with a finger to an area of erythema, the epidermis wrinkles and peels off like wet tissue paper, is positive in SJS–TEN as well as in staphylococcal scalded skin syndrome, pemphigus, and epidermolysis bullosa.
- Skin discoloration and nail dystrophy may persist for years.
- Figures A–E.

Treatment
- Lymphocyte transformation test scan identify the causative agent.
- All medications should be discontinued if possible.

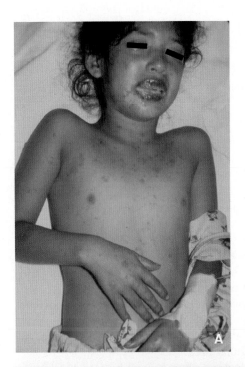

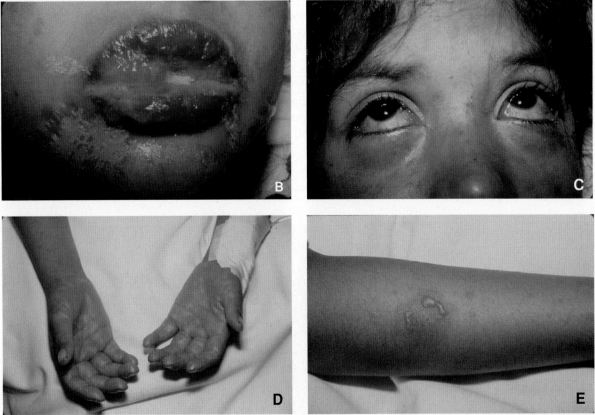

Figures A–E: SJS–TEN in a young girl, 2 weeks following a course of trimethoprim–sulfamethoxazole for the treatment of UTI. Note the pain and discomfort, macules and targetoid rash, erythema of the face, injected conjunctivae, swelling and erosion of the lips, and the thick mucus at the mouth **(Figures A, B, and C)**. Erythema of the palms **(Figure D)** and erythema and bulla **(Figure E)**.

- Supportive care, wound care (much like a burn case), rehydration, control of the electrolytes, and special eye care are necessary. Frequent mouth wash and oral antihistamines are helpful.
- The administration of corticosteroids and IVIG are controversial.

STOMATITIS (ACUTE HERPETIC GINGIVOSTOMATITIS)

Definition
- Acute herpetic gingivostomatitis is the most common cause of stomatitis in children from 1 to 3 years of age.

Etiology
- Herpes simplex virus.

Symptoms and Signs
- The virus can cause disease at any age; yet the most common age of onset is from 10 months to 5 years.
- The incubation period is 3 to 7 days.
- Fever, drooling, refusal to eat or drink, and crying (from pain and hunger).
- Shallow, painful erosions, swelling and ulceration of the gingiva (with bleeding from the gums), oral mucosa, palate, and the tongue, fetor oris, and dehydration.
- The initial lesions are vesicles 2 to 10 mm in diameter on an erythematous base, covered with a grayish-yellow membrane.
- Perioral lesions may be seen on the lips, cheeks, and chin.
- Lymphadenopathy in the neck and the submandibular area.
- Secondary bacterial infection (a rare occurrence) is most often caused by group A β-hemolytic streptococci and *Staphylococcus aureus*.
- The clinical picture leaves little doubt as to the diagnosis. If needed, direct fluorescent antibody studies and viral culture can be confirmatory studies.

Treatment
- Supportive therapy, rehydration, analgesics, local application of lidocaine, oral diphenhydramine, Maalox, and Kaopectate.
- Acyclovir may shorten the course and severity of the disease if given during the first 3 days of onset of disease.
- Figures A and B.

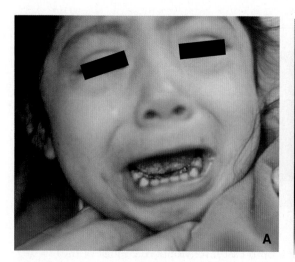 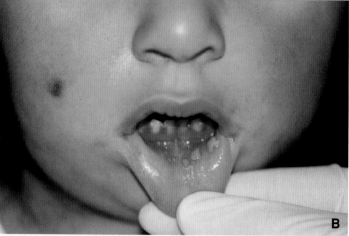

Figure A: A severe case of herpes gingivostomatitis in a 2-year-old with numerous vesicles on her tongue and oral mucosa.

Figure B: Herpetic ulceration on the oral mucosa, the perioral area, and the right cheek.

STOMATITIS, APHTHOUS

(See Aphthous Stomatitis).

STREPTOCOCCAL PHARYNGITIS

Definition
- Infection of the pharynx and tonsils by group A β-hemolytic streptococcus.

Etiology
- There are over 100 serotypes of group A β-hemolytic streptococci (*Streptococcus pyogenes,* GAS).
- Serotypes 49, 55, 57, and 59 are associated with pyoderma and acute glomerulonephritis.
- Serotypes 1, 6, and 12 are associated with pharyngitis and acute glomerulonephritis.
- Direct contact, and not fomites, is required for the transmission of streptococci.
- Overcrowding as well as close contacts (such as seen in schools and the military) contribute to the spread of infection.
- Contaminated food can cause streptococcal pharyngitis.

Symptoms and Signs
- The incubation period is 2 to 5 days.
- Streptococcal pharyngitis is less common in children under the age of 3 years and is quite rare under 1 year. The infection is more common among the school age and is infrequent during the summer months.
- Invasive GAS infections are more common during infancy and old age.
- Fever, sore throat, palpable or visible anterior cervical lymph nodes, vomiting, exudate and/or petechia on the tonsils and/or the palate.
- *Clinical* diagnosis of GAS is *not acceptable*. GAS diagnosis can only be made using laboratory tests.
- Diagnosis is by throat culture on sheep blood agar with a bacitracin disc by the rapid diagnostic test (if negative, culture is necessary to confirm) and by optical immunoassay.
- Throat culture is considered as a "tonsillectomy procedure" by some, as a good quality throat culture requires a vigorous swab of the entire surface of both the tonsils and pharynx.

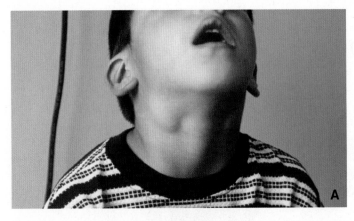

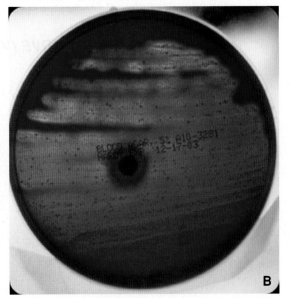

Figure A: Visible anterior cervical lymphadenopathy in streptococcal pharyngitis.

Figure B: A positive throat culture on sheep blood agar. Note the hemolysis, consumption of most of the hemoglobin by streptococcus, and the intact area around the bacitracin disc, resistant to streptococcus (the zone of inhibition) which differentiates group A β-hemolytic streptococcus from other types.

Treatment

- Penicillin V has remained the drug of choice (a 10-day course of 250 mg, three times a day for children <27 kg and 500 mg for others).
- Amoxicillin and alternatively, first-generation cephalosporins are acceptable.
- Macrolides can be used for patients allergic to penicillin (e.g., erythromycin estolate 20 to 40 mg/kg and divided two to four times a day for 10 days).
- Untreated and inadequately treated patients may develop complications of acute glomerulonephritis or a tonsillar abscess or cellulitis.
- Patients are no longer contagious after 24 hours of treatment with the appropriate antibiotics.
- Figures A–B.

STREPTOCOCCAL VULVOVAGINITIS

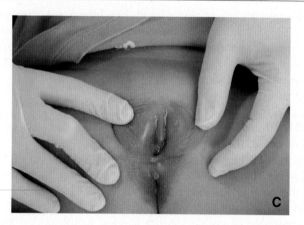

Figure C: This 2-year-old girl had itching and irritation of vagina of a few days duration. No fever or other symptoms. There was erythema of the labia and of the perianal area. No discharge. A swab from the erythematous skin was positive for GAS **(Figure B)**. This young girl responded well to oral amoxicillin. She had refused taking the oral penicillin due to its bad taste.

STURGE–WEBER SYNDROME (SWS, ENCEPHALOFACIAL ANGIOMATOSIS, OR ENCEPHALOTRIGEMINAL ANGIOMATOSIS)

Definition

- The Sturge–Weber syndrome is a neuroectodermal lesion with a port-wine stain (PWS) distributed in the first ophthalmic branch of the trigeminal nerve (V1 n.) and with leptomeningeal angiomatosis.

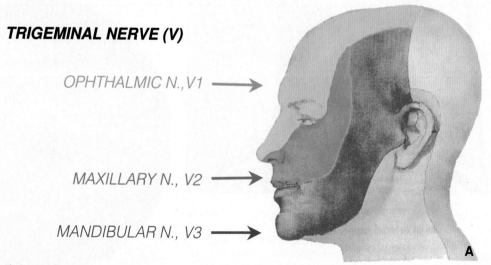

Figure A

figures continues

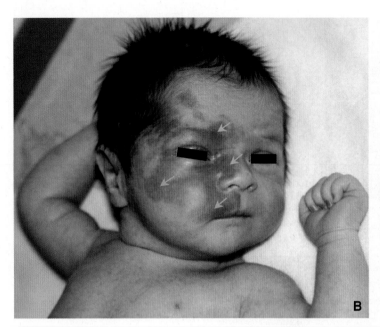

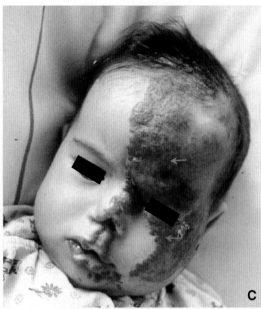

(figures cont.) **Figure B:** Distribution of port-wine stain in an infant with SWS. Ophthalmic nerve, V1. Maxillary nerve, V2. Both branches of the trigeminal nerve are involved.

Figure C: Involvement of the trigeminal nerve in port-wine stain. Ophthalmic nerve, V1. Maxillary nerve, V2. Mandibular nerve, V3.

Etiology
- Unknown.

Symptoms and Signs
- Port-wine stain (PWS) distributed in the region of the V1 nerve, at times with more cutaneous and multidermatomal involvement (Figures A–C).
- CNS findings: Seizure, mostly during the first year of life and difficult to control.
- There is an increased probability of CNS complications when V1 nerve involvement is complete as well as more cognitive and developmental delay.
- The risk of leptomeningeal angiomatosis and glaucoma increases with bilateral involvement of PWS.
- Ophthalmologic findings: Glaucoma, unilateral or bilateral, involvement of episclera, conjunctiva, choroid and retina, nevus of Ota, buphthalmos, and blindness.
- There is a greater probability of having SWS when both eyelids are affected.
- Patients with lesions involving the cutaneous distribution of the ophthalmic division of the trigeminal nerve are at risk of associated neuro-ocular complications and require repeated ophthalmologic examination as well as CT or MRI scans.

Treatment
- Multidisciplinary approach is important. A team including a neurologist, ophthalmologist, and dermatologist should work closely with the pediatrician.
- Surgery and hemispherectomy are often helpful in the control of intractable seizures.
- Anticipatory guidance and support is a very important part of the management.

SUBCUTANEOUS FAT NECROSIS (SCFN)

Definition
- SCFN is a rare, benign, self-limited, and inflammatory reaction of the subcutaneous fat in the newborn.

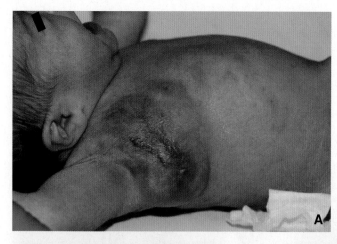

Figure A: This 2-day-old newborn boy was delivered by normal spontaneous vaginal delivery to a gravida 3, para 2 young woman. He had this large plaque since birth. He was breastfed and had no other complications. There is a firm, indurated 6 × 8 cm, purplish-brown, nontender plaque on the right side of the chest extending to the right axilla. The discoloration is not homogeneous.

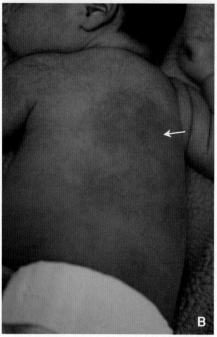

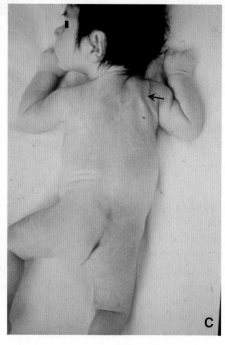

Figure B: Mother noted an area of discoloration on the back of this 12-day-old newborn girl. She was doing well and had no other problems. She was afebrile and had normal weight, height, and head circumference. There was an 8 × 8 cm, reddish, nontender, thickened, and palpable area with clear edges on the back.

Figure C: There was an area of reddish, hard skin, and subcutaneous tissue on the back of this infant, mostly on the right shoulder.

Etiology
- Unknown.
- Possible factors are perinatal trauma, hypothermia, asphyxia, maternal gestational diabetes, preeclampsia, cocaine or calcium blocker use, meconium aspiration, newborn anemia or thrombocytosis, and hypercalcemia.

Symptoms and Signs
- SCFN is often seen during the first few weeks of life.
- It can be single or multiple well-circumscribed, erythematous, indurated, often painless, nodular areas of fat necrosis.
- Cheeks, back, buttocks, arms, and thighs are the sites most affected.

Treatment
- SCFN is a self-limiting disease. However, infants should be seen regularly and monitored for possible hypercalcemia, thrombocytopenia, hyperglyceridemia, and hypoglycemia.

SYRINGOMA

Definition
- Syringomas are benign tumors which originate from the sweat glands.

Etiology
- Unknown, but seems influenced by hormones.

Symptoms and Signs
- Small 1- to 3-mm papules, mostly multiple, and rarely solitary, flesh-colored to yellow, firm, translucent, and are more common in females and during puberty.
- They are found mostly around the eyes and especially the lower eyelids, neck, chest, abdomen, genitalia, arms, and legs.

Treatment
- Treatment is difficult. CO_2 laser ablation, trichloroacetic, surgical excision, cryosurgery, and electrodesiccation.
- Figures A–C.

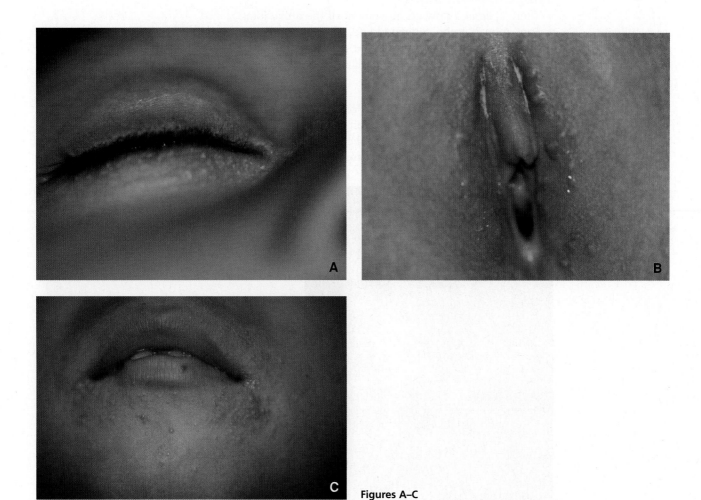

Figures A–C

TALIPES EQUINOVARUS (CLUB FOOT)

Definition
- Talipes equinovarus is a congenital deformity in which the ankle appears to be internally rotated without any flexibility.

Etiology
- Occurs in 1:1,000 live births. Twice as common in males.
- The cause remains unknown. It may be an isolated defect or part of a syndromic association.
- Genetics play a role, as there is usually a previously affected family member.
- It is not related to intrauterine positioning or oligohydramnios.

Symptoms and Signs
- There is limited upward movement of the ankle joint.
- Foot appears to be supinated and adducted. Attempts to reposition the foot in dorsiflexion, and eversion will be unsuccessful.
- Approximately 50% of patients have bilateral involvement.

Treatment
- Serial casting (currently via the Ponseti method) which involves a series of six casts over a 2-month period. Casting is often followed by heel-cord tenotomy and bracing.
- Botulinum toxin injections into the calf muscle.
- Surgical correction in resistant cases.
- Figure A.

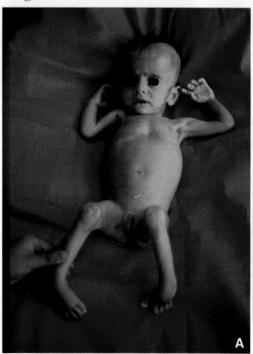

Figure A: A 6-month-old girl with bilateral talipes equinovarus (club foot). The deformity includes plantar flexion (equinus) of the ankle, fixed hindfoot inversion (varus), and supination of the forefoot.

TETANUS (Gr. to stretch)

TETANUS NEONATORUM (TETANUS OF THE NEWBORN)

Definition

- Tetanus is an acute infection of the nervous system. It is characterized by spasmodic contractions of voluntary muscles, trismus, and seizures.

Etiology

- Tetanus is caused by *Clostridium tetani,* a ubiquitous, anaerobic, gram-positive rod with terminal spores.
- The spores may enter the body through a wound and transform into bacteria which release neurotoxins that reach the spinal cord and the brainstem via retrograde axonal transport.
- The toxin then blocks the transmission of inhibitory signals, leading to prolonged, powerful, and painful muscle activity.
- Although tetanus neonatorum is almost eradicated from the Western world, newborns in developing countries remain highly vulnerable to tetanus.
- It is difficult to ascertain the true incidence of tetanus neonatorum since most deaths in developing countries occur prior to issuance of birth certificates.
- In the majority of newborns, the umbilicus serves as the port of entry for *C. tetani.* Circumcised penis and pierced ear lobes may also serve as ports of entry.
- A large number of newborns in the developing countries are born at home, their umbilical cords may be cut by contaminated and nonsterile scissors, knives, or blades.
- Certain cultural practices such as tying a string around the cord or covering the cord with turmeric, henna, or coal ash "to make the cord fall off faster," create ideal environments for the growth of *C. tetani.*
- The author has seen close to 1,000 babies with tetanus neonatorum, the majority of whom could not be saved.

Symptoms and Signs

- The incubation period is classically between 5 and 14 days. However, shorter and longer incubation periods have been observed. Shorter incubation periods are associated with the worst outcome.
- Refusal to feed, trismus (locked jaw). Trismus is an early sign of tetanus and it is caused by the spasm of the masticatory muscles, leading to difficulties in opening the mouth.
- Any attempt to forcibly open the mouth will increase the trismus. However, a gentle pressure on the chin may open the mouth. This finding may disappear with the onset of seizures.
- Hypertonicity and muscular rigidity which may be aggravated by any stimuli (tactile, light, or sound).
- Opisthotonos (Gr. Opistho, behind, at the back). Defined as strong, backward arching of the spine. It can be spontaneous or it may be precipitated by any stimuli. In severe cases, the patient may break his/her spine.
- Convulsions which may increase in severity and frequency as the disease progresses. Seizures can lead to apnea, cyanosis, aspiration, and death.
- Flexion of the wrist may develop during the end of the third week of treatment.
- Prolonged apneas, which may lead to cardiac arrest, and death.
- Figures A–E.

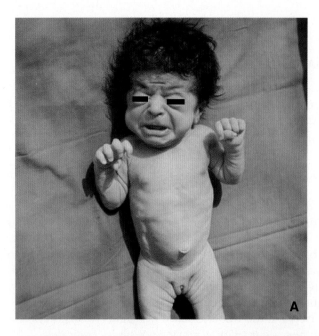

Figure A: The typical facies of tetanus neonatorum in a 7-day-old female who was brought in for feeding difficulties. Note the wrinkled forehead, spasms of the facial and abdominal muscles, and the clinched fists.

The sequence of events in tetanus of the newborn.

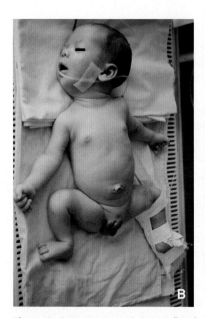

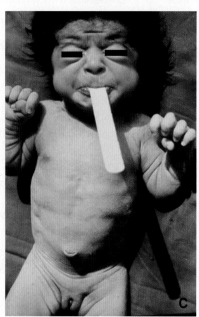

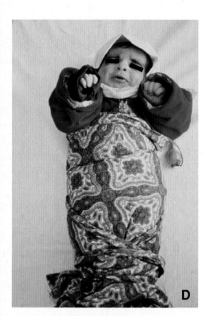

Figure B: Gangrenous penis in a well-sedated 8-day-old male who was circumcised at home and developed tetanus 6 days later. *Clostridium tetani* was recovered from his wound.

Figures C–D: Trismus in a newborn infant with neonatal tetanus **(Figure C)**. A swaddled 6-day-old female was brought in secondary to inability to feed. On examination it was noted that she was unable to open her mouth. Further history revealed that she was born in a public bath and her umbilical cord was cut with a used razor-blade, covered by lard and henna, and subsequently tied by a piece of string. She developed seizures and apnea in the hospital **(Figure D)**.

figures continues

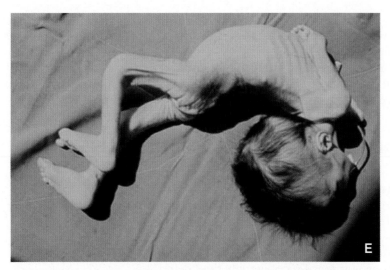

(figures cont.) **Figure E:** Opisthotonus in a 16-day-old, malnourished baby who was born in a taxi prior to arrival at the hospital. The taxi driver cut the umbilical cord with his pocket knife. Six days later, the baby developed excessive crying and developed trismus.

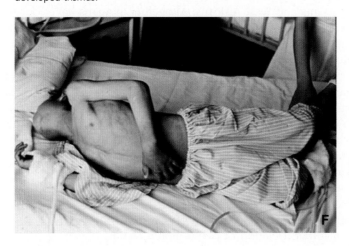

Figure F: Opisthotonus in a 7-year-old boy with tetanus. He had told his parents that he had a sore throat and could not swallow. His trismus was noticed when the ER physician tried to examine his mouth. The source of the infection remained unidentified.

Treatment

- Prevention is the most important and effective means of controlling this disease.
- Appropriate wound care, cleansing and removal of dead tissues, which ultimately addresses the source of spores and bacteria.
- Intramuscular injection of the human tetanus immune globulin (TIG) 500 IU. TIG neutralizes the free toxin in the system. Currently, there is no effective method for neutralizing toxins which are attached to neurons.
- Sedation: A poorly sedated patient may develop status epilepticus. However, it is very important to avoid excessive sedation as this may lead to aspiration, hypothermia, and death.
- Anticonvulsants: There is no ideal drug for this purpose. Phenobarbital, diazepam, and chlorpromazine have been tried. None is sufficiently effective.
- Antibiotics: Oral or IV metronidazole, 30 mg/kg/day (maximum 4 g/day) for 10 to 14 days for the eradication of *C. tetani*. Penicillin is a second-line agent.
- Feeding and proper nutrition are critical parts of proper and effective management. Tube feedings in frequent, slow, and small volumes.
- Prevention and treatment of possible aspiration pneumonia.

- The treatment of choice is complete sedation of the infant and mechanical ventilation. However, these resources are scarce in developing countries where tetanus neonatorum is prevalent.
- Treatment of tetanus is difficult, costly, and in most cases, leads to a disappointing outcome. Prevention of tetanus, on the other hand, inexpensive, and almost a universal success in the developed world.

THALASSEMIA SYNDROME (Gr. Thalassa, sea; Hemia, blood)

Definition
- The thalassemias refer to a group of inherited blood disorders that are characterized by defective synthesis of one of the hemoglobin chains.

Etiology
- It is an autosomal recessive inherited defect.
- They are divided into α and β thalassemias with varying degrees of ineffective globin chain synthesis resulting in hemolysis.
- α thalassemia results from defective α-globin chain synthesis and occurs predominantly in Southeast Asians and West Africans. Altogether, humans have four α-globin genes located on chromosome 16. The severity of the symptoms depends on the number of genes that are affected.
- β thalassemia results from defective β-globin chain synthesis. It occurs predominantly in children of Mediterranean origin. There are two β-globin genes that are located on chromosome 11. The severity of symptoms in β thalassemia depends on the effect of the specific mutation on the β-globin gene expression.
- A reduction of either α- or β-globin chains leads to formation of an unstable hemoglobin tetramer (which is normally composed of two α and two β chains), leading to symptoms of thalassemia.
- Major clinical variations include:
  - β+ thalassemia: Reduced β chain synthesis.
  - β0 thalassemia: No β chain synthesis.
  - α thalassemia silent carrier: Deletion of one α-globin chain.
  - α thalassemia trait: Deletion of two α-globin chains.
  - Hb H disease: Deletion of three α-globin chains.
  - Hydrops fetalis: Absence of four α-globin chains.

Symptoms and Signs
- Depend on the severity of α- and β-globin malfunction. Symptoms may range from asymptomatic carriers, mild microcytic-hypochromic anemia, and significant anemia with need for regular blood transfusions to hydrops fetalis.
- Both α and β thalassemia result in hemolysis, which in turn leads to increased bone marrow activity.
- The marrow space enlarges with the increase in marrow activity, leading to the characteristic growth in skull, face, and other long bones. Figures A–E.
- Failure to recognize and treat thalassemia may result in the following: Failure to thrive, growth retardation, delayed puberty, jaundice, hepatosplenomegaly, and anemia.

Treatment
- No specific therapy is required for mild thalassemias.
- Regular blood transfusions and iron chelation therapy in severe cases.
- Bone marrow transplantation may be curative.

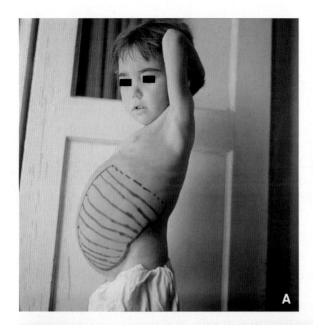

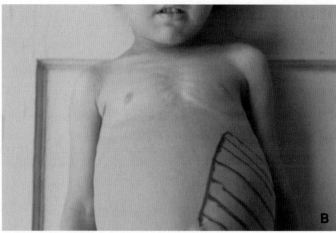

Figures A–B: Characteristic "thalassemia facies" resulting from bone marrow hyperplasia. Note the splenomegaly, frontal bossing, maxillary hyperplasia, and prominent cheekbones.

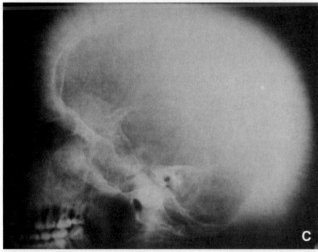

Figure C: Radiographic features of thalassemia. Note the increased marrow activity indicated by the "hair-on-end" appearance in a plain skull radiograph of a patient with β thalassemia.

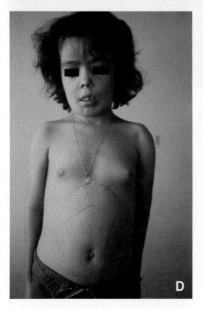

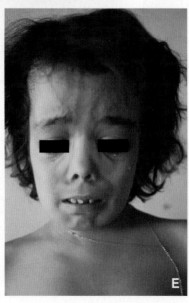

Figures D–E: Typical thalassemic facies in a 12-year-old girl. Frontal bossing, prominent maxillary bones, and skull are secondary to an increase in marrow activity. Pallor, slight jaundice, and hepatosplenomegaly are caused by chronic hemolysis.

THRUSH (ORAL CANDIDIASIS)

Definition
- Candida infection of the oral cavity.

Etiology
- Thrush is caused by a yeast-like imperfect fungus, *Candida albicans* (L. Candida, glowing; Albicans, white).
- It is a common infection in newborns. It may be transmitted from the mother during labor if mother has vaginal colonization.
- Incidence increases with the use of broad spectrum antibiotics.

Symptoms and Signs
- Oral thrush is characterized by painless or painful, white-to-gray, irregular plaques on an erythematous base.
- In oral thrush, the lips, oral mucosa, tongue, and palate may be covered with white spots or a white membrane.
- Thrush is mainly seen in children less than 1 year of age, when cell-mediated (T-cell) immunity is immature (especially during the first 6 months of life).
- There may be concomitant *C. albicans* infection of the diaper area.
- Figures A–C.

Treatment
- Good hygiene including the sterilization of bottles and pacifiers.
- Oral nystatin to be given after feedings.
- If the infant is breast-feeding, then consider treatment of mother's breasts with nystatin.

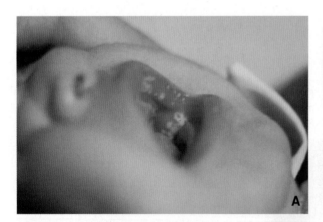

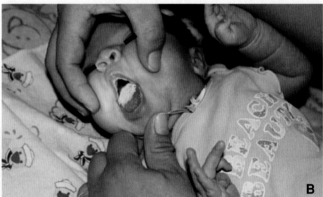

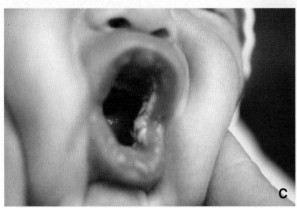

Figure A: The early stage of oral thrush in an infant.

Figure B: Advanced thrush covering the tongue and the oral mucosa in a bottle-fed baby.

Figure C: White spots of thrush on the lips, tongue, and oral mucosa. These patches are only partially removable. This finding distinguishes thrush from milk which can be easily scraped off.

THYMUS HERNIATION

Definition
- Thymus herniation is a rare occurrence. It is defined as an intermittent, superior herniation of mediastinal thymus into the suprasternal notch during maneuvers which increases intrathoracic pressure.

Etiology
- It is thought to be secondary to the loosening of the connective tissue which limits the normal movement of the thymus.

Symptoms and Signs
- Must rule out other causes of midline neck masses in children including thyroglossal cysts, laryngocele, thyroid masses, dermoid cysts, and teratomas.
- Tracheal compression from herniation of the thymus has been reported.
- Figures A–C.

Treatment
- This is a self-limiting condition. Over time, the thymus shrinks in size and no longer herniates.

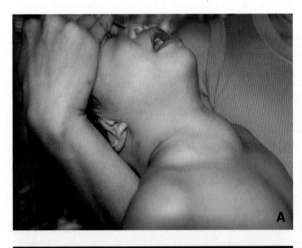
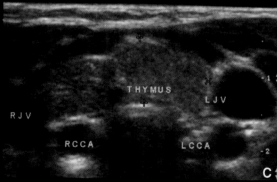
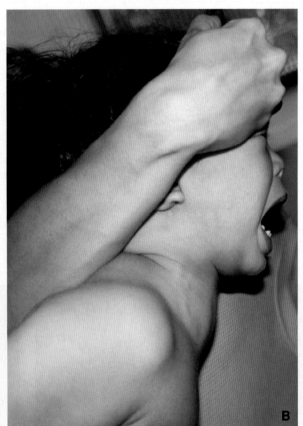

Figures A–B: This 3-year-old girl presented with severe otitis media. On examination, an incidental swelling in her anterior neck was noted. The swelling became appreciably larger while she was crying, and seemed to disappear when she stopped crying. An ultrasound confirmed the clinical diagnosis of thymus herniation.

Figure C: This ultrasound study demonstrates herniation of a normal-appearing thymus through the suprasternal notch. This finding was elicited by an increase in intrathoracic pressure.

TINEA

- Tinea are a group of fungal skin infections. Fungal infections may be superficial or deep and systemic. There are three common types of superficial tinea infections:
  1. Dermatophytes, also called tinea or ringworm due to the annular shape of the lesions.
  2. Pityriasis versicolor (tinea versicolor).
  3. Candidiasis (moniliasis).

TINEA CAPITIS (RINGWORM OF THE SCALP)

Definition
- Deep-seated, fungal infection of the scalp and hair follicles.

Etiology
- *Trichophyton tonsurans* is the most common fungi responsible for tinea capitis.
- Other responsible fungi include *Tricholosporum violaceum, Microsporum canis,* and *Microsporum audouinii.*
- Tinea capitis is more common in males.
- Other risk factors include overcrowded living conditions, large families, and low socioeconomic backgrounds.
- Humans, animals, and fomites (combs, hats, and contaminated barber's instruments) can transmit tinea capitis.
- Puberty leads to an increased resistance to tinea capitis infections.

Symptoms and Signs
- The incubation period is 1 to 3 weeks.
- Milder forms present with minimal erythema, scaling, and patchy alopecia.
- There is a "salt-and-pepper" appearance of the shortened residual hairs which lie among the hairless background.
- The hair may break at the beginning of the follicle. This is referred to as "black dots."
- More severe infections with an inflammatory response may lead to the formation of a kerion, a large, boggy, abscess-like mass with pustule formation and purulent discharge.
- Posterior auricular, posterior cervical, and occipital nodes are often enlarged.
- Fungal culture is diagnostic and 100% specific.
- Diagnosis may also be made by Wood's light examination or visualization of yeasts on potassium hydroxide mounts.
- Figures A and B.

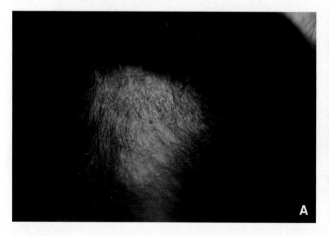
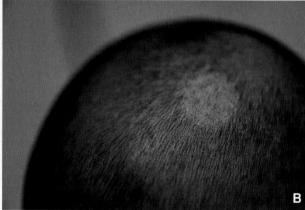

Figures A–B: Tinea capitis in two patients. Areas of alopecia, scaling, and the typical "salt-and-pepper" appearance.

Treatment
- Long-term oral antifungal medications are needed due to the deep nature of these infections.
- Systemic or topical steroids may assist with severe inflammation associated with kerion formation.
- Griseofulvin is the "gold standard." The recommended pediatric dosage is 10 to 25 mg/kg/day for 6 to 8 weeks.
- Absorption of medication is enhanced by fatty meals.
- Photosensitivity, headache, and gastrointestinal disturbances are among the rare side effects of griseofulvin. Unusual side effects include hepatic toxicity and development of a morbilliform rash.
- Use of antifungal shampoos (ketoconazole) for approximately 2 to 3 times a week helps with the destruction of scales and viable spores.
- Terbinafine, fluconazole, ketoconazole, and itraconazole are newer, promising drugs.

TINEA CORPORIS (L. Tinea, gnawing worm; Corporis, of the body)
Definition
- Superficial dermatophyte infection of hairless skin excluding the inguinal, palmar, facial, and plantar surfaces.

Etiology
- *Microsporum audouinii, Microsporum canis,* or *Trichophyton mentagrophytes.*
- In adults, *Trichophyton rubrum, Trichophyton verrucosum,* or *Trichophyton tonsurans.*

Symptoms and Signs
- Tinea corporis initially presents with asymmetric, small, erythematous papules.
- Subsequently, there is gradual spread of the erythematous lesions that are raised, annular, sharply circumscribed with scaly borders and which may contain microvesicles.
- There is central clearing as the infection spreads, hence the common name "ringworm."
- Infection may occur as the result of direct contact with an infected individual or via contact with contaminated clothing, linens, or surfaces.
- Autoinoculation via scratching is often responsible for multiple lesions.
- Diagnosis is typically based on the clinical findings. Appearance of hyphae on KOH preparations of skin scrapings and fungal cultures confirms the diagnosis.
- Figures A–C.

Treatment
- Treatment with antifungal creams for 2 to 3 weeks is typically effective.
- Oral therapy is reserved for patients with widespread infections.

TINEA CRURIS
Definition
- Dermatophyte infection of the skin in the inguinal region.

Etiology
- *Trichophyton mentagrophytes, Trichophyton rubrum,* and *Epidermophyton floccosum* are the most commonly involved dermatophytes.
- Tinea cruris is more frequently seen in adolescent males and adults.
- Risk factors include obesity, excessive sweating, and tight-fitting clothes.

Symptoms and Signs
- Tinea cruris is a common superficial infection. It typically begins on the medial thigh with small, erythematous, scaly, and pruritic papules.

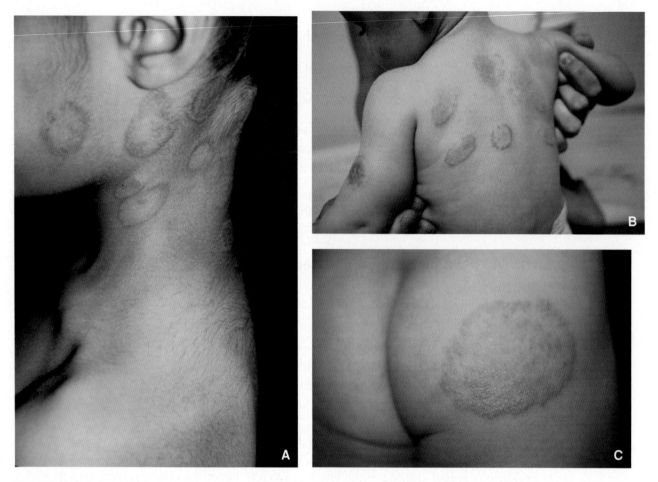

Figure A: Typical plaques of tinea corporis noted on the face and neck. The lesions are round or oval, scaly, with slightly raised margins, and a central clearing.

Figure B: Erythematous plaques with scaly borders and microvesicle formation. The ring-like appearance is due to the central clearing. Auto-inoculation from scratching or repeated exposure to contaminated linens will result in the spread of infection.

Figure C: A 3-year-old girl with a rapidly expanding, plaque-like rash on the right buttock. The area of central clearing is surrounded by a raised erythematous rim.

- Localized spread of the infection involves the intertriginous folds and often leads to bilateral involvement.
- The penis remains spared. This finding differentiates Tinea cruris from a candidal infection.
- Figures A and B.

Treatment
- Topical antifungal creams.
- Patients should be advised to wear loose-fitting and comfortable clothes.

TINEA FACIEI

TINEA MANUUM (TINEA OF THE HAND)
Definition
- Superficial dermatophyte infection of the hands.

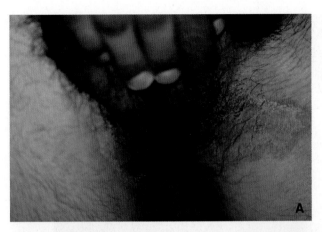

Figure A: Tinea cruris in a 15-year-old male with a pruritic rash of the groins and the scrotum. Note the extent of the erythema and scaling which covers the scrotum, groins, and the adjacent thigh.

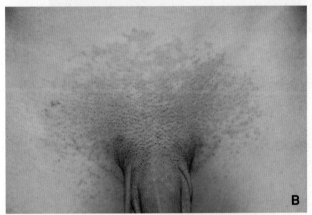

Figure B: Tinea cruris in an adolescent male patient. Confluent erythema, papules, and minimal scaling of the groin and the intertriginous folds. Note the relative sparing of the penis. Hyperpigmentation of this patient's lesions is a result of the long-standing infection.

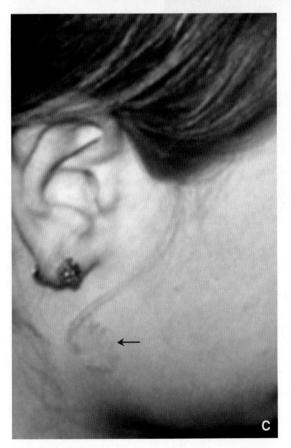

Figure C: A single tinea ring with central clearing in a teenage girl.

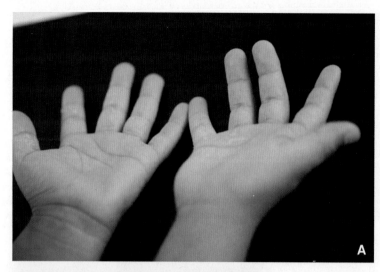

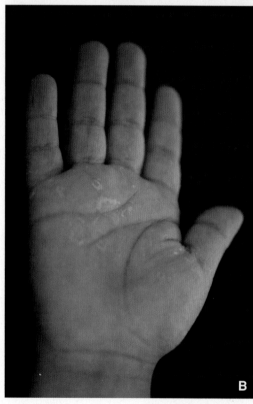

Figures A–B: Bilateral and unilateral tinea manuum in two male teenagers. Note the hyperkeratosis, desquamation of the palms, ruptured vesicles, and erythema of the fingers.

Etiology

- *Trichophyton rubrum, Trichophyton mentagrophytes,* and *Epidermophyton floccosum.*

Symptoms and Signs

- Tinea of the hand is most commonly seen in postpubertal children.
- Diffuse hyperkeratosis of palms and fingers. Patchy inflammatory or vesicular reaction of the fingers and palms, and onychomycosis.
- It is mostly unilateral and can be associated with tinea of the feet.
- Tinea of the dorsum of the hand is called tinea corporis.
- Onychomycosis of all the fingers may suggest psoriasis.
- Diagnosis is clinical and can be confirmed by potassium hydroxide scrapings or fungal culture.
- Figures A and B.

Treatment

- Topical antifungal preparations.

TINEA PEDIS (ATHLETE'S FOOT)

Definition

- Superficial dermatophyte infection of the feet.

Etiology

- *Trichophyton rubrum, Trichophyton mentagrophytes, Epidermophyton floccosum,* and *Trichophyton tonsurans.*
- Infection often occurs in damp, communal locations such as pools or locker rooms.

Symptoms and Signs

- Findings may include erythema; scaling; hyperkeratosis; and maceration of the soles, toes, or the webbing between the toes.
- Vesicles and bullae may be the only dermatologic findings in tinea pedis.
- Painful, burning sensation and pruritus.
- Less commonly, it may spread to the dorsum of the foot or the plantar surface with involvement of the arch.
- Diagnosis is made by clinical findings. Potassium hydroxide scrapings and fungal cultures are confirmatory.

Treatment

- Treatment includes topical antifungal sprays, ointments, or powders.
- Patients should be advised to wear clean, dry, cotton socks with shoes in order to decrease the amount of moisture around the feet.
- Oral antifungal therapy is rarely needed. Griseofulvin or terbinafine may be used in such cases.

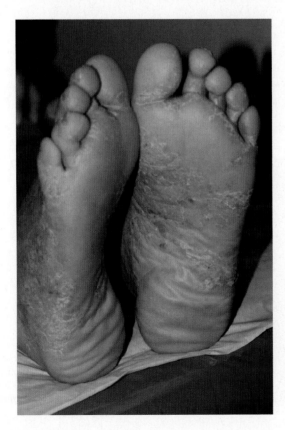

Tinea pedis superimposed on atopic dermatitis in a 17-year-old male. Maceration and inflammation involve the webbing between the toes and feet. Note the dry, scaly, and erythematous skin.

TINEA UNGUIUM (ONYCHOMYCOSIS)

Definition

■ Tinea unguium is a dermatophyte infection of the nail bed of the fingers or toes.

Etiology

■ *Trichophyton rubrum, Epidermophyton floccosum, Trichophyton mentagrophytes,* and *Candida albicans.*

Symptoms and Signs

■ It is rarely seen in prepubertal children.
■ Onychomycosis can be associated with tinea of the feet or tinea of the hands.
■ Involvement of the toes is much more common than that of the fingers.
■ Initially presents with minimal thickening of the nails with white scales and paronychial inflammation.
■ Infection of the underlying nail bed and lower part of the nail plate leads to detachment of the nail plate and thickening of the subungual tissues.
■ The progression of the infection leads to discolored, brittle, and yellow nails.
■ More severe infections can result in black discoloration and detachment of the nail.
■ The clinical diagnosis can be confirmed by visualizations of hyphae via potassium hydroxide scrapings and fungal cultures.
■ Figures A and B.

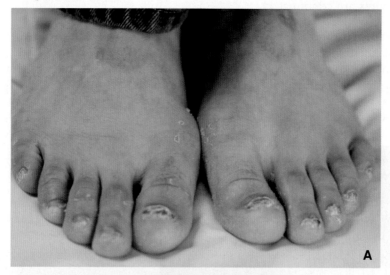

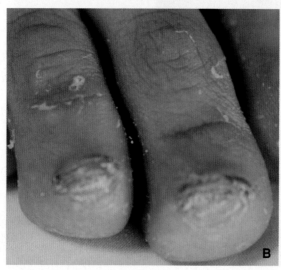

Figures A–B: An 18-year-old athletic male with a 2-year history of tinea unguium. There has been a recent darkening and thickening of the toenails and subungual tissues **(Figure A)** and close-up view **(Figure B)**.

Treatment

- Due to the deep nature of these infections, topical antifungals are ineffective and long-term oral antifungal treatment is required.
- Oral griseofulvin, terbinafine, and fluconazole are typically used for treatment of onychomycosis.

TINEA VERSICOLOR (PITYRIASIS VERSICOLOR)
(Gr. Pytron, BRAN + IASIS)

Definition

- Tinea versicolor is a common superficial, opportunistic, skin infection.

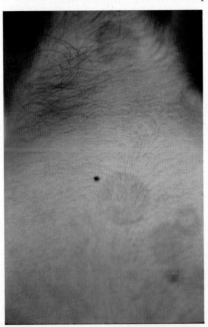

Tinea versicolor in a male teenager.

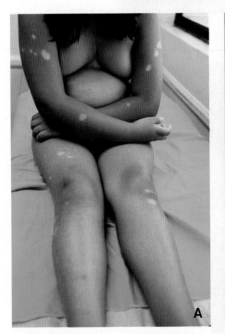

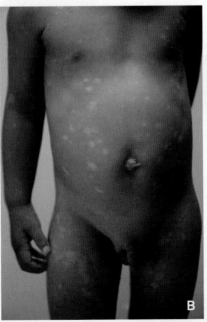

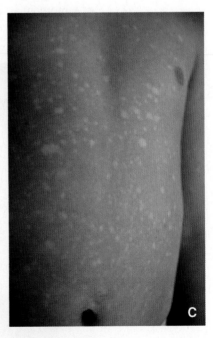

Figures A–C: Postinflammatory hypopigmentation following tinea corporis infection in two children. Disorders of pigmentation, particularly on visible areas of the body, can be devastating to children. However, most inflammatory changes resolve spontaneously over time.

Etiology

- It is caused by any of the yeast forms of the *Malassezia furfur, Pityrosporum orbiculare,* and *Pityrosporum ovale.* These organisms are part of the normal cutaneous flora.

Symptoms and Signs

- Tinea versicolor is more common in adolescents.
- It is often characterized by round areas of scaly hypopigmentation or hyperpigmentation.
- It occurs most commonly on the trunk, but can be on other areas of the body.
- A powdery scale can often be obtained by scraping the skin.
- Potassium hydroxide preparations demonstrate the typical, short, fungal hyphae and spores in clusters that appear like a "spaghetti and meatball pattern."

Treatment

- There is a high recurrence rate.
- Tinea versicolor can be treated with a topical agent, but the hypopigmentation may persist for a period of time after the treatment.
- Topical treatments include 2.5% selenium sulfide shampoo, 2% ketoconazole shampoo, and 1% terbinafine spray.
- Oral therapy is recommended for severe, resistant, or recurrent cases.
- Oral antifungals in single dose or various dose regimens may be used.

TOE TOURNIQUET SYNDROME

Definition

- Circumferential strangulation of digits by hair or fiber.

Etiology

- Entanglement of a toe by a loose piece of hair or thread.
- A moment of inattentiveness is all that is needed for a curious child to accidentally strangulate her finger or toe.
- Maternal hair loss can be a risk factor.

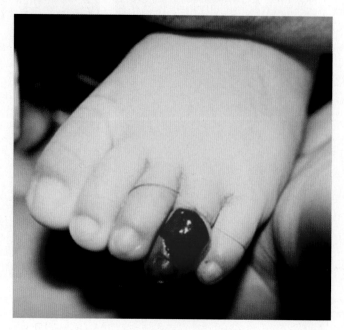

This infant presented with inconsolable crying for hours. On physical examination, a tight hair was noted around the base of this swollen and inflamed toe. The toe was saved by incision and removal of the hair.

Symptoms and Signs
- Edematous, pale, and necrotic appearing digit.

Treatment
- Management includes removal of the constricting hair or fiber to allow reperfusion of the digit.
- Fully necrotic digits may require amputation.

TORTICOLLIS (L. Tortus, twisted; Collum, neck)

Definition
- Stiff neck associated with muscle spasms. It can be congenital or acquired.

Etiology
- Congenital torticollis is usually due to shortening or contracture of the sternocleidomastoid muscle on the side to which the head is tilted.
- The cause is believed to be the abnormal positioning within the uterus, fibrosis from venous occlusion of the sternocleidomastoid muscle, or trauma that results in a hematoma within the muscle itself.
- Rarely associated with syndromic findings (Klippel–Feil syndrome).
- Acquired torticollis may be secondary to posterior fossa tumors, strabismus, infections of the posterior pharynx or the ear, or medication side effects (Reglan).

Symptoms and Signs
- Tilting of the neck toward one side of the head, while the chin is turned to the opposite side.
- Occasionally, a mass may be felt on the affected sternocleidomastoid muscle in newborns.
- Plagiocephaly, metatarsus adductus, and congenital hip dysplasia are associated findings.
- It occurs in approximately 1:300 live births.

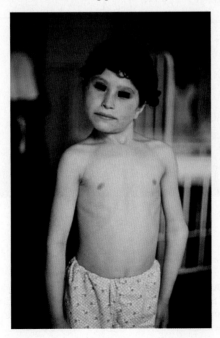

A child with untreated left-sided torticollis. Note the head is tilted toward the left neck and the chin is rotated toward the right. The child also has a left cubitus varus deformity of the elbow, likely related to a malunion of a supracondylar fracture.

Treatment

- Stretching exercises and physical therapy until resolution of torticollis.
- Untreated torticollis may result in the following complications: Facial asymmetry, abnormal position of the head, as well as limited motion of the neck.
- Surgical release of the muscle may be required, if there is no improvement by 18 months of age.

TOXOPLASMOSIS

Definition

- Toxoplasmosis is a parasitic disease in which the parasite infects most warm-blooded mammals including humans; however, the primary host is cat.

Etiology

- Toxoplasmosis is caused by an intracellular protozoan, *Toxoplasma gondii*. It is a single-celled organism which occurs globally.
- Transmission of the disease is through direct contact with cat feces or litter, consumption of contaminated and undercooked meat, transplacental exposure to contaminated blood products, or organ transplantation.

Symptoms and Signs

- Initially, toxoplasmosis may be asymptomatic or cause flu-type symptoms.
- It is a serious disease in the fetus, the pregnant women (due to potential effects on the fetus), and immunocompromised hosts.
- Congenital toxoplasmosis infection may be devastating. Presenting features may include microcephaly, hydrocephalus, intracranial calcifications, seizures, chorioretinitis, deafness, and mental retardation.

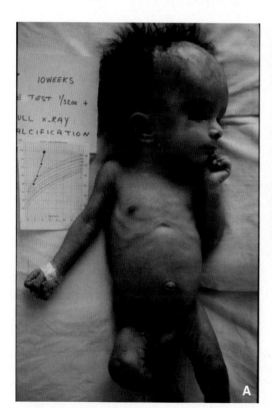

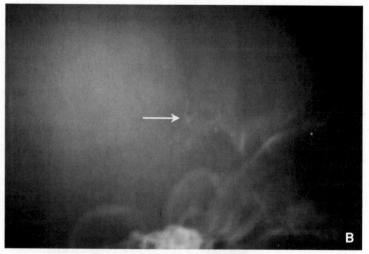

Figure A: This 3-month-old male presented with hydrocephalus, enlarged anterior and posterior fontanelles, hepatosplenomegaly, and high antibody titers to *Toxoplasmosis gondii*. Note the head circumference chart. His skull x-ray showing intracranial calcifications (*arrow*) in **Figure B**.

- Non-CNS manifestations of this disease include jaundice, hepatosplenomegaly, maculopapular rash, generalized lymphadenopathy, and thrombocytopenia.
- Approximately 70% of children born with congenital toxoplasmosis are asymptomatic at birth.
- Up to 80% of the asymptomatic children develop learning or visual difficulties later in life.
- Diagnosis is by polymerase chain reaction (PCR), serologic tests of newborn or cord blood, or lymph node biopsy.

Treatment
- Termination of pregnancy for early and documented fetal infection with evidence of hydrocephalus on ultrasound examination is an option.
- Combination drug treatment options for congenital toxoplasmosis include pyrimethamine–sulfadiazine and folinic acid for 1 year.
- Ongoing ophthalmologic and developmental follow-up is needed.
- Treatment of acute infections in immunocompromised hosts and pregnant women. Pyrimethamine–sulfadiazine, clindamycin, and spiramycin may be used in various combinations.

TRISOMY 18 (L. Tres, three; Gr. Soma, body)

Definition
- Trisomy 18 (Edwards syndrome) is the second most common autosomal trisomy, after trisomy 21. It consists of many life-threatening congenital abnormalities.

Etiology
- Trisomies are the most frequent chromosomal abnormalities.
- Trisomies are caused by meiotic nondisjunction or the failure of a chromosome pair to separate.
- Trisomy 18 may occur in the mosaic form, affecting some, but not all cells of the body.
- The incidence of trisomy 18 is 1:6,000 live births. However, the overall incidence may be higher since the majority of infants with trisomy 18 die in utero.

Symptoms and Signs
- Small for gestational age status, small facies, low-set and structurally abnormal ears, prominent occiput, micrognathia, clenched hands with overlapping fingers, short sternum, and rocker bottom feet. Congenital heart disease.

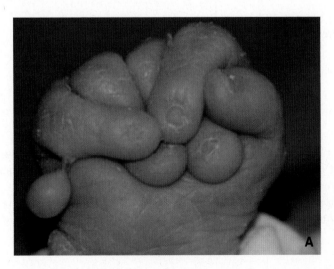

Figure A: Clenched hand, overlapping fingers, and a supernumerary digit in a newborn with trisomy 18.

figures continues

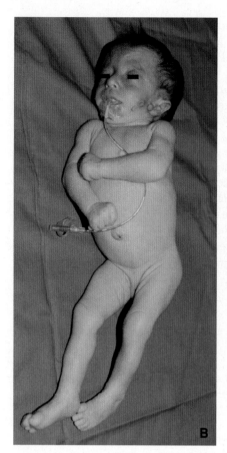

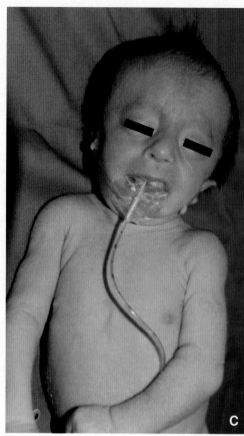

(figures cont.) **Figures B–C:** Abnormal facies in a female diagnosed with trisomy 18. Note the small facies, bilateral ptosis, multiple preauricular skin tags with deformed low-set ears and micrognathia. Other findings include ventricular septal defect, spasticity, and clenched hands. She was tube-fed and died within the first month of life.

- Severity of the disease varies according to the extent of the chromosomal abnormalities, that is, complete or partial trisomy of chromosome 18 or mosaicism.
- Approximately 50% die within the first week of life.
- Five to ten percent may live to their first birthday. Survivors are mostly females who have less structural abnormalities.
- Significant and profound mental retardation is seen in all patients including those with mosaicism.

Treatment
- Children with trisomy 18 have an extremely poor prognosis.
- There is no treatment for trisomy 18.
- Figures A–C.

TUBERCULOSIS

Definition
- Tuberculosis (TB) is a common and potentially lethal disease. Recently, there has been a resurgence of tuberculosis in the industrialized countries due to the increased number of immunocompromised, HIV positive patients.
- There were approximately 1.5 million TB-related deaths in 2010. During the previous centuries, numerous notable deaths were attributed to TB, including Eleanor Roosevelt,

King Louis XIII and XVII, and King Henry VII of England. Frederic Chopin, the composer, died during a performance from TB-related hemoptysis.

Etiology

- Tuberculosis is an infectious disease caused by *Mycobacterium tuberculosis,* a weak gram-positive bacilli. It is transmitted by the inhalation of small airborne droplets from an individual with contagious, active pulmonary TB.
- Immigrants from highly endemic regions, homeless individuals, health-care professionals, residents of correctional facilities or institutions, and immunocompromised individuals are at greatest risk of acquiring TB.
- The source of infection in infants and children is usually the parents, close relatives, or caretakers.

Signs and Symptoms

- TB is asymptomatic in approximately 90% of patients (latent TB). These patients are not infectious, but they have a small risk of developing active TB later in life.
- Fever, chills, night sweats, cough, hemoptysis, and weight loss are common symptoms in patients with active TB.
- Pulmonary TB is the most common and the best known form of tuberculosis. However, tuberculosis may become disseminated and present with extrapulmonary manifestations including cervical adenitis, meningitis, abdominal presentations, and skeletal disease.
- Examples of some of these manifestations are illustrated in the images that follow.
- A "Ghon focus," is the primary site of tuberculosis. It is located either in the upper part of the lower lobe or the lower part of the upper lobe.
- Initial screening studies include tuberculin skin test (TST) or the Mantoux skin test which utilizes five tuberculin units of purified protein derivative (PPD) and chest radiographs.
- A positive PPD is identified by measuring the area of induration and not the area of erythema.
- A positive PPD test is indicative that a person has previously been infected with TB. It does not indicate that the person has active or latent TB.
- A definitive diagnosis of active tuberculosis may be made by a combination of the following: Patient's history and clinical findings, positive gram stain, and culture for acid-fast bacilli. The culture may be taken from sputum, CSF, pleural effusion, ascites, and biopsy specimens.
- In younger children, early morning gastric lavage samples are more likely to produce positive gram stains and culture results.
- BCG vaccine is used as a preventive measure in many countries with a high prevalence of TB in order to prevent childhood tuberculous meningitis and disseminated disease. However, BCG is not routinely recommended in the United States. Often times, previous BCG vaccination may interfere with PPD skin test reactivity.
- Figures A–P.

Treatment

- Latent TB infections (positive PPD, no signs or symptoms of active TB disease, and normal x-ray findings) should be treated with Isoniazid (INH) or rifampin based on local sensitivity patterns.
- INH, rifampin, and pyrazinamide for active pulmonary and extrapulmonary TB.
- INH, rifampin, pyrazinamide, and an aminoglycoside for TB meningitis.
- Treatment of patients with a positive PPD and a previous history of BCG vaccination should be considered based on CDC guidelines.

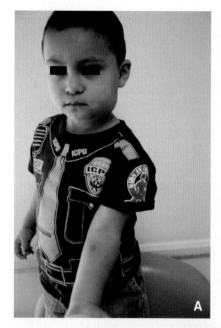

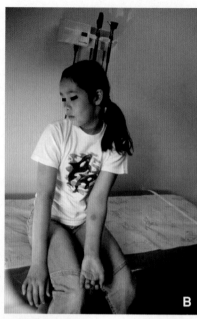

Figures A–C: Positive tuberculin skin test in a child with visible cervical lymphadenopathy. Tuberculous cervical lymphadenitis (scrofula) is the most common form of extrapulmonary tuberculosis in childhood.

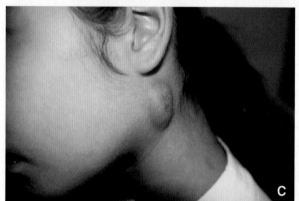

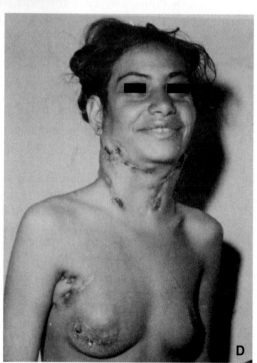

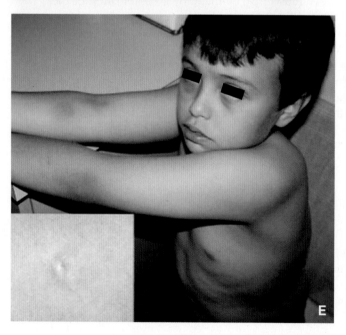

Figure D: Advanced tuberculous lymphadenitis (scrofula).

Figure E: Positive tuberculin skin test (PPD) is not uncommon in many asymptomatic, healthy children who have immigrated to the United States from countries in which the BCG vaccine is routinely administered during childhood. The insert in **Figure E** is a close-up view of the BCG scar on this patient's left deltoid.

figures continues

TUBERCULOSIS OF THE FINGERS (TB DACTYLITIS)

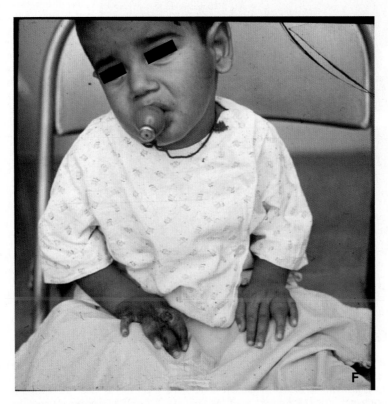

(figures cont.) **Figure F:** This patient presented at 18 months of age due to the inability to walk. On examination, his fingers appeared ulcerated and deformed. There was a strong family history of TB-related morbidities **(see Figure I)**. Maternal PPD testing was positive, but her chest x-ray did not reveal evidence of active pulmonary TB. Paternal testing, however, revealed a positive PPD and extensive pulmonary TB. The child had a strongly positive PPD as well. Bone biopsy confirmed the clinical and radiologic diagnosis of TB dactylitis. He was treated successfully with antituberculosis drugs.

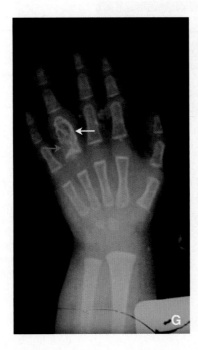
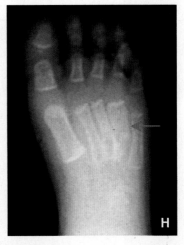

Figures G–H: Radiographs of the child in **Figure F** revealed the destruction and sclerosis of the proximal phalanx of the fourth digit **(Figure G)** and the fourth metatarsal **(Figure H)**. The red arrow in **Figure G** represents the biopsy site.

figures continues

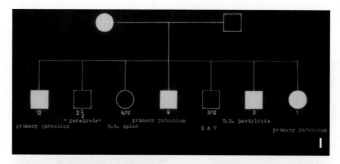

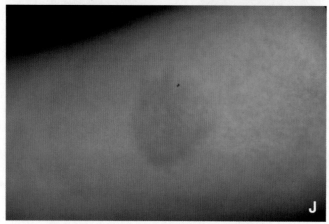

(figures cont.) **Figure I:** The family history of the child was strongly suggestive of TB**.** His 12-year-old brother, 6-year-old brother, and 1-year-old sister were all diagnosed with primary TB. He had lost a 2 ½-year-old brother and a 6-month-old sister with what appeared to be spinal TB. Incidentally, his 3-month-old sister died due to vomiting and diarrhea, possibly intestinal TB.

Figure J: Positive PPD. Note the central erythema and induration which is surrounded by a larger, less erythematous area. Once a PPD is properly placed, it should be read within a 24 to 36 hour period. When reading a PPD, it is important to measure the area of induration (and not just erythema). An induration which is greater than 15 mm is considered positive in children who are 4 years or older. For children who are younger than 4 years or in older children in high-risk categories, an induration greater than 10 mm is considered positive. A 5-mm induration in an immunocompromised child is considered a positive test. False-negative PPD tests may be caused by malnutrition, dehydration, fulminant tuberculosis, immunosuppressive medications, measles, and HIV.

TUBERCULOSIS, LYMPHOHEMATOGENOUS (DISSEMINATED) DISEASE

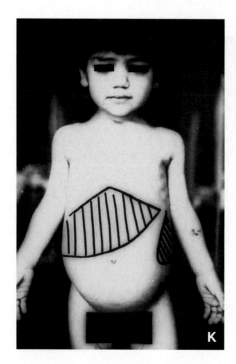

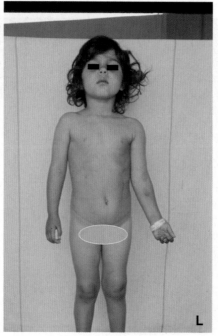

Figures K–L: This 3-year-old female **(Figure K)** was brought in for insidious onset of loss of appetite, low-grade fever, abdominal pain, and irregular bowel movements. On physical examination, she was noted to have a distended abdomen and marked hepatosplenomegaly. There was no palpable ascites or lymphadenopathy. She had a strongly positive PPD test with a negative chest x-ray. Marked improvement was noted after antituberculosis therapy **(Figure L)**.

figures continues

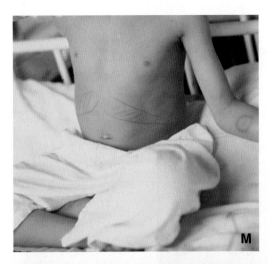

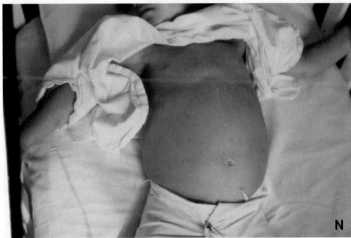

(figures cont.) **Figures M–N:** Abdominal TB. These two patients presented with low-grade fever, abdominal pain and distention, and hepatosplenomegaly. Note, positive PPD tests on their left and right forearms (**Figures M** and **N,** respectively). Both patients responded well to antituberculosis therapy.

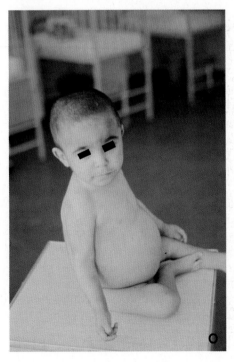

Figure O: Patient with abdominal distention and a positive PPD. Abdominal TB may be caused by hematogenous spread of pulmonary TB or by ingestion of unpasteurized milk of a cow infected with TB.

SPINAL TUBERCULOSIS

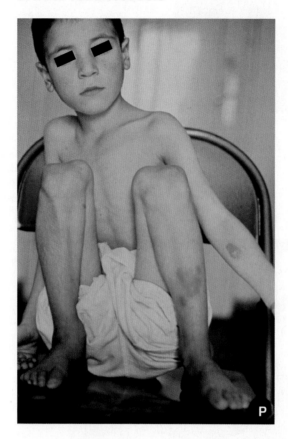

(figures cont.) **Figure P:** A 10-year-old male who presented with neck pain and torticollis. He had a positive PPD test and radiographic changes consistent with TB of the cervical spine. Tender, erythematous nodules, consistent with erythema nodosum, erupted on his shins while he was hospitalized.

TUBEROUS SCLEROSIS (TS)

Definition
- Tuberous sclerosis is a rare multisystem disease that causes growth of hamartomatous tumors in the brain and other vital organs.

Etiology
- Tuberous sclerosis is an autosomal dominant neurocutaneous disorder caused by deletions of the hamartin protein in chromosomes 9 and 16. There is variable penetrance and expressivity of the mutations.
- Approximately two-thirds of the new cases arise from de novo mutations.

Symptoms and Signs
- Cutaneous manifestations
  - Ash leaf spots: White macules that are often better visualized with Wood's lamp.
  - Adenoma sebaceum: The pathognomonic lesions of TS. These fibroangiomatous tumors usually appear during the preschool years as pink or flesh-colored papulonodular eruptions on the cheeks, nose, forehead, and chin.
  - Shagreen patches: Large skin-colored, collagenous plaques with a cobblestone texture. They are commonly located in the lumbosacral area.
  - Periungual fibromas: Small, flesh-colored, firm, protruding nodules that grow around the lateral and posterior nail folds from under the nail plate.
- Neurologic manifestations
  - Seizure disorder: Often associated with infantile spasms.

- Mental retardation including learning difficulties, autism, ADHD, and self-injurious behavior.
- Cerebral calcifications.
- Sclerotic patches (or "tubers") scattered throughout the cortical matter.
- Whitish-yellow areas in the retina called astrocytic hamartomas. Nonretinal findings may include colobomas and angiofibromas of the eyelid.
  - Cardiac manifestations
    - Benign tumors called rhabdomyomas which may be noticed during echocardiography. Rhabdomyomas are the most common cause of an intracardiac tumor in a newborn. They may cause outflow obstruction, arrhythmia, or murmurs.
  - Renal manifestations
    - Benign hamartomatous tumors of the kidney which may cause hematuria.

Treatment
- Symptomatic management of seizure and other problems as they arise.

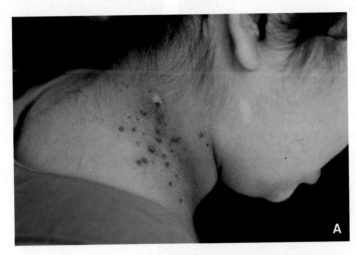

Figure A: A 9-year-old female with tuberous sclerosis who presented with seizures, autism spectrum disorder, developmental delay, obesity, and hemihypertrophy **(Figures A–G)**. White, ash leaf macules, noted on the right shoulder and cheek. Adenoma sebaceum can be seen on the neck.

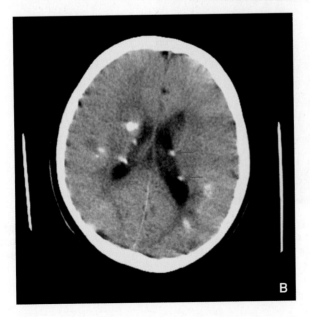

Figure B: Axial CT scan of the brain without contrast demonstrates multiple subependymal calcifications (hamartomas) (red arrows) as seen in tuberous sclerosis.

figures continues

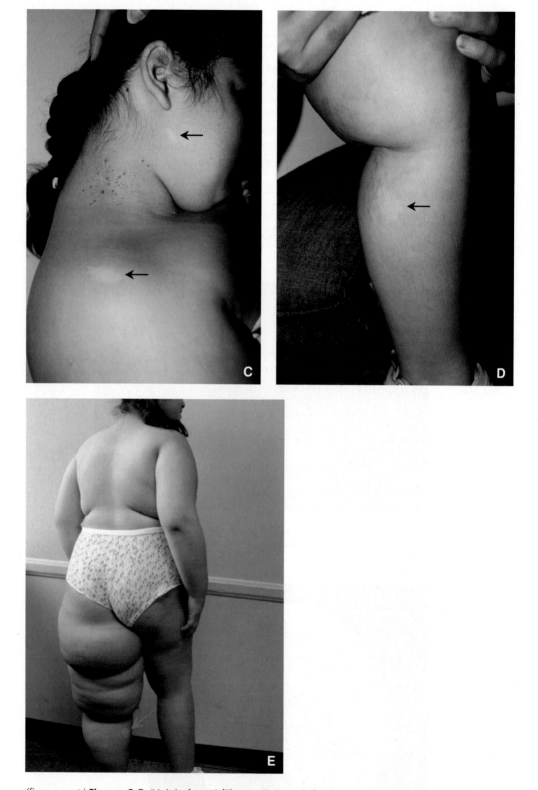

(figures cont.) **Figures C–E:** "Ash leaf spot" **(Figures C, D,** and **E)**. These hypopigmented macules are present in 90% of cases. They are easier to identify in dark-skinned individuals. Wood's lamp examination may be required to identify these lesions in fair-skinned individuals. Hemihypertrophy is a rare finding in TS **(Figure E)**.

figures continues

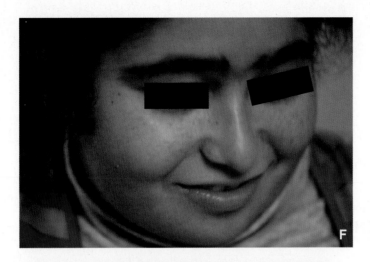

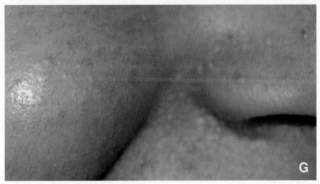

(figures cont.) **Figures F–G:** Angiofibromas in a characteristic butterfly pattern.

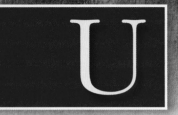

UMBILICAL HERNIA

(See Hernia).

UNILATERAL LATEROTHORACIC EXANTHEMA (ASYMMETRICAL PERIFLEXURAL EXANTHEM OF CHILDHOOD)

Definition
- A benign, self-limited skin eruption of unknown etiology, which affects mostly children 2 to 3 years of age; more common in girls.

Etiology
- Unknown, possibly viral in view of prevalence in spring and winter.

Symptoms and Signs
- Unilateral laterothoracic exanthema is at times preceded by fever, upper-respiratory symptoms or gastrointestinal symptoms.
- It may begin with small erythematous papules with a surrounding white halo on the lateral chest wall or near a flexural area, which can coalesce into small plaques and then spread centrifugally.
- The rash can be macular, papular, morbilliform, scarlatiniform, annular, reticular, or eczematous.
- The lesions may spread to the contralateral side.

Treatment
- Symptomatic.
- Most lesions resolve within a week, but can rarely last up to 8 weeks.

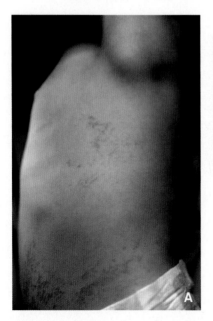

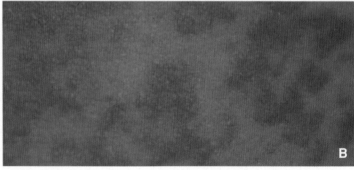

Figures A–B: A 2-year-old boy with a rash for 18 days which started following 3 days of cold symptoms. Most of his left lower abdomen and part of his left axilla were covered with an erythematous rash involving many papules **(Figure A)** and a close-up view **(Figure B)**.

U

URTICARIA (Urtica L., the nettles)

Definition
- Urticaria is a cutaneous vascular reaction as a manifestation of a systemic disease.

Etiology
- Urticaria is mostly a type 1 hypersensitivity reaction triggered by a protein (like milk) or a nonprotein (like aspirin).
- Drugs, food and food additives, almost any infection (including malaria parasite—see Malaria) but mostly viral infections in younger children, insect bites, physical factors, autoimmune disease, contact allergens, and inhalants.
- The cause of urticaria in many children remains unknown.

Symptoms and Signs
- It can be acute (<6-week duration) or recurrent and chronic (>6-week duration).
- Intense itching with skin lesions that can appear anywhere, and change shape and location constantly, in less than 24 hours.
- Urticaria lesions can be pinpoint in size, pale red, small papules, large wheals with central clearing, bullae, well circumscribed, annular, oval, or serpiginous, and occasionally with odd shapes.

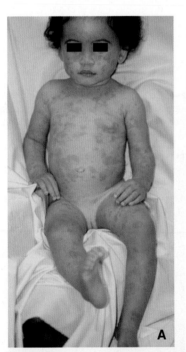
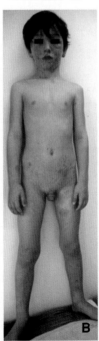
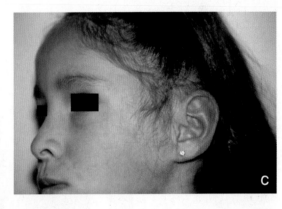

Figures A–B: Generalized wheals surrounded by erythema and central clearing (in some) in two children.

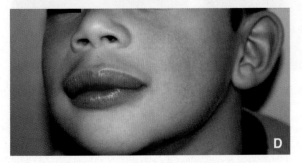

Figures C–D: Redness of the left ear and cheek with itching in a 6-year-old girl **(Figure C)**. Note redness and edema of the left ear, redness of the left cheek (urticaria), and edema of the upper lip (his main concern for visiting our office) which is also a feature of angioedema **(Figure D)**.

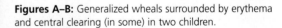

figures continues

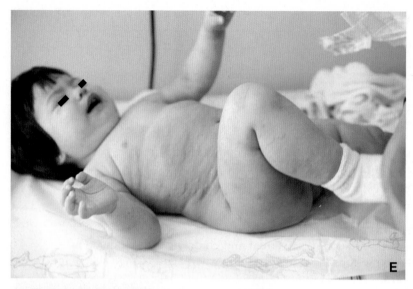

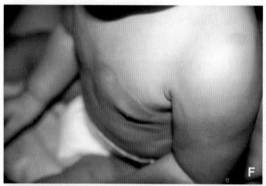

(figures cont.) **Figures E–F:** Generalized urticaria in a 14-month-old girl. She has pinkish wheals throughout her body **(Figure E)**. A large plaque of urticaria on the chest and abdomen as well as a few smaller plaques and hives on the arms, legs, and the trunk **(Figure F)**.

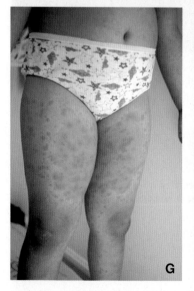

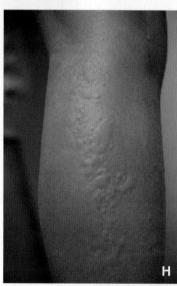

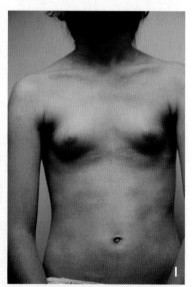

Figure G: This 2-year-old girl developed this rash 7 days after she had been taking Augmentin (amoxicillin and clavulanic acid). Generalized pinkish, flat papules of varying size surrounded by erythema mostly on the legs and arms.

Figure H: Pale-red wheals of different sizes and shapes, some with central clearing, on the legs of this 7-year-old girl. The cause could not be determined.

Figure I: This 11-year-old girl with a previous history of urticaria developed severe urticaria 2 days following the start of Augmentin. She had taken amoxicillin without any reaction in the past. This outbreak could be a recurrence of her urticaria, hypersensitivity to clavulanic acid, or even to amoxicillin.

Treatment
- The cause of urticaria should be investigated and, if found, treated.
- Symptomatic treatment with nonsedating H1 blockers such as loratadine (Claritin) and levocetirizine (Xyzal) in higher doses is sufficient in the majority of cases.
- Sedating H1 blockers such as diphenhydramine (Benadryl) and hydroxyzine (Atarax) can be used in others for whom the sedating side effect may be an advantage.
- Paradoxical hyperactivity and irritability, although rare, can be seen in children.
- H2 blockers such as cimetidine and ranitidine and leukotriene receptor antagonists such as montelukast (Singulair) can be used with or without H1 or H2 blockers.
- Epinephrine gives immediate and urgent relief from urticaria or for signs or symptoms of airway compromise. Doxepin, intravenous immunoglobulin, cyclophosphamide, cyclosporine, methotrexate, and plasmapheresis have all been used for chronic urticaria.
- Corticosteroids should rarely be used due to side effect profile.
- Aspirin and NSAIDs should be avoided as they may exacerbate chronic urticaria.

URTICARIA, CHOLINERGIC

Definition
- Cholinergic urticaria is a cutaneous vascular reaction as a manifestation often associated with stress, exertion, or change in weather.

Etiology
- Physical stimulus precipitated by exercise, hot showers, and sweating can cause urticaria in susceptible patients.

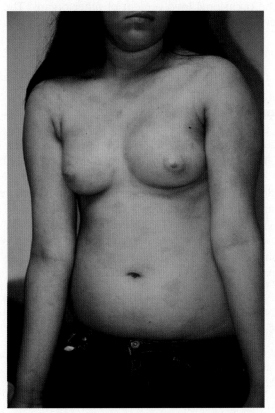

During the last few months, this 12-year-old girl developed shortness of breath and this rash and is forced to stop 5 minutes into the exercise during school PE (physical education). No wheezing or syncope. No history of asthma or previous urticaria. She developed generalized, discrete, erythematous papules within a few minutes of going up and down the stairs in the office. No wheezing or change in the blood pressure. The rash faded within 10 minutes of an injection of epinephrine.

- Action of acetylcholine on mast cells seems to be involved in cholinergic urticaria.
- Elevated histamine levels can be detected 5 minutes after exercise, reaching a peak of 25 ng/mL at 30 minutes in persons with cholinergic urticaria.

Symptoms and Signs
- Generalized, discrete papular wheals, smaller than the eruptions seen in urticaria, mostly on the arms and trunk, with or without surrounding erythema.
- Occasionally symptoms of more generalized cholinergic stimulation such as lacrimation, wheezing, salivation, and syncope may be observed.
- Some persons report cholinergic urticaria symptoms only during the winter months. They apparently have a reaction only when exposed to heat or heat-producing exercise, while not adapted to heat in the winter months.
- Occasionally an attack of cholinergic urticaria can be eliminated by rapid cooling.
- Cholinergic urticaria usually begins during adolescence, can recur for months (years), and then spontaneously resolves.

Treatment
- Antihistamines, mostly cyproheptadine, cetirizine, and hydroxyzine are useful.
- Diet modification may be helpful because cholinergic urticaria attacks can sometimes result from hot foods and beverages, spicy foods, and alcohol.

URTICARIA PIGMENTOSA (MASTOCYTOSIS)

Definition
- Mastocytosis is a group of clinical disorders characterized by the accumulation of mast cells in the skin with the occasional involvement of other organs. The most common presentation of mastocytosis is urticaria pigmentosa.

Etiology
- Some are caused by a mutation.

Symptoms and Signs
- Most common during the first 2 years of life.
- Tan-red or brown macules or papules can be just a few or thousands in number, and anywhere on the skin, uncommon on the mucous membranes, and rarely seen on the palms and soles.
- Bullous mastocytosis: Some urticaria pigmentosa lesions progress to vesicles and bullae, which can be painful and can get infected.
- Darier sign: A stroke on the lesion causes mast cell degranulation and may become pruritic and erythematous. This sign is common in urticaria pigmentosa.
- Resolution of the lesions at puberty is common.
- Symptoms and signs may worsen and include systemic involvement.

Treatment
- Supportive with antihistamines and corticosteroids.

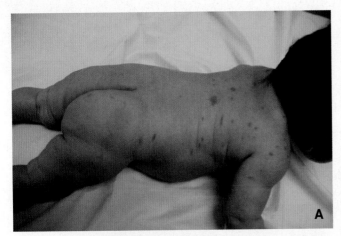

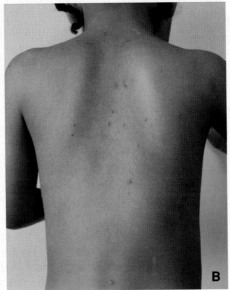

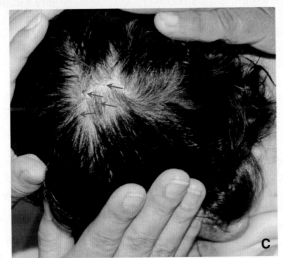

Figure A: Multiple hyperpigmented macules and papules in this 6-month-old girl.

Figure B: Brownish macules and papules on the back of a 6-year-old girl with urticaria pigmentosa.

Figure C: Several brownish-red macules and papules on the scalp of this 7-year-old girl.

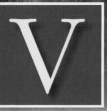

VAGINITIS AND VULVOVAGINITIS

Definition
- Vaginitis is an inflammation of the vaginal mucosa.
- Extension of the irritation or infection to vulva causes vulvovaginitis.

Etiology
- Prepubertal: The thin vaginal epithelium, with a relatively low-estrogen environment, is susceptible to infection. Need to rule out sexual abuse.
- Postpubertal: Poor perineal hygiene, candida infection, gonorrhea, chlamydia, enterobiasis, giardiasis, streptococcal and staphylococcal infections, shigellosis, molluscum contagiosum, pediculosis pubis, scabies and foreign body.

Symptoms and Signs
- Vaginal discharge, foul odor, erythema, pruritus, and at times dysuria and frequency.

Treatment
- Is dependent on the etiology. Azithromycin or doxycycline for chlamydia, cefixime for gonorrhea, metronidazole for trichomonas infections, penicillin for streptococcal infections and cephalexin for staphylococcal infections, and clotrimazole or single dose fluconazole for adolescents and adults with yeast infection.
- For simple irritation without an infection, a steroid cream can work well.

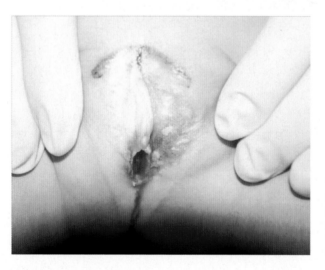

This 4-year-old had pain, irritation, and redness of the vulvo-vaginal area for 1 week. No fever or exudate. Labia majora and labia minor are swollen, irritated, and tender. A vaginal swab was negative for herpes and chlamydia.

VARICELLA (L., chicken pox)

Definition
- Varicella is a viral infection manifested by mild constitutional symptoms and a rash, typical for this disease.
- Varicella is much less common today due to the successful immunization program.

V

Etiology

- Varicella zoster virus (VZV) is a double-stranded DNA genome, neurotrophic human herpes virus.

Symptoms and Signs

- Incubation period is 14 to 16 days.
- Prodromal symptoms if present are mostly mild consisting of low-grade fever, anorexia, malaise, headache, and mild abdominal pain.
- Varicella lesions are initially intensely pruritic, erythematous macules, which evolve into papules and vesicles, which appear a day or two later, on the scalp, face, and trunk.
- The two main characteristic features of the varicella rash are the following:
  1. Fresh new crops of papules and vesicles erupt, as some vesicles are crusting, and the three stages of rash can be seen on the skin at the same time.
  2. Lesions, unlike variola, are centripetal (mostly on the trunk).

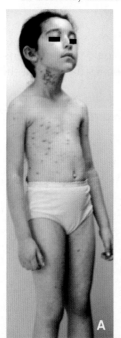
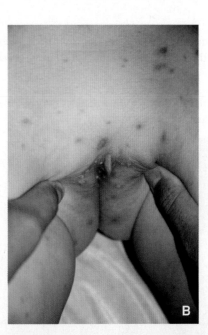

Figures A–C: Varicella in a 12-year-old girl. Macules, papules, and vesicles (one crusted lesion) are visible on the neck.

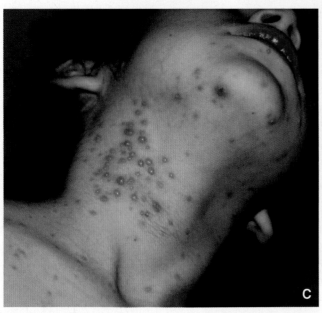
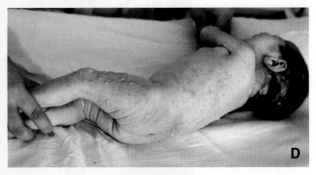

Figure D: Varicella in a newborn.

- Vesicles on the oropharynx and vagina are common.
- Hyperpigmentation or hypopigmentation of the skin lesions may last for weeks.
- *Breakthrough varicella* is when a person develops varicella despite immunization. In such cases, the disease is mild with fewer lesions and symptoms. This disease is, nevertheless, highly contagious.
- *Progressive varicella* is a dangerous complication of varicella and may present with hemorrhage, coagulopathy, and intestinal involvement.

Treatment
- Acyclovir: It is not recommended for otherwise healthy children.
- *Neonatal varicella* is a more serious disease with a high mortality rate. Birth within 1 week before or after the onset of maternal varicella may cause varicella in the newborn.

VARIOLA (SMALL POX)

Definition
- A viral infection, eradicated in 1978, with dermatologic manifestations unique to this disease and the cause of several devastating epidemics throughout the centuries.

Etiology
- Variola is a member of the Poxviridae family. Monkeypox, vaccinia, and cowpox are some other members of this family.

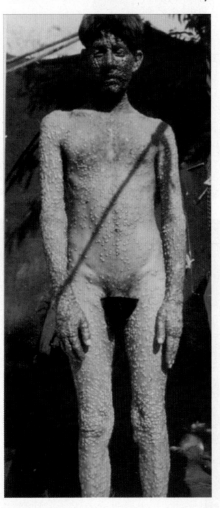

A young man with severe small pox from a tribe in Iran during an epidemic which killed many and terrified many more in 1954.

Symptoms and Signs

- Incubation period is 7 to 17 days, followed by severe prodromal symptoms, high fever, malaise, severe headache, backache, abdominal pain, and prostration which may last 2 to 5 days and can be accompanied by some oral lesions.
- The next stage is the rash which appears on the face, forearm, trunk, and legs.
- The sequence of the skin lesions evolves from macules to papules and then to vesicles. The vesicles then evolve into firm pustules which crust in 8 to 10 days.
- Some of these crusts leave permanent scars.
- Skin lesions are centrifuge (mainly on the face and extremities).
- The crops are always in the same stage anywhere on the skin.

Treatment

- Supportive.

VELOCARDIOFACIAL SYNDROME (VCFS), SHPRINTZEN SYNDROME

Definition

- A congenital abnormality with characteristic craniofacial abnormalities, congenital heart disease, and hypocalcemia.

Etiology

- Autosomal dominant monosomy 22q in 15%, and new mutation in approximately 85%.

Symptoms and Signs

- VCFS and DiGeorge syndrome have so much in common that they are considered as a phenotypic variation of a single genetic defect and collectively given the acronym CATCH 22, with DiGeorge syndrome at the severe end of the spectrum and VCFS at the mild end.

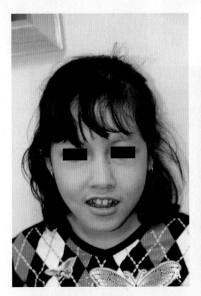
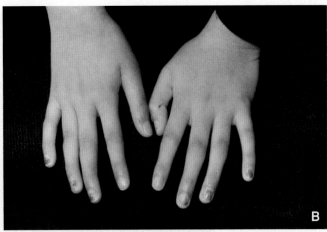

Figures A–B: A 13-year-old girl, the fourth child of a healthy couple. She has some developmental delay, learning disability, bifid uvula, ankyloglossia, cleft palate, a long face, narrow palpebral fissures, prominent nasal root, flat malar bones, long-tapered digits, overriding of the right fourth toe, bilateral flexible flat feet, and femoral anteversion. Chromosome analysis and fluorescence in situ hybridization (FISH) study demonstrated 22q microdeletion and normal karyotype of 46 XX. Also normal CBC, electrolytes, EEG, and renal ultrasound. Her thyroglobulin was 105 (normal <20 IU/mL), thyroid peroxidase antibodies >1,000 (normal <35 IU/mL), and free T4 0.9 (normal 0.9 to 1.6 ng/dL) 2 years ago. She has VCFS, bipolar disorder, attention deficit hyperactivity disorder (ADHD), femoral anteversion, and flat feet.

- The characteristic phenotype of VCFS is divided into three clinical areas:
  1. Velo: Abnormalities of the palate or pharynx.
  2. Cardio: Congenital abnormalities of the heart.
  3. Facial: Craniofacial abnormalities such as microcephaly, narrow palpebral fissures and abnormalities of the nose and chin (prominent bulbous nose and micrognathia).
- Other abnormalities include long-tapering fingers, short stature, nasal speech, conductive hearing loss, hypotonia and hypocalcemia in the newborn, and psychiatric diseases such as schizophrenia and bipolar disorder in older children and adults.

Treatment
- Corrective surgery.
- Speech and physical therapy.
- Treatment of the psychiatric comorbidities.

VITILIGO (L.)

Definition
- A chronic, mostly progressive abnormality of the skin characterized by depigmentation and white patches that can be surrounded by a darker skin.

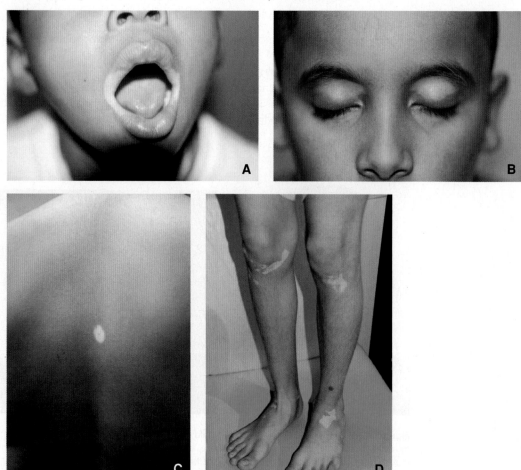

Figures A–F: show diffuse, flat areas of hypopigmentation with sharp borders of vitiligo in several patients. Note the hypopigmentation of the left upper eyelid and eyelashes in **Figure F** and location of many lesions on sun-exposed and high-friction areas such as the fingers and knees. Bilateral, irregular distribution is common.

figures continues

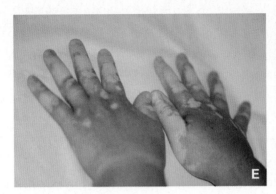
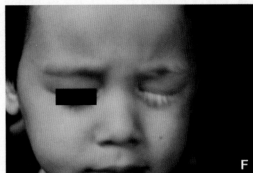

(figures cont.) **Figures E–F**

Etiology
- A suspected autoimmune process due to the higher incidence in those with other autoimmune disorders, resulting in the absence of melanocytes within the affected epidermis.
- Potentially triggered by trauma but also with predilection for areas of skin with sun exposure and frequent friction (elbows, knees, and face).

Symptoms and Signs
- Affected areas present with hypopigmentation of irregular shape, size, and distribution with characteristic sharp borders.
- Nearly 50% of cases present before the age of 20 and up to 40% of the cases are familial.
- The lesions are painless, flat, and may coalesce into broad areas.
- Approximately 20% will spontaneously repigment.

Treatment
- Phototherapy may improve some affected areas and high-concentration topical steroids can decrease the appearance of early, small lesions.
- Patients should be advised to use sunscreen as the hypopigmented lesions are vulnerable to sunburn.

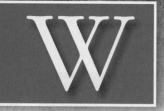

WART (L. Verruca)

Definition
- A lobulated benign epithelial hyperplasia is characterized by papules and plaques with a horny surface.

Etiology
- Human wart virus of the papova group.

Symptoms and Signs
- Asymptomatic, but can be painful on the palms and soles.
- They are found mostly on sites of trauma and contact: Hands, feet, and knees.
- Warts manifest as hyperkeratotic round vegetations looking like red dots as a single or multiple lesions.

Treatment
- Liquid nitrogen, 40% salicylic, laser therapy, and electrocautery.
- Duct tape takes longer, but works in the majority of cases.

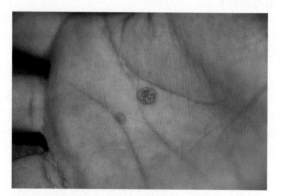

WART, FLAT

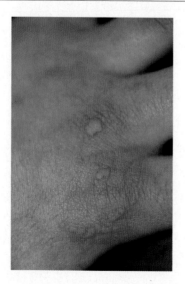

PLANTAR WART

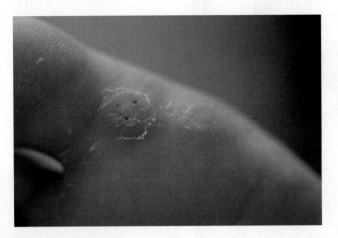

WHITLOW (FELON)

Definition
- Herpetic whitlow is a herpes simplex virus (HSV) infection of the digits frequently involving the thumb and nail bed.

Etiology
- The viral inoculation often follows trauma, burns, or an abrasion to the nail bed of the digit.
- Auto-inoculation can occur in thumb-sucking infants suffering from herpetic gingivostomatitis.

Symptoms and Signs
- Infection results in groups of painful and erythematous spreading vesicles often associated with erythema and edema of the affected digit.

Treatment
- Lesions typically resolve within 2 to 3 weeks. Treatment with oral antiviral medications may shorten the course.
- Figures A–E.

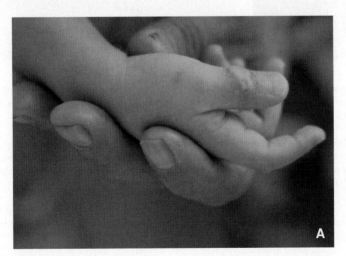

Figures A-C: Images of herpetic whitlow in two young infants. A coalescing area of vesicles on the first finger **(Figure A)**. Note the erythema and edema of the digits associated with the infection especially in **Figures B** and **C**.

figures continues

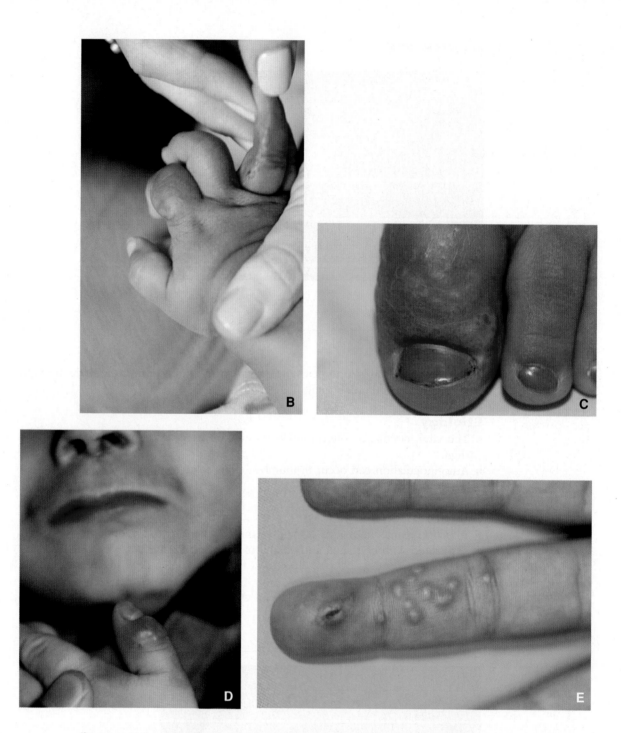

(figures cont.) **Figure C:** A 3-year-old girl with a 2-day history of increasing redness and swelling of the left big toe. The big toe is swollen, erythematous, has a few vesicles and is slightly tender. An aspirate of the larger vesicle is culture-positive for the herpes simplex virus.

Figure D: This 7-year-old boy has Cornelia de Lange syndrome. He is severely delayed and his thumb is in his mouth most of the time. He had a viral stomatitis last week. His parents noted swelling of his left thumb 5 days after the onset of the viral stomatitis. Note the swelling of the left first finger with a large vesicle covering the erythematous swollen finger and the vesicles on his left nostril and chin.

Figure E: Some "rash" on the finger of this 8-year-old girl, 2 days following a rose thorn cut her finger. There was a longitudinal laceration on the left third finger with raised edges and another 13 vesicles. No fever, itching, or constitutional symptoms. Herpes simplex virus type 1 was cultured from the vesicles.

ZONA

(See Herpes Zoster).

Index

Note: Page numbers followed by "f" indicates figure only.